Further praise for *The Adaptation Diet*

"If you have no hope you can ever lose weight and feel at peace, read *The Adaptation Diet*. It provides clear, concise suggestions that can help you shed not only the pounds but also many of your other health concerns. Yes, you are holding the book that has proven, sensible recommendations and explanations to resolve many medical challenges. Turn your life around today by simply trying this diet."

—**Doris J. Rapp**, MD, author of *Our Toxic World: A Wake Up Call*

"*The Adaptation Diet* offers a unique perspective on weight loss, pointing out the weight-gaining effects of 'dietary stress,' and how to deal with them. Going way beyond just calorie control, Dr. Charles Moss points out that dietary stress reduction—with or without calorie reduction—will result in significant and sustained weight loss. He tells us which foods and supplements actually reduce the food-stress-induced, over-active cortisol response, allowing that elusive goal, weight loss, to happen while at the same time improving your health. If you want to lose weight, *The Adaptation Diet* is an excellent place to start!"

—**Jonathan Wright**, MD, Editor, *Nutrition & Healing Newsletter*

"Dr. Moss is a colleague I've admired for decades for his competence, compassion, clarity, and communication style. His latest book reflects his considerable accomplishments in ways accessible for all those interested in better health. With epigenetics or lifestyle and environment determining 92 percent of health due to what we eat, drink, think, and do, the healthier choices recommended in this guide can add years to life and life to years."

—**Russ Jaffe**, MD, PhD, Founder/Chief Executive Officer Fellow, Health Studies Collegium Perque Integrative Health Elisa/Act Biotechnologies

"Too tired to exercise? Is your willpower ambushed by unrelenting food cravings? Start reclaiming your health with *The Adaptation Diet*. Patients self-prescribing this book can consider it as a toehold for scaling impediments to optimal wellness. They can be confident in the medical science and in Dr. Moss."

—**Ingrid Kohlstadt**, MD, MPH, FACPM, FACN, Faculty, Johns Hopkins Bloomberg School of Public Health; Executive Director, NutriBee National Nutrition Competition, Inc.; Editor, *Advancing Medicine with Food and Nutrients*, CRC Press, December 2012

"As a colleague of Dr. Charles Moss in integrative medicine since the 1970s, I can attest to his pioneering work in nutritional medicine, and to his wide-ranging knowledge and contemporary application of Traditional Chinese Medicine (TCM), the world's oldest mind-body medicine model. In this book he blends the wisdom of the latter with his thirty-five years of practical clinical experience with cutting-edge nutritional medicine. The result is a book that helps the reader deal with modern health risks with clear and practical suggestions and with the wider understanding of how our diet itself directly affects our stress levels."

—**Ronald Puhky**, MD, BAc, Dip Ac. Medical Director, InspireHealth Integrative Cancer Center, Victoria, BC

THE
ADAPTATION
DIET

A Three-Step Approach to
Control Cortisol, Lose Weight,
and Prevent Chronic Disease

CHARLES A. MOSS, MD

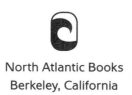

North Atlantic Books
Berkeley, California

Published by
North Atlantic Books
P.O. Box 12327
Berkeley, California 94712

Cover and book design by Suzanne Albertson
Printed in the United States of America

The Adaptation Diet: A Three-Step Approach to Control Cortisol, Lose Weight, and Prevent Chronic Disease is sponsored by the Society for the Study of Native Arts and Sciences, a nonprofit educational corporation whose goals are to develop an educational and cross-cultural perspective linking various scientific, social, and artistic fields; to nurture a holistic view of arts, sciences, humanities, and healing; and to publish and distribute literature on the relationship of mind, body, and nature.

North Atlantic Books' publications are available through most bookstores. For further information, visit our website at www.northatlanticbooks.com or call 800-733-3000.

MEDICAL DISCLAIMER: The following information is intended for general information purposes only. Individuals should always see their health care provider before administering any suggestions made in this book. Any application of the material set forth in the following pages is at the reader's discretion and is his or her sole responsibility.

Library of Congress Cataloging-in-Publication Data

Moss, Charles A., 1947–
    The adaptation diet : a three-step approach to control cortisol, lose weight, and prevent chronic disease / Charles A. Moss, MD.
        pages cm
    Summary: "Based on his 35 years of clinical experience, Dr. Charles Moss presents an easy-to-implement approach to normalize cortisol (the main stress hormone), lose weight, and reduce your risk for diabetes, heart disease, and cancer"—Provided by publisher.
    Includes bibliographical references and index.
    ISBN 978-1-58394-611-4 (pbk.)
    1. Weight loss. 2. Reducing diets—Recipes. 3. Health. I. Title.
    RM222.2.M654 2013
        613.2'5—dc23   2012033900

1 2 3 4 5 6 7 8 SHERIDAN 18 17 16 15 14 13
Printed on recycled paper

*Dedicated to my mother, Helen Moss,
for her unconditional love and many
nutritious home-cooked meals.*

ACKNOWLEDGMENTS

Over the course of my practice experience, I have learned more about stress and diet from my patients than from any book or medical conference. I am indebted to their commitment to improve their lives through the ideas presented in this book.

I have had many colleagues over the past thirty years who have shared their own clinical experiences and helped me to refine my approach with patients. A partial list includes Jonathan Wright, MD, Jeffrey Bland, PhD, Theron Randolph, MD, Doris Rapp, MD, David Buscher, MD, as well as other members of the following professional organizations, of which I am a member: the American Academy of Environmental Medicine, the American College for Advancement in Medicine, the Institute for Functional Medicine, and the American Academy of Medical Acupuncture.

I want to thank Kate Jordan, Deb Blotner, and Kathy Sartain for their professional help in organizing this information and making this book possible.

CONTENTS

PREFACE

When I started my practice in integrative medicine in 1978 there was no organized teaching about the impact that nutrition had on well-being and very little understanding of the connection between diet and disease. There were no road maps on how to practice nutritional medicine—the field was wide open for physicians like me to find a way to use diet to make a difference in people's lives. Over the years, practicing this new type of medicine has brought its share of challenges but also incredible satisfaction and excitement.

One of the keys to practicing nutritional medicine is a physician's willingness to suggest to people that they make significant dietary changes and utilize nonpharmaceutical approaches including herbs, antioxidants, vitamins, and minerals to help them recover from illness. Most importantly, the careful observation of the effect of these therapies and the feedback from my patients taught me what was useful and effective. Whenever I found significant improvement in symptoms like fatigue, joint and muscle pain, digestive problems, allergies, arthritis, headaches, or other conditions, either diagnosed or mysterious, I took notice. I wanted to understand why people got better, even if medical research could not explain these beneficial effects at the time.

In the 1980s, the field of psychoneuroimmunology revolutionized the understanding of the mind/body connection and provided a window into the connection between diet and changes in stress hormones. I realized that stress from poor dietary habits had a similar effect on the brain as did emotional and social stress. I began to research how diet and specific nutrients can improve the function of the brain and of cortisol, the key hormone from the adrenal glands that influences metabolism and, ultimately, weight gain and risk for diabetes, heart disease, and cancer.

Recent breakthroughs further clarified the changes that can occur in the midbrain, the area of the brain that directly controls stress-hormone secretions. Concepts such as allostasis and allostatic load describe how stress alters cortisol production and provide an understanding of why so many people have trouble recovering their health after stressful experiences and prolonged poor dietary habits. These ideas helped me to appreciate the widespread effect of stress on my patients' symptoms and led me to focus on methods to improve adaptation. This new information further refined my approach with patients and led to the information in this book.

In the past couple of years, one issue has become increasingly critical for the health of the world's population: obesity. In a study that looked at population data from 106 countries, Kelly and colleagues (2008) reported that if present trends continue, by the year 2030 there will be more than 2.16 billion overweight and 1.2 billion obese people in the world, many of whom will suffer from cortisol-driven disease. One aspect of the obesity epidemic that has received little attention in the popular press and is extensively discussed in this book is epigenetics, which describes the effect that diet and environmental toxins have on the gene expression that controls all cell function and is linked to weight gain and overall health. The book also contains important new information on the connection between cortisol and obesity and the importance of maintaining healthy gut bacteria (microbiota) to prevent diabetes and to lose weight, including key nutrients needed for the gut bacteria to thrive. In addition, the latest research on the key brain-protecting nutrients is detailed.

Findings from the emerging field of epigenetics will have a dramatic effect on the practice of medicine in the future. Epigenetics describes heritable changes in gene expression—passed from generation to generation of cells and at times from parents to children—influenced by diet and environmental toxins. Epigenetic studies (more than sixteen thousand research articles are published every year) also show the beneficial effect of certain foods (bioactive foods) and dietary practices on normalizing gene expression, reducing the risk for obesity, cancer, diabetes, and many other diseases. The bioactive foods include curcumin from turmeric, sulforaphane from broccoli, green tea, and genistein from soy. Epigenetic research has also identified specific deficiencies in the diet, such as lack of folic acid that can lead to increased risk of abnormal gene expression and obesity. These findings add another dimension to the Adaptation Diet program designed to control cortisol, lose weight, and prevent chronic disease.

In addition, common pollutants including polychlorinated biphenyls (PCBs), bisphenol A, and mercury, to name a few, greatly impact gene expression and increase the risk for obesity and cancer. A group of chemicals called persistent organic pollutants (POPs) include several toxins that are termed obesogens because of their dramatic effect on weight gain. Reducing exposure to these toxicants provides an additional tool in protecting the genome and maintaining normal weight, adaptation, and high-level wellness. Making people aware of this essential new research, so critical to controlling the obesity and diabetes epidemics, is one of my main goals for this book.

The Adaptation Diet is the result of working with thousands of patients over the past thirty-five years, a culmination of what I have learned about regaining adaptation, optimizing weight, and preventing disease. Especially in today's stressful climate, everyone needs to reduce stress in the areas that they can control. The place to start is at the dinner table.

La Jolla, California
July 23, 2012

1

Adaptation
and Health

The ability to adapt to changing circumstances is critical to maintaining health and aging well. Adaptation requires the right set of physical, emotional, and spiritual tools to manage stress and the challenges that life has in store for everyone. My patients who adapt well stay healthy; those who don't are at greater risk for major disease. Often overlooked is the critical effect diet has on the biochemistry of adaptation. In my practice over the past thirty-five years, I have found that eating habits and nutritional therapies play an enormous role in a patient's capacity for adaptation by keeping his or her body's chemistry better balanced and preventing excessive production of stress hormones from inappropriate dietary practices.

The biochemistry of adaptation starts in the midbrain, the crossroads of thought and emotions and the center of control over production of stress hormones: cortisol from the adrenal glands and epinephrine from the adrenals and autonomic nervous system. Hans Selye, the father of modern stress research, identified the three stages of the stress response: alarm, adaptation, and exhaustion or maladaptation. (Selye originally described this third stage as exhaustion because of his initial findings that the adrenal glands no longer produce adequate amounts of cortisol after chronic stress. Later research found that this is often not the case, so a more accurate term for the third stage is maladaptation.) In acute stress, such as a car accident or other threat to survival, the body immediately responds with the alarm reaction, secreting epinephrine (adrenaline) from the adrenal glands and norepinephrine (noradrenaline) from the brain and adrenals. Sweaty palms, increased heart rate, hypervigilance, and rapid breathing prepare the fight-or-flight response to ensure survival, reflecting the activity of the sympathetic nervous system (part of the autonomic nervous system not under voluntary control, originating in the brain and spine and branching out to all organ systems). Though the alarm reaction is often described as short-lived and occurring only in the context of immediate life-or-death situations, I have observed many of my patients remaining in this stage chronically, leading to enormous discomfort and anxiety. Caffeine, excessive intake of processed sugars and grains, and other foods that trigger maladaptation contribute to continued and inappropriate production of epinephrine.

If stress continues beyond a few minutes, cortisol (from the adrenal glands) is produced to raise blood sugar, move blood to muscles and away from digestion, lower levels of sex hormones, and break down protein stores for energy. Continuation of a stressful state is described as the adaptation stage, since it promotes short-term survival even at the cost of long-term health. The adaptation stage with elevated cortisol levels is maintained as long as there is the perception of a threat, real or imagined. During this stage, inflammation is suppressed and the immune system is inhibited by increasing cortisol levels. Appetite is often stimulated, and a person is more likely to increase energy consumption in the form of higher caloric intake. Increasing weight and the effect of cortisol on inhibiting insulin's action to bring blood sugar into cells can lead to insulin resistance, a condition that is the starting point for many chronic illnesses. Continued stress eventually leads to the maladaptation stage in which the body starts to break down from the effects of elevated cortisol. The maladaptation stage is marked by immune system suppression, poor wound healing, thinning bones, insulin resistance, loss of muscle mass, weight gain around the midsection, depression and anxiety, poor sleep, and elevated blood pressure—all courtesy of elevated levels of cortisol and epinephrine. Another key negative impact of excess cortisol is the loss of muscle mass from the catabolic effect of this hormone. Research has shown that maintaining a healthy amount of lean muscle mass is the single best prevention against premature aging and diseases such as diabetes and heart disease. What I have discovered is that the long-term stress that leads to these dire consequences can arise not only from emotional and situational states but also from what is eaten on a daily basis.

Cortisol is one of forty stress hormones from the adrenal glands called glucocorticoids. The adrenals sit atop the kidneys and are divided into two areas: the adrenal medulla and adrenal cortex. The medulla produces epinephrine and norepinephrine (noradrenaline) used for immediate fight-or-flight response. The cortex has several zones that produce the glucocorticoids (including cortisol) and mineralocorticoids, which regulate electrolytes and fluid balance and impact blood pressure. Along with cortisol, the other key hormones are dehydroepiandrosterone (DHEA) and aldosterone.

Cortisol production is tightly regulated by feedback mechanisms in the midbrain, hypothalamus, and pituitary gland, with rising cortisol shutting down further stimulation of the adrenal glands. This feedback loop is called the hypothalamic-pituitary-adrenal (HPA) axis. However, in a state of continued stress, including the wrong foods and eating habits, the feedback loop between the brain and the adrenal glands' cortisol production breaks down, leading to inappropriate levels of cortisol.

Elevated cortisol, from poor dietary habits or other chronic stress, leads to a change in the brain and endocrine system called allostasis. This revolutionary new concept describes the stress response as not simply a short-term adjustment that eventually returns the body to a preset level of cortisol secretion, but a more permanent change in the control over stress-hormone production. Even if the original stressful event has been resolved, a new set point might continue, leading to ongoing excess cortisol production. The damage that occurs from this new set point of cortisol production is called allostatic load, made even worse by poor dietary habits and nutritional deficiencies. Eventually, the wear and tear of poor adaptation and allostatic load, coupled with the brain's fail-safe shutdown of chronic cortisol elevation, lead to a failure of normal cortisol regulation, inhibiting additional cortisol secretion by the adrenal glands. This leads to fatigue, anxiety, depression, poor resistance, and an inability to recover effectively from life's challenges.

Emotional states impact adaptation and cortisol levels as well. The brain, through the limbic lobe (the emotional center), connects

---

Stages of Stress Response

- The brain experiences or thinks of something stressful.
- An immediate release of norepinephrine and epinephrine from the adrenal medulla and sympathetic nervous system occurs.
- This raises heart rate, blood pressure, and respiration rate and shunts blood from the digestive tract to the muscles.
- If stress is not resolved immediately, the brain secretes CRH (corticotropin-releasing hormone).
- CRH causes the release of ACTH (adrenocorticotropic hormone) within fifteen seconds and the subsequent release of cortisol from the adrenal glands.
- The pancreas releases glucagon, which raises the circulating levels of glucose for use by the brain and muscles for energy during the stress.
- The pituitary gland releases prolactin to suppress reproductive activity and reduce testosterone, estrogen, and progesterone.
- Thyroid function and growth-hormone production are inhibited.
- Endorphins, enkephalins, and vasopressin are secreted to suppress pain and improve cardiac function.
- If the stress continues, many of these effects become chronic and cause continued alterations in physiology.
- Chronic stress leads to elevated blood glucose, insulin resistance, depressed sexual function, weight gain, suppressed immunity, and elevated blood pressure and heart rate.

emotions and perceptions of the world with the appropriate level of cortisol production and nervous system stimulation. Fear, worry, anxiety, or the anticipation of a stressful experience is enough to trigger the brain to initiate the biochemistry of stress. Poor diet, lack of exercise, and obesity also increase cortisol levels and allostatic load. Many people are more prone to be emotionally stressed because of poor dietary habits, which change the brain's chemistry and reduce their ability to adapt, leading again to more cortisol. Even more problematic is the fact that elevated cortisol itself alters the emotional stress response, increasing allostatic load, obesity, and disease.

One of the consequences of chronic cortisol elevation is the impact on how stressful events are perceived. The emotional memory of any significant trauma or stress, whether from a car accident, abuse in a relationship, or any other chronically stressful situation, is stored in two parts of the midbrain (as well as the cerebral cortex): the amygdala and the hippocampus. The memory in the amygdala is implicit and nonspecific, a remembrance that stress occurred, but not of the details of the specific event. When stress continues over time, the amygdala literally grows new neuronal connections to ensure the survival of these memories. The identification of new neuronal growth, called long-term potentiation, is a major breakthrough in the understanding of brain function. (Until recently it was believed that no new cell growth could occur in the central nervous system.) The amygdala contributes directly to elevated cortisol levels through secretion of corticotropin-releasing hormone (CRH). Poor diet could also add to the neuropotentiation of the amygdala.

The amygdala has connections to many parts of the brain and is a major source of corticotropin-releasing hormone (CRH), which controls secretion of cortisol and epinephrine, impacting both the fight-or-flight response and later allostasis. In addition, the amygdala sends neurons to the sympathetic nervous system to further activate the fight-or-flight response (rapid heart rate, shallow breathing, hypervigilance). Most importantly, it sends "emotional" information to the frontal cortex, which colors perceptions of events and memories, allowing past trauma to influence the present.

Repeated stressful events lead to long-term neuropotentiation in the amygdala, creating increased levels of neurotransmitter chemicals and new growth of neurons that reinforce the stressful memories. However, the implicit memories associated with the amygdala are not necessarily associated with specific events or people, but contain a nonspecific and preconscious response, which often involves fear or other stressful emotions. It is because of the generality and vagueness of this type of memory that the amygdala is so often involved in maladapted chronic stress response. This is one of the reasons that people have trouble disengaging themselves from their illness and their stress; the memories and connections from the amygdala keep the stress going, though the details might be lost and perceptions altered. This is at the root of poor adaptation.

The other part of the midbrain that is involved with memories of stressful events is the hippocampus, also a major player in controlling cortisol and epinephrine output. The hippocampus is the seat of declarative memory, a detailed and specific recollection of actual stressful events. The hippocampus is also the site of the regulatory mechanism that measures cortisol levels and influences adrenal secretion of this hormone. Unfortunately, elevated levels of cortisol actually damage the hippocampal neurons, impair long-term potentiation in this part of the midbrain, and degrade the declarative memory.

We are left with an enhanced preconscious and implicit, nonspecific stress memory and response from the amygdala, while lacking the accurate conscious and declarative memory of the hippocampus to modify the stress response. Over time, with ongoing stress, the nonspecific memory of the amygdala becomes more entrenched while the details of what the stress actually was, stored in the hippocampus, are lost. This keeps us from being in the present. Although specific memories may not be accessible, perceptions continue to be colored by past events, continuing the stress response.

Long-term stress, whether from situational issues, emotional challenges, or poor dietary habits, can lead to maladaptation and damage from allostatic load through these changes in the brain. Cortisol and CRH from the amygdala are the chemicals that produce these changes. In studies of depressed patients, the hippocampus is 10 to 20 percent smaller than normal, the result of elevated cortisol production. Stress-induced inhibition of new neuron formation in the hippocampus impacts the cortisol control mechanism and declarative memory.

Another outcome of long-term dysregulation of cortisol is the depletion of norepinephrine levels in the brain (especially in an area called the locus coeruleus, which is involved with attentiveness and activity). This is another aspect of the connection between stress and depression (along with the depletion of serotonin and dopamine from the frontal cortex of the brain, which is also caused by elevated cortisol levels). In fact, in animal studies, stress-induced elevated cortisol during pregnancy has been shown to affect the fetuses by reducing the size and structure of the hippocampus as the offspring become adults. This could explain why family traits of depression are frequently found. So many of my patients with stress-related medical problems come from dysfunctional families, often with depressed or anxious mothers who did not create a safe and nourishing environment for their children. It's possible that these early experiences affected the midbrain, increasing the vulnerability for stress-induced illness.

These changes in the midbrain explain why some people develop chronic anxiety, depression, or post-traumatic stress disorder. It is now recognized that with treatment—psychotherapy, acupuncture, and possibly medication—the amygdala can remodel and reduce the chronic stimulation of CRH and cortisol. What has been overlooked is the effect of diet and food choices on the biochemistry of stress.

Poor dietary choices—whether they are excessive processed sugars and carbohydrates, inflammation-causing fats, or chemicals in the food chain in nonorganic vegetables, fruits, and proteins—impact cell signaling and increase biochemical stress. This leads to a greater cortisol response and all its negative consequences. Like emotional traumas or physical illness, daily choices about what is on the dinner plate are a major trigger for increased allostatic load, enhanced amygdala neuropotentiation, and the slippery slope of stress-induced chronic disease.

Cortisol and other stress hormones, which are essential for survival and adaptation to stress, become just as dangerous as the external threats themselves when they are chronically elevated and maladapted. Cortisol levels also increase with age, unlike all other hormones, leading some to call cortisol the "death hormone" because of its connection to so many degenerative diseases. Cortisol imbalance can lead to fatigue, weight gain, immune suppression, susceptibility to colds and flu, joint pains, mood swings, anxiety, depression, insomnia, and digestive symptoms such as reflux and heartburn. (See list below.) These symptoms are a message of poor adaptation, not necessarily a message to take antidepressants, stomach acid blockers, or pain medication! Because people often ignore the real meaning of these common complaints, we are in an epidemic of diseases of maladaptation, such as obesity, cancer, heart disease, hypertension, stroke, diabetes, Alzheimer's disease, depression, anxiety, and premature aging.

Markers of Allostatic Load

- Abdominal obesity, increased waist/hip ratio
- Fatigue
- Elevated blood pressure or pulse
- Poor concentration and memory
- Poor resistance to infections
- Elevated blood sugar, cholesterol, LDL
- Inflammation, including headaches, muscle pain, joint pain
- Digestive symptoms, reflux

Cortisol and Obesity

Obesity and cortisol are inexorably linked. Higher levels of cortisol directly contribute to obesity while obesity itself leads to increased cortisol. In addition, increased levels of cortisol have many physiologic costs. To provide energy to deal with a stressful situation—whether it's running from a tiger, dealing with your obnoxious neighbor, or eating a hot dog and chips (pro-inflammatory foods)—cortisol mobilizes fats and sugars from storage sites in the body, resulting in an increase of glucose, proteins, and fats in the blood to fuel muscles. Chronic increase in cortisol leads to elevated blood sugar and free fat production that can result in not only obesity but insulin resistance (a state in which insulin, needed to bring blood sugar into cells, is not effective because of changes in cell-membrane receptors) and increased risks for heart disease, cancer, and diabetes.

Studies of patients with small adrenal tumors (called incidentalomas, causing subclinical Cushing's disease) have shown that even a slight increase in cortisol production over a long period of time leads to abdominal obesity, diabetes, high blood fats, and hypertension. Elevated cortisol and obesity set up a vicious cycle. Obesity itself causes elevated cortisol—as shown in a 2010 study where Roelfsema and colleagues found higher twenty-four-hour cortisol levels in obese women compared to lean controls—increasing the risk for insulin resistance and other unhealthy consequences. Elevated cortisol and HPA (hypothalamic-pituitary-adrenal) axis activity was also shown to be greater in type 2 diabetics with abdominal obesity compared to controls (Prpic-Krizevac 2012).

Cortisol is a major cause of obesity because it stimulates increased appetite and food-seeking behavior to support the energy requirements of the stress response. Cortisol elevation is strongly linked to abdominal fat accumulation, reduced synthesis of muscle protein, and increased weight. In addition, fat cells in the abdomen (visceral fat) have an enzyme that converts inactive cortisone to active cortisol, contributing to the vicious cycle of stress and poor diet, causing elevated cortisol, which leads to more fat deposition, which leads to higher cortisol and even more abdominal obesity. For many people, insomnia, depression, anxiety, and fatigue—all symptoms initiated or made worse by cortisol dysregulation—are linked to excessive caloric intake and obesity.

In a healthy state, cortisol levels should decline prior to sleep onset and peak in the morning. I have found through salivary cortisol measures that many of my patients with sleep disturbance and obesity have an elevated cortisol level prior to sleep and a low level in the morning. This dysregulated cortisol pattern is a hallmark of poor adaptation, insomnia, fatigue, and weight gain. This pattern also leads to lower levels of leptin—a hormone made in fat cells needed to suppress appetite—making weight loss even more difficult.

Another hormone that contributes to cortisol excess is ghrelin, a powerful appetite stimulant made in the stomach. Ghrelin production is suppressed by healthy food choices, but many aspects of the typical American diet, including high-fat meals, fewer and larger meals, and excess sweets, do not effectively reduce ghrelin, further increasing cortisol levels. In obese individuals there exists a faulty regulation of ghrelin with less dietary suppression even with the same caloric intake, leading to more cortisol production.

Insulin resistance from excess dietary sugar also contributes to faulty regulation of ghrelin, contributing to more cortisol and weight gain. Protein intake (up to 35 percent of daily calories) is associated with less hunger and lower ghrelin levels and, therefore, lower cortisol levels and a better chance for weight loss. Breakfast, the most important meal in terms of hormonal control, should contain at least 25 percent of its calories from protein to suppress ghrelin and reduce cortisol. Beware of the high-carbohydrate breakfast, such as cereals and baked goods, which raises cortisol from poor suppression of ghrelin, blood-sugar spikes, and high insulin levels.

There is a great deal of research connecting cortisol and obesity. Wallerius and colleagues (2003) studied middle-aged men in Sweden and found that morning cortisol levels were directly correlated with body mass index (a measure of body fat), waist/hip ratio, and abdominal diameter. The higher the cortisol level, the more weight and fat were carried. In another study, from 2012, Himeno and colleagues measured morning cortisol levels and inflammatory markers in eighty-three obese Japanese patients. After a three-month weight-loss program he found that lower baseline cortisol predicted a better outcome in terms of weight loss while higher cortisol was associated with inflammation and arterial stiffness, a risk for heart disease and hypertension. The higher the cortisol the more difficult the weight loss as well as the more likely a person would be overweight.

Studies have shown that cortisol drives energy (calorie) consumption and increases appetite especially for carbohydrates and fats. In 2010 Shi and colleagues found that cortisol reduces the level of adiponectin, the key hormone that decreases appetite and caloric intake. This is another way cortisol excess can increase obesity in many individuals. In a study of more than six hundred children, Hill and colleagues (2011) found that an increased waist circumference was associated with higher morning cortisol levels; the higher the cortisol, the greater the weight gain during the nine-month period of the study.

In addition to cortisol adding to the risk of obesity, the stress response (increased cortisol and epinephrine levels) itself is heightened in individuals who are overweight, setting up a vicious cycle of continued weight gain and poor adaptation. In 2008 Farag and colleagues discovered that in the seventy-eight women in their study the more obese the person, the greater the perceived stress response. Results of the study showed that the body mass index (BMI) alone predicted higher cortisol secretion independent of stress levels. A study by Lasikiewicz and colleagues in 2012 found that men with greater waist/hip ratios secreted higher amounts of cortisol under a stressful memory task and had poorer performance compared to normal-weight individuals.

There is yet another aspect of the cortisol/obesity connection: the direct effect of stress—whether psychological or physical—on the inflammatory pathways, which ultimately results in elevated cortisol and greater abdominal fat. We all assume that weight gain in times of stress occurs from "comfort" eating as a stress-reducing behavior. However, many of my patients still gain weight in times of stress even if they do not consume excess calories. Recent scientific findings have begun to shed light on the connection between stress and weight gain, and it is more involved than eating that extra serving of dessert.

It turns out that the stress response includes not only increased cortisol and adrenaline (epinephrine) production, but also the release of several cellular messengers called cytokines that induce an inflammatory response. These mediators include interleukins (IL-6, IL-1), tumor necrosis factor (TNF), and C-reactive protein (CRP). IL-6, like cortisol, is associated with increased appetite and visceral fat. In addition, any increase in inflammation prompts the HPA axis to upregulate cortisol production, leading to all of its many effects on weight gain and greater visceral fat accumulation.

The biochemistry of visceral fat also contributes to the obesity/cortisol connection. Visceral fat has a greater density of cortisol receptors than does subcutaneous white fat, leading to a preferential increase in this fat mass when there is a greater energy supply from elevated cortisol or excess caloric intake. There is also greater blood supply in visceral fat, contributing to its many hormonal effects. It appears that circulating glucose and free fatty acids, which are used for energy, are shunted more to visceral fat for storage and greater triglyceride synthesis, increasing the size and number of fat cells in the abdomen. Greater amounts of visceral fat lead to the increased release of inflammatory molecules like IL-6 and TNF-alpha as well as the hormones leptin, resistin, and adiponectin, continuing a vicious cycle of weight gain and inflammation. All of these changes increase the likelihood of greater abdominal girth, more visceral fat, more cortisol, and obesity.

The common thread in all of these complex biochemical and hormonal responses is increased cortisol, not only from psychological stress, but also from the heightened inflammatory state and increased visceral fat. Once excess fat is established in the abdomen, the slippery slope toward obesity, diabetes, metabolic syndrome, and heart disease has begun. The way out of this dilemma, detailed in the following pages, is to effectively control cortisol through dietary and behavioral means and to reverse the accumulation of visceral fat.

Elevated cortisol also inhibits thyroid function, adding to weight gain and fatigue. The immune system is suppressed in a variety of ways by excess cortisol, leading to a greater chance for serious infections, causing more maladaptation. Cortisol excess has been linked to bone loss, lowered sex hormones, and greater inflammation. Elevated stress hormones inhibit digestion and have been associated with ulcers, intestinal disorders, and irritable bowel syndrome (a condition of abdominal pain, bloating, and alternating diarrhea and constipation). With these and other stress-induced digestive

Early Signs and Symptoms of Maladaptation

Emotional and behavioral signs	Physical signs and symptoms
Fatigue	Weight gain, especially in abdomen
Nervousness	
Anxiety, agitation	Hypoglycemia, low blood sugar
Little resilience, stress intolerance	Headaches
	Frequent colds and flu
Noise sensitivity	Muscular pain and tenderness
Worries and fears	Joint pain and tenderness
Inability to concentrate	Heart palpitations, elevated heart rate
Alcohol craving or intolerance	
Sweets and fats cravings	Menstrual irregularity
Lower sex drive	Back or neck pain
	Abdominal discomfort

problems, poor functioning of the small intestine and colon can lead to malabsorption of nutrients and nutritional deficiencies. These resulting nutritional deficiencies open the door to many other medical problems, worsening maladaptation, allostatic load, and poor weight control. To avoid the consequences of excess cortisol and to lose weight, the goal has to be to do everything possible to normalize cortisol.

Later Signs and Symptoms of Maladaptation

Emotional and behavioral signs	Physical signs and symptoms
Poor wound healing	Allergies
Increased blood pressure	Sexual dysfunction, impotency
Apathy	Loss of muscle mass
Life seems difficult, unfair	Depression
Salt craving	Facial swelling, fluid retention
Worsening premenstrual tension	Glucose (sugar) intolerance, insulin resistance
Generalized weakness	Loss of bone density (osteoporosis)
Poor memory	Moon (swollen) face

The Adaptation Diet gives you control over your cortisol secretion and a method to stop the biochemical stress that leads to weight gain. The key to adaptation and control over cortisol through diet is threefold: (1) reducing inflammation through healthy food choices, including the use of good fats, (2) preventing insulin resistance and metabolic syndrome through the use of low-glycemic-index carbohydrates and organically grown whole food, and (3) identifying and avoiding food allergens to reduce many nagging symptoms and decrease cortisol production. This book describes in detail the dietary changes needed to achieve normal cortisol levels and improve the biochemistry of adaptation, reduce allostatic load, and reduce the likelihood of premature aging. Following these guidelines has helped many of my patients achieve adaptation, lose weight, and improve well-being.

2

Food and Adaptation

During my thirty-five years of practice, I have seen the remarkable effects diet can have on reducing stress and regulating cortisol levels. I first became aware of the impact of diet on health when I was in medical school in the late 1960s. What I learned came not from my professors (in 1969 there was no instruction on nutrition; even today there still is little taught) but from personal research my classmates and I performed. I had been eating a standard American diet (SAD) heavy on meat, cheese, bread, and sweets. It left me a bit overweight and very sluggish. When my roommates and I decided to adopt a macrobiotic diet (a Westernized application of a traditional Asian diet popularized by Michio Kushi), my life changed.

Our version of the macrobiotic diet included brown rice, cooked vegetables, tofu, fish, and chicken. There was no red meat, sweets, fruits, sweeteners, dairy, corn, or wheat. The results were remarkable—I lost weight effortlessly, my energy improved, I was more relaxed, and I felt mentally sharper. Aches and pains disappeared, and my digestion improved as well. It was then that my orientation toward what I was being taught in medical school changed. I realized, as Hippocrates said, that food is your best medicine, and that I would have to teach myself how best to help my patients. My practice today is consistent with that personal epiphany in 1969.

Current research demonstrates convincingly that diet contributes to 35 percent of all cancers and the majority of heart disease. The standard American diet not only is implicated in these chronic diseases but is the biggest factor in premature aging. Not appreciated, however, is the mechanism by which diet directly causes maladaptation and cortisol dysregulation. To counteract the maladaptive effects of eating habits, I developed the Adaptation Diet, a template to regain adaptation and robust health. Every aspect of the Adaptation Diet is aimed at cortisol regulation and reduction of allostatic load, leading to weight loss, enhanced well-being, and disease prevention.

Diet and Adaptation

Shane looked at me in disbelief. He was a strapping man in his mid-forties with wide-open eyes that made him appear as if he had just been startled. His main complaints were insomnia, anxiety, and a mind that raced like that of a NASCAR driver. Luckily, he had not yet developed any heart disease or diabetes. I had measured his salivary cortisol levels, and they were off the chart. He was expecting me to reach for my prescription pad; instead, I told him that if he wanted to eliminate his problems, he needed to normalize his cortisol and the place to begin was changing what he ate.

I recommended that Shane stop eating all processed foods: white flour products and, most importantly, all sugar, desserts, candy, and other sweets. He was put on a program to keep his blood sugar stable throughout the day by having a protein-rich breakfast and snacks of nuts, seeds, nut butter, or protein powder. In six weeks he repeated his cortisol test. He came in to my office soon thereafter, his demeanor drastically changed. He sat calmly in his chair, not fidgeting but able to focus on what I was saying.

Within a week of changing his diet, Shane was sleeping better, he was calmer, and, most surprising to him, he felt more positive about life in general. Over the next six weeks, he started to feel like his old self, was more pleasant to be around (according to his wife), and was more productive at work. His salivary cortisol levels had come down to normal.

Another patient, Beth, had just completed her food allergy skin testing when she saw me for a consultation. She was markedly overweight, fatigued, irritable (especially during the week prior to her menstrual period), and a poor sleeper. Beth, a thirty-two-year-old mother of two, felt like she was eighty. Her joints hurt every day, her muscles were weak, and she had no stamina. As a child, Beth had a history of hay fever and a touch of asthma, which she had outgrown. Most of her doctors had assumed she was depressed and treated her with antidepressants, which only made her feel more tired and out of sorts.

Beth looked a bit panicked when we started to talk about her test results. The first words out of her mouth were "What am I going to eat?" Her skin testing revealed significant reactions to wheat, dairy, baker's yeast, corn, and tomatoes. Her cortisol test showed a dramatic deficit in cortisol production, especially in the morning. (She was in the later stages of cortisol dysregulation; after decades of elevated levels, her brain had shut down the cortisol response.) With the help of our nutritionist, we created a well-balanced diet including a small amount of grains other than wheat and corn and the elimination of tomatoes, dairy, and yeast.

It took only a few days for Beth to see the change. The first thing she noticed was that her aches and pains disappeared. Gradually she began to sleep better, was less irritable, and lost some of her extra weight. When I retested her cortisol levels two months later, her morning measurement was in the normal range. She came in after that with a smile as wide as her whole face. She had not felt this good since she was a youngster and thanked me for giving her a chance to be happy again.

What happened for Beth and Shane? They had regained adaptation, reducing their allostatic load, rapidly normalizing their cortisol levels. The foods that Shane ate that caused low blood sugar, as well as the unhealthy fats that he was exposed to daily, had raised his cortisol to dangerous levels. Yet, within a short period of time, his hypothalamic-pituitary-adrenal (HPA) axis, with help from this change in eating habits, reverted to a normal pattern. In Beth's case, she reduced her inflammatory response by avoiding foods that she was allergic to, allowing her HPA axis to reset normal cortisol levels.

Fortunately, I have been able to help many patients improve their allostatic load simply by making dietary changes. For some, avoiding food allergens is the key. For others, it is maintaining normal blood sugar and avoiding hypoglycemia. For all my patients, a key component is reducing foods that trigger inflammation, such as refined sugar and flour products, fried foods, and animal protein that is not free range or fed organically. (For example, free-range chicken eggs have one-tenth the omega-6 inflammatory fatty acids as industrially produced eggs.)

The common denominator for all these patients is finding a way to regain biochemical adaptation through limiting their body's abnormal cortisol response to the wrong foods. I call this approach the Adaptation Diet because the goal is to control the abnormal production of cortisol and the cascade of hormonal changes that characterize maladaptation.

The components of the Adaptation Diet are:

- Emphasizing anti-inflammatory foods rich in phytonutrients such as flavonoids, carotenoids, and omega-3 fatty acids, and eliminating inflammation-causing foods, especially the pro-inflammatory fats, including omega-6 fatty acids and trans fats
- Identifying food allergies and avoiding allergy-causing foods
- Avoiding gluten-containing grains if gluten sensitive
- Using low-glycemic-index carbohydrates, maintaining normal blood sugar and insulin levels, and avoiding hypoglycemia and insulin resistance
- Using foods, herbs, and supplements that normalize cortisol
- Detoxifying to reduce inflammation and cellular damage
- Protecting the genome through bioactive foods (see Chapter 9)

Five aspects of dietary habits directly link to elevated cortisol levels. The first is food composition. Studies have shown that excess intake of protein and fat (especially the "wrong" fats) and simple carbohydrates increases cortisol production significantly in stressful situations. On the other hand, consumption of whole grains and omega-3 fatty acids can lower the cortisol response. In a study performed by Markus and colleagues (2000), people identified as high stress responders (you probably know if you are in that category) showed lower cortisol responses and less depression when fed a complex-carbohydrate-rich and protein-poor diet as compared to a typical high-protein diet. (The protein in this study was not defined but probably contained excessive amounts of red meat, dairy, and eggs. If the protein was mainly fish and vegetable based, cortisol levels would not have been adversely affected.)

The second key to lower cortisol is maintaining normal blood sugar and avoiding spikes in insulin production that can lead to insulin resistance. Insulin resistance is an increasingly common finding in overweight individuals. In insulin resistance, the receptors on the cell surface become dysfunctional, leading to the production of more and more insulin. Inflammation is thought to be one cause of this cell-membrane dysfunction. Repeated use of refined sugars and simple carbohydrates can lead to metabolic syndrome (high blood pressure, elevated blood fats, and increased risk for heart disease), obesity, and diabetes.

High-glycemic-index (a measure of how rapidly a food causes a spike in blood sugar) and refined and processed foods such as white flour products (white bread, cookies, pastas, candy, muffins), refined sugar, juices with added sugar, soft drinks (especially with high-fructose corn syrup), most breakfast cereals, and chips are the main culprits in poor control of blood sugar. Using foods that are high in fiber slows digestion of carbohydrates and improves blood-sugar maintenance, preventing blood-sugar spikes, increased insulin production leading to obesity, and hypoglycemia. Beans, brown rice, steel-cut oatmeal, buckwheat, and green vegetables like broccoli and spinach are some of the good sources of fiber.

Another concern regarding high-glycemic-index meals is the impact they have on appetite and eating behavior. Because low blood sugar often follows the spike in glucose from high-glycemic-index foods, eating behavior is enhanced and people will consume more calories throughout the day after a high-glycemic-index meal. Without adequate protein, ghrelin production will not be suppressed after a meal, another reason for increased caloric intake. This is a setup for weight gain, abdominal obesity, and eventually insulin resistance and all its subsequent health risks.

On a flight recently, I listened carefully to the list of drinks and snacks that were offered to the passengers. As I watched the majority of my seatmates consume sodas, juices, crackers, and other high-glycemic-index foods, it wasn't hard to imagine what was happening to their physiology and allostatic load while they silently flew toward their destination. The blast of sugar triggered a spike in blood glucose, activating a potent release of insulin to drive the glucose into the cells, which then led to hypoglycemia and a release of the counter-regulatory hormones, including cortisol. This soft-drink-induced event ended with a release of free fatty acids in the form of triglycerides and other fats and increased adiposity in the abdominal cavity.

Repeated sodas later, the sequence changes. No longer does the insulin effectively bring down the glucose from the sudden burst of sugar, because insulin resistance has occurred. The adipocytes (fat cells) secrete inflammatory hormones, including resistin, that interfere with the cell-membrane signaling from insulin, impacting the cell's ability to absorb glucose from the bloodstream for energy. The result is more allostatic load, cortisol, free fats, obesity, and inflammation. The cycle repeats with every high-glycemic-index meal, leading to first being overweight with a body mass index (BMI) of 25–30, then obese with a BMI of 30–35, then morbidly obese (over 35 BMI), and finally super morbid obesity with a BMI over 50.

The third key to lower cortisol is choosing the right fats: foods rich in omega-3 and gamma linolenic omega-6 fats. Salmon, walnuts, almonds, halibut, flaxseed, pumpkin seeds, and other sources of these good fats reduce inflammation and prevent excess cortisol production. Avoidance of the omega-6 fats found in vegetable oils, including corn oil, safflower oil, and sunflower oil; the trans fats found in most processed foods; and the saturated fats in red meat and whole dairy products also lowers inflammation and the demand for cortisol.

The fourth key to lower cortisol is to include foods that are rich in flavonoids, carotenoids, and other phytonutrients that can help to detoxify the body and protect cellular health. Green tea, garlic, onions, red wine, blueberries, broccoli, tomatoes, bell peppers, and kale are just a few of these superfoods that reduce the need for cortisol by controlling cellular damage.

The fifth and most overlooked key in controlling cortisol is identifying food allergies and food intolerance. Reactions from food allergies trigger a dramatic rise in cortisol; in my clinical experience food allergies are one of the most frequent causes of depression, fatigue, anxiety, insomnia, aches and pains, and digestive problems. The most common food triggers are the most commonly overused foods: wheat, beef, yeast, corn, dairy, sugar, and soy.

When I look back at my early experiment with macrobiotics, it amazes me that most of these five keys to lower cortisol were accomplished through that diet. Today I know much more about the mechanisms of food-triggered cortisol response and have helped many of my patients regain adaptation through diet. Let's look at another of my patients with a common story.

Sara was always feeling stressed. She was anxious, light-headed, tired, and depressed. No longer able to hold a job, she was in a doctor-shopping frenzy. Sara had a history of episodic depression and fatigue as well as hay fever and other allergies. At thirty-six, she felt that life was passing her by, was rarely feeling well, and was always on the verge of overreacting to whatever challenges life presented.

Her complaints made me suspicious of cortisol dysregulation. I ordered a salivary cortisol test that showed highly elevated cortisol levels, typical for someone in a chronically stressed state. Though Sara was well versed in stress-management techniques, including meditation and exercise, it did her little good. What did matter was her diet.

Every day when waking, her level of dread and anxiety was at its highest, calming down after breakfast. Sara had always had an enormous sweet tooth; her breakfast was usually a sweet roll, juice, and coffee. She snacked on chips and pretzels throughout the day. She also liked red meat; one of her favorites was a carne asada burrito at a local Mexican fast-food restaurant. Without knowing it, Sara had multiple food allergies that we later identified through intradermal skin testing. This technique involves placing a small amount of a food antigen under the skin and observing the wheal growth over a period of ten minutes. According to the American Academy of Environmental Medicine, this is the gold standard for food allergy tests.

Sara's diet contributed to elevated cortisol in several different ways. She had reactive hypoglycemia—low blood sugar as a result of eating foods rich in simple sugars and white flour products. Sara felt so dreadful in the morning because her late-night desserts first caused a spike in her blood sugar and insulin, then a dip, triggering a compensatory response to raise her blood-sugar levels back up. The hormones that accomplish this include cortisol and norepinephrine. As a result of this all-night hormonal chaos, she awoke with anxiety. (One of cortisol's roles is to elevate blood sugar if it drops too low from excess insulin production, often the result of eating processed foods.)

Throughout the day, Sara's blood sugar would bounce up and down—her simple-carbohydrate-rich breakfast and lunch (a sandwich and some chips) led to low blood sugar in the mid-afternoon and additional increases in cortisol and norepinephrine. She would feel tired, out of sorts, thickheaded with poor concentration, anxious, and jittery. (Most people with reactive hypoglycemia have their worst slump after lunch, probably because they eat little at breakfast and lack the right foods at lunch, whereas dinner is typically higher in protein and more substantial.)

Unfortunately, low blood sugar was not the only trigger for Sara's elevated cortisol. Her snacks often included foods with unhealthy omega-6 fats, processed from corn or soy oils, as well as trans-fatty acids. These fats trigger cellular inflammation, though there are few signs or warnings that this is occurring. The inflammatory response to these foods is a significant biochemical process affecting the coronary arteries, brain neurons, joints, and the digestive tract. The body's antidote for inflammation is cortisol. The chips, pretzels, cookies, and fast foods create a clarion call to the adrenal glands to help rescue the body from the onslaughts of the modern food industry.

One more factor contributing to Sara's medley of cortisol triggers was food allergy. Sara had a history from her teenage years of respiratory allergies, a hint that food allergies were playing a role. She had other signs including digestive complaints, fatigue, headaches, and dizziness, all occurring after meals. When she avoided the foods we eventually identified as her triggers—corn, soy, wheat, and dairy—she improved quickly.

Here's what Sara needed to do to resolve the cortisol overload from her diet:

1. To improve her hypoglycemia:

   - Eat a protein-rich breakfast (choose from eggs, low-fat unsweetened yogurt, oatmeal, nut butter, nuts, seeds, fish); use only complex carbohydrates (whole grains, especially steel-cut oatmeal); avoid all high-glycemic-index foods (see Appendix A).

   - Have protein snacks between breakfast and lunch, and eat a protein-rich lunch and dinner (nuts, seeds, nut butter, beans, unsweetened yogurt, turkey, chicken, fish).

- Avoid all processed sweets, white sugar, white flour, processed grains, and fruit-sweetened food and drinks—use whole fruit as dessert.

- Supplement with protein powder as needed between meals or as a meal replacement (when in a rush).

- Avoid sweets late at night—use complex carbohydrates and protein instead.

2. To improve the types of fatty acids in her diet:

- Avoid snack foods such as pretzels, chips, cookies.

- Never use margarine, corn oil, or polyunsaturated oils.

- Use olive, grapeseed, or canola oil for cooking or salad dressing.

- Avoid fried foods, especially deep-fried fast foods.

- Increase intake of wild salmon, avocados, walnuts, almonds, flaxseed (powder and oil), halibut.

- Decrease red meat intake; use only low-fat organic dairy.

- Never use trans fats.

3. To improve the food allergies:

- Follow the avoidance and challenge program of the Adaptation Diet to identify the main food triggers.

- If she has access to a physician experienced in food allergy management, get skin tested or blood tests that are approved by the American Academy of Environmental Medicine.

- If not sure about which foods are triggers, avoid the big seven of delayed food allergy: wheat, corn, soy, dairy, yeast, beef, and tomatoes.

- Adopt a rotation diet, eating foods no more often than twice a week that are causing symptoms.

Once these suggestions were adopted, Sara improved quickly. Her cortisol levels returned to normal. She slept more deeply and awoke refreshed. Her anxiety and fatigue during the day were much reduced. She was thrilled by a weight loss of twelve pounds over six weeks.

As many of my patients have proven, what is on the dinner plate has as much an influence on adaptation and aging well as anything else that a person can control. Cortisol production increases when there is inflammation from the wrong fats in the diet, hypoglycemia in response to eating high-glycemic-index foods, food allergy reactions, increased abdominal girth and insulin resistance, and exposure to toxins. If you think these triggers are not common in the typical American diet, you are wrong. Obesity rates are now approaching 50 percent of all Americans, including children. Food allergies and food intolerance affect nearly that many. Inflammation is the result of eating the wrong fats—omega-6 (packaged and processed foods, red meat, eggs, and whole-fat dairy) instead of omega-3 (cold-water fish, walnuts, and almonds)—as well as the result of exposure to pollutants in the food chain.

The Adaptation Diet is the answer to adaptation and aging well. Most Americans' eating habits contribute to premature aging through triggers that raise cortisol levels. Perhaps we should rename the standard American diet the maladaptation diet, because most people are doing themselves harm by increasing their stress hormones through their dietary habits.

3

Detoxification
and Adaptation

The first step of the Adaptation Diet program in reclaiming adaptation is a three-week detoxification program to assist the body's ability to remove toxins and pollutants and reduce allostatic load. The concept of detoxification goes back to Hippocrates, considered the founder of Western medicine, who believed that cleanliness was key to health and advocated fasting, steam baths, bathing in springs, and gymnastics. The Chinese Taoist physicians also were aware of the need to detoxify, employing herbal remedies to clear poisons from the system. Detoxification occurs primarily through the liver, kidneys, and digestive tract. The liver, the principal organ of detoxification, converts toxic chemicals, drugs, hormones, and products of metabolism such as free radicals to inert substances that can be eliminated through the gut or the kidneys.

Repeatedly, my patients have dramatic improvements in a host of symptoms by simply "cleaning up" their diets during the detox phase. Headaches, joint pains, constipation, abdominal discomfort, and fatigue are just a few of the problems that consistently begin to resolve, often within the first ten days of the program. Symptoms improve because of the use of more nutritious foods, the avoidance of simple sugars and starches and other toxic foods, the elimination of the foods that are most likely to trigger an allergic response, and the improvement in the detoxification pathways to clear chemicals and other toxins from the body. All of these aspects have one thing in common: the normalization of the cortisol response.

Modern life presents an enormous challenge to the detoxification system. For example, to make shelf life longer, a Twinkies cake has thirty-nine ingredients, including polysorbate 60 replacing real cream, artificial vanillin instead of the real thing, diacetyl instead of butter, yellow no. 5 and red no. 40 for coloring, and industrial chemicals such as corn dextrin (used as a thickener, and also used in glues) and calcium sulfate (food-grade plaster of Paris). The shelf life of a cake made with only natural ingredients would be a few days; the shelf life of a Twinkie is many months if not years. The food industry, to meet the demands of the American diet, has loaded the average American with thousands of chemicals, every one of which needs to be detoxified. Though alone each of these chemicals is not necessarily toxic, when combined with unintentional additives to the food chain such as pesticide residues, and industrial chemicals found in air and water pollution, any breakdown in the detoxification system, from stress or poor nutritional status, can lead to disastrous results and biochemical maladaptation.

Annually, almost one billion pounds of pesticides are sprayed on food crops in the United States. The average American consumes one gallon of food additives a year. There are also more than ten thousand incidental additives found in the food chain, including pesticides, fumigants, solvents, colorings, stimulants, chlorine bleach, and plastic polymers. In 1970, the Food and Drug Administration (FDA) began assessing the problem of chemicals in the food chain. Through a combination of lack of funding and a lack of political will because of industry economic influences, the FDA created the Generally Recognized as Safe list, consisting of chemicals that were never studied but were assumed to be safe. Twenty-seven hundred chemicals were placed on this list in 1970, and the number of untested chemicals has continued to grow.

Using similar assumptions as those made about environmental chemicals, the FDA allowed chemicals in the food chain if they did not prove to be carcinogenic, even if there were other effects on the immune system. In the few chemicals that were studied, additive effects of the chemicals were not considered. For example, when a study showed a minority of animals became ill, but most were not affected, the chemical was deemed safe. This translates into millions of people being at risk from the additive effects of the thousands of chemicals in the food chain. To survive this onslaught of man-made chemicals, the detoxification system must be operating efficiently. Unfortunately, the detoxification process requires an adequate intake of phytonutrients, sorely lacking in the typical American diet.

It is not just the food chain that provides challenges to the detoxification system. The U.S. Environmental Protection Agency estimated that more than two billion pounds of potentially toxic chemicals are released annually into the environment in the United States. Six hundred pounds of air pollution are released for every person in America per year. There are more than 83,000 chemical compounds in use in the United States, but only 200, or less than 1 percent, have been adequately studied under the Toxic Substances Control Act. In addition, assessment of many chemicals is prevented due to industry's claims that those chemicals are proprietary and that an assessment would negatively impact trade secrets. Of those chemicals that were studied, the only tests done looked for carcinogenicity and not other subtle effects on the immune system and allostatic load. A 2009 survey by the Centers for Disease Control and Prevention (CDC) found traces of 212 environmental chemicals in Americans, including arsenic, cadmium, PCBs, bisphenol A, and phthalates.

Classes of Toxins

- Airborne industrial chemicals and combustion pollutants, including PCBs, as well as halogenated hydrocarbons that are airborne
- Pesticides: more than eight hundred different chemicals, including herbicides, fungicides, and insecticides
- Endocrine disruptors such as DDT and PCBs; phthalates in plastic; and synthetic steroids in meats and poultry
- Toxic metals, including lead, mercury, cadmium, and arsenic, which accumulate in the body and are difficult to remove
- Additives, preservatives, and drugs that are intentionally added to or inadvertently end up in food and water

The Detoxification System

Diets rich in phytonutrients support detoxification by providing cofactors for the liver to convert toxins to inert materials. The liver does this through two steps: Phase I deactivates the toxic substance through the cytochrome P450 pathway, and Phase II clears the toxin by linking with another compound through either conjugation, sulfation, methylation, or acetylation. Once this occurs, the chemical is removed through the kidneys or colon.

These reactions are dependent on adequate supplies of nutrients such as B vitamins, glutathione, amino acids, flavonoids and phospholipids, zinc, copper, selenium, coenzyme Q_{10}, vitamins A, C, and E, and other plant-derived nutrients. Proper functioning of both phases of detoxification is needed to avoid the buildup of intermediary metabolites that can cause free-radical damage to cell membranes. The activities of the Phase I and Phase II systems have to be coordinated; otherwise, an excess or deficiency of one versus the other can lead to significant medical problems.

The body protects against free-radical and oxidant damage through the action of antioxidants. Some of the key antioxidants are made by the body and include uric acid, albumin, and bilirubin. The body, however, can produce only a small portion of the required antioxidants, which otherwise must come from the diet. The key food-based antioxidants are vitamin C, vitamin E, carotenoids (vitamin A, beta-carotene, lycopene, lutein), selenium, zinc, coenzyme Q_{10}, bioflavonoids, manganese, molybdenum, copper, and sulfur. These antioxidants work in concert with each other, and high doses of one without the others can be counterproductive.

The intestine is also an organ of detoxification. It is estimated that more than twenty-five tons of food per person are processed over a lifetime, with exposure to a large number of xenobiotics (chemicals that destroy good bacteria) and antigens in the digestive tract. Detoxification enzymes are found in the wall of the intestine to reduce the toxic load of the body. Beneficial bacteria in the gut, such as acidophilus and bifidobacter, also are protective. Reduction of the good bacteria levels in the intestines due to antibiotics or other medications allows overgrowth of unhealthful bacteria that undo the Phase II reactions and allow reabsorption of toxic substances into the body, furthering the toxic load, creating inflammation, and elevating cortisol levels.

Problems with the barrier function of the intestines will also lead to increased toxin load. The so-called leaky gut, or increased intestinal permeability, is the result of poor nutrition, stress, poor oxygenation, and medications such as antibiotics that can lead to overgrowth of *Candida albicans,* a yeast organism responsible for vaginitis in women and digestive symptoms such as bloating and generalized fatigue. A "leaky gut" increases absorption of toxins and food allergens, leading to a host of inflammatory states and higher cortisol levels.

Nutritional support of the detoxification process involves specific foods and nutrients that are required for Phase I and Phase II of the process. Phase I detoxification involves the cytochrome P450 enzyme system found in the mitochondria (small organelles inside the cell that are involved in energy production). The end product of Phase I detoxification is often free radicals, which are products of oxidation (combustion) of the toxic substances and are themselves injurious to the cell. They include singlet oxygen, peroxides, and other charged molecules. When free radicals come in contact with cells, they can damage the mitochondria and cause deficiency in the energy production of the cells as well as cause neuromuscular problems.

Free radicals can injure any organ in the body, especially the liver. The exposure of the cell nucleus to free radicals can alter the genetic code of the cell and be a precursor of cancer. The creation of these toxic intermediaries in the detoxification process is influenced by a number of factors, including the use of medications. Certain drugs—such as the acid blockers Zantac, Pepcid, and Tagamet; antidepressants including fluoxetine, paroxetine, and sertraline; antibiotics such as erythromycin, clarithromycin, and fluoroquinolones; and antifungals including Nizoral, Diflucan, and Sporonox—inhibit the cytochrome system from detoxifying other medications. Another over-the-counter medication that depletes the sulfur compounds needed for detoxification is acetaminophen, found in Tylenol and other medications. The Phase I process can be dangerous if inhibited by drugs or by creating excessive amounts of free radicals that cannot be converted to nontoxic substances.

Toxins (urea, lactic acid, and others) are also produced from normal metabolism and require detoxification by the liver. Hormones including estrogen, testosterone, thyroid, and especially cortisol require detoxification by the liver, a process that can be compromised by chemical toxins called xenohormones, which mimic the body's own hormones. With excess accumulation of inorganic chemicals, it is possible that hormones themselves become a source of toxicity. Poor dietary habits, nutritional deficiencies, and inadequate intake of protein and carbohydrates can compromise the detoxification pathways, leading to a progressive buildup of toxins and the consequences of greater biochemical stress.

Symptoms of Inadequate Detoxification

- Fatigue and malaise
- Cognitive problems such as poor concentration and memory loss
- Depression and anxiety
- Musculoskeletal symptoms such as fibromyalgia, muscle aches, arthritis
- Sensitivity to odors and medications
- Paresthesias or tingling and nerve problems in the extremities
- Edema and fluid retention
- Worsening symptoms after anesthesia or pregnancy
- Multiple allergies to foods, molds, pollens

Detoxifying the Diet

- Eat vegetables and fruits grown organically.
- Eat fiber-rich foods, including flaxseed powder, oat and rice bran, and legumes.
- Eat antibiotic- and hormone-free meat and chicken, and limit red meat to once a week.
- Drink only filtered or bottled water.
- Eat eggs only from free-range chickens fed on organic feed.
- Avoid farm-raised fish.
- Limit the amount of swordfish, tilefish, tuna, and other fish known to have high mercury levels.
- Avoid all foods that are fried or contain trans-fatty acids and other unhealthy fats.
- Do not drink soft drinks or excessive fruit juice.
- Restrict caffeine, including coffee and black teas.
- Eliminate refined sugar, including candy, pastries, sweetened canned fruits, ice cream, cookies, and cakes.
- Eat live-culture, unsweetened yogurt or kefir to increase beneficial bacteria.

Food choices also make a difference in the detoxification of toxins. A diet rich in vegetables, fruits, nuts, seeds, legumes, whole grains, and seafood reduces the toxic effect of pesticides, carcinogens, and over-the-counter drugs. However, proteins that are pro-inflammatory with high levels of arachidonic acid (red meat, pork, dairy, eggs—especially not organically raised) or other unhealthy fats (fried foods, trans fats in baked goods) generate greater toxic loads on the liver. High-glycemic-index foods, including white flour and processed sugars, can depress the cytochrome P450 system, as well as increase the prostaglandins and leukotrienes that generate more free-radical stress. Good fats such as omega-3 fatty acids from fish and walnuts, and monounsaturated fatty acids from olive oil, grapeseed oil, almonds, and avocados, are helpful in the detoxification process.

Increased fiber intake benefits detoxification in many ways. Fiber promotes the removal of conjugated toxins (from Phase II) that are excreted in bile into the intestines. With adequate dietary fiber, fewer of these toxins are reabsorbed. Fiber can directly bind toxins that are mutagens (those that cause cell mutation and cancer) and remove them from the body. Fiber also supports the growth of beneficial bacteria in the gut that play a significant role in detoxification. These bacteria, including lactobacillus and bifidobacter, directly detoxify hormones as well as xenobiotics arising from contaminants in the food chain. Improved colon function with adequate fiber goes a long way toward detoxifying the whole body.

Fasting

Over the centuries therapeutic fasting has been employed as a means to detoxify and purify the body. In my practice, I suggest either a short juice fast, a more extended raw-food diet, or the use of medical foods designed to detoxify while placing less stress on the body. I do not recommend water fasting for my patients because of the severe ketosis (acidosis and protein breakdown) and rapid release of toxins that occur in a starvation mode. Severe caloric restriction also raises cortisol levels in response to stress from inadequate calories. I suggest that any fasting or detoxification be undertaken with medical supervision.

Juice fasting is best if based on organic vegetable juices such as combinations of celery, spinach, carrot, and parsley. Before any fasting or severely restricted diet, it is necessary that you refrain from as many over-the-counter medications as possible, avoid smoking, and stop all alcohol and caffeine for at least three weeks before undertaking a more restricted program. This avoids a severe detoxification crisis.

If desired, it is possible to juice fast one day a week, or three days in a row every four months. I prefer my patients use the medical food approach that is designed to improve the liver's detoxification pathways while restricting the diet and avoiding "offender" foods.

The Effect of Food on Adaptation and Longevity: A Short List

- One-quarter cup of nuts eaten five times per week lowers the risk for diabetes 21 percent and reduces LDL cholesterol by one-third.
- Five servings of fruits and vegetables per day reduces the incidence of cancer, heart disease, diabetes, and hypertension.
- Twenty-five grams of fiber per day reduces risk of heart disease (by 30 percent), breast cancer, colon cancer, and stroke.
- Intake of omega-3 fatty acids from fish, oleic acid from olive oil, and avoidance of trans-fatty acids reduces the risk of heart disease, stroke, and diabetes.

All the foods listed above, as well as many others rich in flavonoids, carotenoids, and other phytonutrients, improve detoxification, reduce inflammation, and help maintain healthy levels of cortisol. Despite the enormous number of toxic exposures that are part of modern life, with the right dietary approach, the detoxification system is able to cope. Improved detoxification reduces inflammation, thereby decreasing allostatic load and cortisol production. To begin this journey back to adaptation, a three-week detoxification program is helpful to jump-start the process. In my practice, I use a diet limiting the trigger foods that can induce an allergic response and emphasizing foods without additives, chemicals, and toxic fats. In addition, these foods are rich in detoxifying and anti-inflammatory phytonutrients. Adding nutritional supplements improves the liver detoxification systems and accelerates the process.

The Adaptation Diet program is divided into three phases:

Phase One: Weeks One to Three: Detoxification and elimination of allergens

Phase Two: Weeks Four and Five: Food allergy challenge

Phase Three: Week Six On: Maintenance with an anti-
inflammatory, low-allergy, phytonutrient-rich, blood-sugar-
balancing diet

Most of my patients by week six are feeling better and are on
their way to regaining adaptation, losing weight, and reducing cortisol and allostatic load.

4

Phases One and Two of the Adaptation Diet

Detoxification and Identification of Food Allergies

Phase One: Dietary Detoxification:
Weeks One to Three

Surprisingly, the body's ability to detoxify and reduce allostatic load is quickly activated through dietary changes. I have used several diets in my practice to help people detoxify and have found the approach detailed here the easiest to adopt. Success requires a willingness to follow the program precisely. There often is a struggle over giving up desserts, alcohol, coffee, and other comfort foods; however, after the first three to four days, most people don't even miss these foods. My patients have shown me that if given a chance, the body will respond and recover from maladaptation.

Any person who has medical issues, including diabetes, heart disease, cancer, or any chronic or acute medical condition, has to be under the care of a physician before undertaking the detoxification phase of the Adaptation Diet. Withdrawal from alcohol in people who habitually drink can be life threatening and must be closely supervised. Caffeine-withdrawal symptoms are also very common in habitual coffee or tea drinkers. Symptoms often include headaches, fatigue, and irritability. I suggest that caffeine withdrawal be accomplished before starting Phase One of the diet so that no over-the-counter pain medications are required. Some people on an elimination diet for the first time will feel significant symptoms from the detoxification effect and withdrawal from their normal food patterns. Some of my patients felt quite badly during this phase of the program and needed my guidance to adjust how they went through the dietary change. Therefore, any person with health concerns should not attempt this diet unless supervised by their physician.

One of my patients illustrated what can occur with sudden caffeine withdrawal. Benita was a patient with fibromyalgia (severe, widespread muscle pain), headaches, and fatigue. Within a week of starting the detoxification diet, she developed major headaches and eye pain. Unfortunately she went to her ophthalmologist without first consulting me. He thought she had developed a problem with her visual system, ordered several tests, and treated her with pain medications. Benita, a heavy coffee user, had abruptly stopped her coffee intake, resulting in migraine-type headaches from caffeine withdrawal. However, even in the face of the caffeine-withdrawal symptoms, her generalized muscle pain and fatigue had greatly improved from removing the toxins in her diet and avoiding her probable food allergy triggers. If Benita had gradually withdrawn from caffeine, her symptoms would have been much less severe and her detoxification would have gone smoothly.

Some people will actually experience withdrawal symptoms from sugars, wheat products, and other food allergens, including headaches, fatigue, and mood changes. These symptoms are typically short-lived and generally do not require intervention, though short-term (one or two days) use of acetaminophen or aspirin is allowed if needed. If symptoms of fatigue, severe headaches, or muscle pain continue past the fourth day, the diet should be terminated and a physician consulted.

I suggest starting the detoxification part of the diet over the weekend to prevent symptoms from taking you away from work. Purchase the foods that are included in the diet ahead of time so that you are not tempted to revert to old habits. If you use caffeinated coffee or teas, gradually withdraw from these foods over at least one week before starting the detoxification diet. Make sure to have adequate water intake, at least sixty-four ounces per day. It is important to use only purified water, either bottled or filtered. Organic foods are best where available. It is especially important that organically raised animal protein is used. Cravings for sweets, starches, and other comfort food will occur for most people, usually resolving within the first four days.

Some people will feel more fatigue during the first week of the diet. It is recommended to cut down on intense exercise and possibly just walk during the first two weeks. If fatigue becomes more intense past the first few days, the diet should be stopped and a health care practitioner consulted.

Table 1 lists the foods to include and those to avoid during the detoxification phase. Introducing foods that are not on the allowed list will slow down the process of detoxification and prevent the resolution of symptoms associated with food allergy. The majority of my patients succeed in the detoxification process because they quickly feel so much better, motivating them to stick with the program. To prevent blood-sugar swings, I suggest snacking between meals on nuts, seeds, nut butters (excluding peanut), or other proteins, including chicken, turkey, and fish. Filtered or bottled water, vegetable juices, and herbal teas are the preferred beverages.

If needed, psyllium seed husks or flaxseed powder can be added to assist detoxification at the first sign of constipation. It is important to avoid hidden refined sugars, including any food with sucrose, fructose, high-fructose corn syrup, dextrose, honey, or other sweeteners. Artificial flavorings and colorings in processed and packaged foods, sodas, and all caffeinated beverages must go!

In addition, all gluten-containing grains, including wheat, rye, barley, spelt, and kamut, are not allowed. Steel-cut, slow-cooking oatmeal is allowed. Substitutes are buckwheat (not related to wheat), rice, tapioca, millet, and amaranth.

Shellfish, red meat, pork, cold cuts, and sausage are eliminated in the detoxification process because of the presence of chemicals added in processing, antibiotics and hormones (used in raising beef), and contaminants in shellfish. Allowed protein includes free-range-fed chicken and turkey, fish other than farm raised (if possible), lamb, and wild game. Cow's milk dairy products, including cheese, yogurt, milk, and ice cream, are not used because of the frequency of allergic response to these foods. Eggs are eliminated for the same reason. Recipes are in Appendix B.

Table 1: Foods for Phase One

	Foods to Include	*Foods to Exclude*
Fruits	Unsweetened fresh, frozen, water-packed, and canned fruits; fruit juices (except orange)	Oranges, orange juice
Vegetables	All fresh, raw, steamed, sautéed, juiced, and roasted vegetables	Corn, creamed vegetables
Grains	Rice, oats, millet, quinoa, amaranth, teff, tapioca, buckwheat	Wheat, corn, barley, spelt, kamut, rye; all gluten-containing products
Bread/Cereal	Products made from rice, oats, buckwheat, millet, potato flour, tapioca, arrowroot, amaranth, quinoa, teff	Products made from wheat, spelt, kamut, rye, barley; all gluten-containing products
Legumes (vegetable protein)	All beans, peas, and lentils (unless otherwise indicated)	Soybeans, tofu, tempeh, soy milk, other soy products
Nuts and Seeds	Almonds, cashews, walnuts, sesame (tahini), sunflower, pumpkin seeds; butters made from these nuts and seeds	Peanuts, peanut butter
Meat and Fish (animal protein)	All canned (water-packed), frozen, and fresh fish, chicken, turkey, wild game, lamb	Beef, pork, cold cuts, frankfurters, sausage, canned meats, eggs, shellfish

	Foods to Include	Foods to Exclude
Dairy Products and Milk Substitutes	Milk substitutes such as rice milk, almond milk, oat milk, coconut milk, and other nut milks	Cow milk, cheese, cottage cheese, cream, yogurt, butter, ice cream, frozen yogurt, non-dairy creamers
Fats	Cold-expeller pressed olive, flaxseed, canola, grapeseed, sesame, walnut, pumpkin, and almond oils	Margarine, butter, shortening, processed and hydrogenated oils, mayonnaise, spreads, sunflower and safflower oil
Beverages	Filtered or distilled water, herbal tea, seltzer, and mineral water	Soda pop or soft drinks, alcoholic beverages, coffee, tea, other caffeinated beverages
Spices and Condiments	All spices unless otherwise indicated. For example, cinnamon, cumin, dill, garlic, ginger, carob, oregano, parsley, rosemary, tarragon, thyme, turmeric, vinegar	Chocolate, ketchup, mustard, relish, chutney, soy sauce, barbecue sauce, and other condiments
Sweeteners	Brown rice syrup, fruit sweetener, blackstrap molasses, stevia	White or brown refined sugar, honey, maple syrup, corn syrup, high-fructose corn syrup, candy, desserts made with these sweeteners

(Adapted from Metagenics UltraClear Patient Guide)

This phase of the Adaptation Diet accomplishes two important goals: avoidance of foods that are contaminated with chemicals, including colorings, preservatives, additives, pesticide residues, hormones, and industrial pollutants; and avoidance of common food allergens. Through reduction in chemical exposure and food triggers of inflammation, the detoxification system can recover and become more efficient, reducing cortisol production. In the long run, this is the bottom line for healthy aging.

In my practice I often use a "medical food" protein powder that enhances the liver detoxification process. Use a powder that is a hypoallergenic, rice-based protein that includes nutrients needed for the two phases of liver detoxification. (It is best if these products are used under medical supervision.) If this powder or a similar product is not used, it is possible to accomplish the same effect by adding the following supplements, listed below, during the first five weeks of the diet. In addition, eat protein-rich snacks between meals.

At the end of three weeks on the detoxification diet, most people will notice improvement in fatigue, anxiety, moodiness, muscle and joint pain, headaches, and digestive problems and will lose between two and eight pounds. The weight loss is from water weight produced by inflammatory reactions to the foods that were eliminated. Some people will not notice much of a change during the detoxification phase, either in weight loss or symptom improvement. In

---

Daily Supplements for Phases One and Two

- A multivitamin/multimineral not containing yeast, soy, wheat, sugar, or corn with at least 200 international units (IU) of mixed tocopherols (vitamin E)
- Vitamin C (buffered with calcium and magnesium): 500–1,000 milligrams (mg)
- N-acetylcysteine: 100 mg
- Alpha lipoic acid: 100 mg
- EPA/DHA (eicosapentaenoic acid/docosahexaenoic acid) fish oils: 700 mg
- Bromelain enzymes (unless allergic to pineapple) twice daily between meals

those cases, if significant symptoms continue, additional medical evaluation is warranted.

The Food Allergy Challenge

Identifying foods that trigger inflammation and a wide range of symptoms is a major step along the path to adaptation and healthy aging. I could cite hundreds of case histories demonstrating the impact food intolerance has on health.

Mary was a good example of the effect food allergy has on adaptation. Mary had chronic headaches, neck pain, and TMJ (temporomandibular joint disorder, a common problem of jaw pain and clicking when chewing that can be quite disabling). She had been to many specialists, who devised mouth guards and treated her with pain medications and physical therapy. None of the therapies had made much difference despite many years of committed treatments. Mary knew that stress was a trigger, but despite her best efforts she had difficulty relaxing.

I put her on the Adaptation Diet and within ten days her pain had disappeared. During Phase Two of the diet, the food challenge, Mary reintroduced corn and found her pain return within two hours of eating corn on the cob and popcorn. Several days later she re-created her pain again after eating tomatoes and drinking tomato juice.

After she adopted a diet eliminating corn and tomatoes and stayed with the anti-inflammatory maintenance phase of the Adaptation Diet, Mary continued to be pain free. If she strayed from her diet and had corn or tomato products, she had symptoms within the next few hours. She also noted an effect that I have seen many times after eliminating food allergens. She was more relaxed and handled stress more easily. This was not surprising, because her allostatic load had been reduced, calming down her cortisol and epinephrine production. Most of my patients are able to reintroduce the food allergen in a rotation diet (see

Appendix D) within three to four months of elimination. Rarely does a food need to be eliminated indefinitely.

Phase Two: Identification of Food Allergies: Weeks Four and Five

By the time Phase Two has been reached, the hard part is over. Often, after avoidance of a food allergen for three weeks, symptoms and allostatic load associated with that food have been reduced. Phase One of the diet has eliminated all the common food allergy triggers. By avoiding these foods, most people will have "unmasked," meaning that the next time they eat the food, if they are allergic to it, symptoms will be more noticeable and quicker to occur. This makes Phase Two of the diet so instructive in realizing the connection between foods and specific symptoms.

There is one caveat to the food challenge: anyone with asthma or a history of severe reactions to foods should not undertake the food challenge without medical supervision. Severe food reactions are typically limited to foods that trigger IgE antibodies (involved with immediate hypersensitivity and anaphylaxis) and include peanuts, Brazil and other nuts, shellfish, and strawberries.

The food challenge part of the diet requires good record keeping while carefully following the rules. Use only the forms of the food listed below to do the challenge. For example, wheat can only be tested using shredded wheat or matzo, not bread, because there are many other ingredients in a slice of bread. Symptoms generally occur within the first few hours; however, they might be delayed as much as twenty-four hours. Reactions to these foods are generally mild and consist of headaches, fatigue, digestive upset, mood changes, poor concentration, or muscle and joint pain.

Use at least two portions of the challenge food with two consecutive meals in addition to the foods from the Phase One diet. If symptoms occur, do not challenge another food until the symptoms resolve, usually within twenty-four hours. Record all symptoms in a diary so that you can review these at a later date if symptoms reoccur. Think of this exercise as empowering, not restricting. Many of my patients are upset to discover food allergies because it restricts their gustatory freedom. However, knowledge of food allergies provides control over symptoms and premature aging. For Mary, the trade-off of not eating corn in order to be free of her TMJ pain was an easy choice.

The Food Challenge

The most common and significant food allergies are to wheat, corn, soy, dairy, beef, tomatoes, and yeast. The two-week period of Phase Two can be extended to test additional foods if needed. Don't deviate from the dietary restrictions of Phase One, especially avoiding sweets, coffee, and any fast foods. Starting with wheat on day one, add each food to be challenged in sizable portions to two consecutive meals. Observe symptoms over the subsequent twenty-four hours and keep a diary of foods introduced and symptoms. If there are no symptoms by the following day, a new food can be tested. As mentioned before, if symptoms occur, no new food should be introduced until the symptoms have cleared. If it is unclear whether there were significant symptoms, challenge the food again after waiting at least four days to retest. To hasten clearing of food allergy symptoms, drink at least sixty-four ounces of purified water every day, increase vitamin C intake to 2,000 milligrams for a few days, and use Alka-Seltzer Gold (only Gold has the right bicarbonate mix) as directed. Wait to challenge the next food until symptoms have cleared. Below are the specifics on food challenge for the major food allergens.

- Wheat: Use shredded wheat, matzo, wheat crackers without yeast, wheat pasta, or pure wheat cereals. Do not use bread, because it contains multiple ingredients. If there is no reaction to wheat, it can be kept in the diet but only in whole wheat or sprouted wheat forms.

- Dairy: Cow's milk (whole), plain unsweetened yogurt, and cottage cheese are recommended for challenging. Ice cream and aged cheeses (such as Swiss, cheddar, and blue) are not to be used. Butter has little or no milk protein, so it is not used as a challenge food. If lactose intolerance is an issue, this challenge should be avoided. Digestive symptoms are common with dairy products in people who have not eaten them in a while. If dairy is tolerated in the food challenge, I recommend using only low-fat yogurts and kefirs, to reduce the inflammatory response to the fats in dairy. Organic dairy products are strongly recommended to reduce the inflammatory fatty acids and chemical contaminants.

- Corn: Fresh corn on the cob, canned corn (not creamed), popcorn (plain without flavorings), or polenta (corn flour) can be used. Corn—including corn syrup, cornstarch, high-fructose sweeteners, cornmeal, and other ingredients—is one of the most common adulterants in prepared foods. If symptoms from corn are identified in the food challenge, then reading labels is essential. Even if there is no allergy, avoidance of foods sweetened with high-fructose corn syrup products leads to better blood-sugar control and less cortisol production.

- Beef: Eating six to eight ounces of beef, preferably organically raised, is the best way to test for beef allergy. If there are no symptoms, most people should use only small portions of beef at most once a week because of the inflammatory fatty acids and saturated fats in beef. Organically raised beef is much better in terms of these fats and toxic chemicals.

- Eggs: Two or three eggs at a serving preferably boiled or poached is the best challenge. Eggs that come from organically fed and free-range chickens have enormous differences in fatty acid composition from industrially produced eggs. Only eggs from free-range and organically fed chickens should be consumed. If eggs trigger symptoms in the food challenge, it is possible that chicken itself is an allergen and should be tested separately. If eggs are tolerated, they are best prepared by boiling or poaching, not breaking the yolk during cooking. Depending on a person's cholesterol levels, eggs can be eaten twice weekly.

- Soy: Challenge with plain soy milk, roasted soybeans, tofu, or tempeh. Do not use sweetened soy milk. With the tremendous increase in soy use during the past several decades, I have seen many more soy allergies. If the test for soy is positive, read labels diligently to avoid the many products with soy as a filler or stabilizer.
- Yeast: Baker's yeast is a common allergen and can be tested by eating bread if wheat and dairy are not problematic. The other option is adding a package of nutritional yeast to water or juice. Yeast allergy is often seen with chronic digestive symptoms or recurrent respiratory infections.
- Other foods that can be tested include tomatoes, pork, sugar, coffee, black tea, potatoes, oranges, chocolate, peanuts (if no history of severe allergic reactions), and food colorings.

When Phase Two is completed, whether it takes two weeks or longer, the maintenance Phase Three of the Adaptation Diet is begun. All foods that tested positive need to be avoided for the next three months. At that point, these foods can be reintroduced one at a time. If no symptoms are noted, they can be used as often as twice a week for the subsequent three months. (See Appendix D for rotation diet examples.)

Food Allergy and Cortisol: A Key to Adaptation

Adaptation and reduction of allostatic load can only be achieved if the biochemical stress from food allergies and food intolerance is taken into account. Food allergies and food intolerance are a major cause of maladaptation. Studies estimate that as many as one in every two Americans might have some level of food allergy or food intolerance. Symptoms triggered by food allergy promote inflammation and changes in the hormonal system leading to an elevated cortisol burden. Most physicians never take into account the possibility that food intolerance can be contributing to a host of symptoms (see below). Every day in my practice, patients report dramatic improvement in a host of symptoms from dietary changes based on food allergy testing.

Symptoms of Delayed Food Hypersensitivity

- Asthma and recurrent respiratory infections
- Nasal congestion and discharge
- Skin rash, eczema, hives
- Recurrent ear infections, fluid in ear, dizziness
- Recurrent yeast vaginitis
- All chronic digestive disorders—bloating, gas, heartburn, reflux, diarrhea, constipation, irritable bowel syndrome, and colitis
- Frequent urination, recurrent bladder infections, burning when urinating, bed-wetting in children
- Fatigue and lethargy
- Depression, moodiness, and anxiety
- Headaches and migraine
- Joint pains, arthritis, unexplained muscle pain
- Hyperactivity and ADD, ADHD
- Cognitive dysfunction—poor concentration
- Eczema and hives
- Obesity and food cravings

Signs of Food Allergy in Children

- Allergic shiners (dark circles under eyes)
- Allergic salute (rubbing the nose and eyes)
- Difficulty sitting still, restlessness
- Red earlobes
- Clearing throat excessively
- Nasal congestion
- Frequent vague abdominal pains
- Impulsivity, distractibility

I have been guiding my patients on their diets since I started my practice in 1978. In 1980, I attended the training program presented by the Society for Clinical Ecology (now known as the American Academy of Environmental Medicine) at a retreat center in the Rocky Mountains outside of Fort Collins, Colorado. It was one of the most important professional decisions I ever made, dramatically changing the way I practiced medicine.

One of my good friends in medical school had spent a year with the founder of clinical ecology, Theron Randolph, MD. Randolph was a traditional allergist who discovered that foods, molds, and chemicals—including natural gas, phenol, and benzene—were triggering a wide range of symptoms in his patients. (Other pioneers in the area of environmental medicine who broke ranks with their allergist colleagues in the 1930s and 1940s included Herbert Rinkel, Albert Rowe, and Arthur Coca.) Randolph painstakingly recorded detailed histories from his patients, identifying the culprits in problems such as fatigue, depression, arthritis, digestive problems, asthma, and other allergic symptoms. He hospitalized his most difficult patients in an environmental control unit where they had no exposure to common food allergies or chemicals that might cause problems. He then challenged his patients with foods that triggered their symptoms, discovering that many of these chronic complaints were caused by commonly eaten foods.

What amazed Randolph and revolutionized the field of food allergy was the wide range of symptoms caused by foods that had previously been unrecognized. Traditional allergy practice limited the scope of symptoms attributed to foods to only those mediated by IgE antibodies, including hives, eczema, allergic rhinitis, asthma, and acute diarrhea. (There are several types of antibodies that contribute to allergic responses. Traditional allergists concern themselves only with IgE, which causes histamine release. A different antibody, IgG, and cell-based responses are associated with delayed sensitivity to foods.) It became gospel that any other symptom could not be triggered by a food. The traditional allergists were wrong. In my own practice, the most common symptoms I find from foods are fatigue, tension, anxiety, insomnia, headaches, migraines, depression, joint pains, and digestive upsets (including heartburn, reflux, bloating and gas, constipation, and diarrhea). Even in patients without major medical issues, symptoms of maladaptation can be triggered by foods.

The controversy surrounding the notion that food allergies cause such widespread symptoms has to do with the difference between delayed and immediate reactions. Symptoms from immediate food reactions are mediated through histamine release and include hives, wheezing, swelling of the face or throat (anaphylaxis when severe), itching eyes or throat, and runny nose. It is obvious to people who suffer from this problem what foods triggered their reaction since it occurs within minutes of ingestion. These reactions are considered fixed food allergies that do not change or vary over a person's life. If you react to Brazil nuts with breathing problems or anaphylaxis as a child, this will probably continue even into adulthood, and Brazil nuts should be avoided. The most common foods that trigger immediate sensitivity include peanuts, shellfish, Brazil and other nuts, and strawberries. Most of the time, these problems can be avoided by identifying the food trigger, reading labels, and asking at restaurants about ingredients.

Delayed food reactions, also called cyclic, can occur up to twenty-four hours after eating a food, though most commonly the response is within several hours. The symptoms are not as dramatic and sudden as those of fixed food allergies, but often involve vague problems, including fatigue, sore muscles, joint pain, headaches, mild depression, and a feeling of general unwellness. Though vague and often not severe, every time a food triggers symptoms, the body responds with increased cortisol and the attending allostatic load. This is why identifying food allergy and changing diets is so important in regaining adaptation.

Part of the difficulty in identifying food triggers for these symptoms is a phenomenon known as masking. When a food is eaten repetitively, even though it might cause an immunological or biochemical response, symptoms can be hidden or masked and not recognized. For example, fatigue, pain, depression, or other symptoms might be triggered by wheat; however, if wheat is eaten every day, a masked state occurs and no cause and effect will be noticed. However, if there is a period of avoidance, such as Phase One of the Adaptation Diet, unmasking will occur, and when the food is reintroduced, symptoms will be more obvious.

John, a patient who is wheat intolerant (he did not know it at the time), traveled to China on vacation, where at that time no wheat products were available. He felt more energetic and less achy and moody during the trip, though he assumed it was because of the vacation and the incredible experience of touring China. When John returned and resumed his normal eating habits, including wheat cereal in the morning and sandwiches daily, the fatigue and muscle aches returned with a vengeance. He never thought that his diet was the culprit.

When he relayed this story to me, I asked him to stop eating wheat for a week and then reintroduce it. The same sequence happened: his fatigue and muscle aches improved when he stopped eating wheat and returned once he ate wheat again. We then skin tested John for food allergy to confirm the sensitivity to wheat. John had unmasked his wheat allergy during his trip and the test period. By doing this, he moved from an adapted state in which there was a hidden price to pay for the wheat intolerance (fatigue and muscle aches) to a preadapted state where the symptoms are gone but when exposed to a food allergen, the reaction will be stronger. This technique of unmasking is the reason that a simple home testing approach (avoidance and challenge), which is Phase Two of the Adaptation Diet, helps to identify food offenders.

When a person eats a food to which they are intolerant (corn, for example), the protein in the corn, after digestion in the gut and absorption through the small intestine wall into the bloodstream, triggers a response in the immune system that causes joint pain (or any one of many other symptoms) through release of immune hormones, including lymphokines, cytokines, interferons, and histamine. The immune cells in the gut, which constitutes nearly half of the entire immune system, can also react to the allergen, leading to inflammation and digestive problems. Symptoms might be delayed up to twenty-four hours (though most commonly they would be seen within six hours), making the connection to corn as the culprit very difficult. If corn was repeatedly eaten, a more continual joint pain might ensue, usually without the characteristics of serious arthritis like rheumatoid or osteoarthritis. (Findings common for inflammatory arthritis such as redness, swelling, and heat are not typically seen with food reactions.)

Using joint pain triggered by corn as an example, let's see how most physicians would approach this problem. A battery of blood tests and X-rays would be ordered to identify the type of arthritis.

Treatment with anti-inflammatory medications would probably follow. In this situation, lab test results would be normal. While initially a response to medications might be favorable, in the long run ironically these medications can actually intensify food allergy.

Most nonsteroidal anti-inflammatory drugs (NSAIDs) work by preventing the enzymes COX-1 and COX-2 from triggering leukotrienes that cause inflammation. Unfortunately, the COX-1 enzyme is also used by the digestive tract to ensure membrane integrity (the reason one side effect of these drugs is stomach ulcers). Another little-known side effect of these medications is an increase in intestinal permeability that allows the absorption of larger-than-normal proteins from the digestion of foods. These proteins are interpreted by the immune system as foreign substances, which can lead to more antibody production by the immune system and intensify food allergy. Therefore, treating joint pain triggered by corn with ibuprofen (or other anti-inflammatory medication) will work for a time, but eventually it will make the problem worse. The solution is to recognize the effect food can have on chronic symptoms and change the diet.

Not surprisingly, the most common foods that trigger delayed food allergy are the ones most Americans eat the most: milk, cheese, wheat, yeast, soy, corn, eggs, beef, and tomatoes. When I put my patients on an allergy-free diet that avoids the major allergens and also takes out all processed foods, sugar, and desserts, remarkable changes occur in most of their main complaints. Headaches, fatigue, joint pain, and digestive problems frequently improve within weeks. To identify the food triggers after an elimination diet, reintroduction of each food one at a time often re-creates a person's symptoms. For people with medical problems or multiple allergies, consulting a physician who specializes in food allergies, such as a member of the American Academy of Environmental Medicine, is the best approach.

How is one to suspect food allergy? Here are some hints. A history of any respiratory allergy including hay fever, asthma, nasal congestion, or itching nose, eyes, or throat makes food allergy likely. Itching in the ear canal, rectal itching, and itching between the shoulder blades also can indicate food allergy. Any family history of allergy increases the likelihood of food intolerance. A childhood history of colic, chronic digestive problems, bed-wetting, car sickness, recurrent ear infections, tonsillitis, and frequent colds is suspicious. Frequent respiratory or urinary-tract infections, or chronic digestive complaints including gas, bloating, constipation, diarrhea, and skin rashes, are usually a sign of food allergy in an adult. Unexplained fatigue, mood changes, and depression can all be caused by food allergy. Probably the most common complaints from my food-allergic patients are fatigue, aches and pains, and the inability to lose weight.

Many of my patients ask why they have developed food allergies. People who have strong genetic predispositions for allergies often have sensitivities to pollens, molds, and dust as well as foods. They typically have respiratory symptoms such as hay fever and asthma. However, the majority of food-intolerant patients have developed this problem over time rather than through a strong genetic component. The digestive tract is often the culprit. As I mentioned earlier, the use of anti-inflammatory medications impacts the integrity of the gut wall, leading to a leaky gut, which in turn causes absorption of larger molecules from food and an allergic response.

Antibiotics also play a major role in initiating food allergy by reducing the number of protective bacterial organisms in the digestive tract. This leads to overgrowth of unwanted bacteria and yeast (Candida albicans) or susceptibility to parasitic organisms. With fewer lactic-acid-forming bacteria, the gut wall is susceptible to leaky gut and food allergy. In addition, abnormal organisms in the gut trigger a brisk immune response that can lead to excessive reactivity to foods. Candida albicans is especially problematic because it adheres to the gut wall and directly contributes to a leaky gut.

Acid-blocking medications (Zantac, Prilosec, Tagamet, to name a few) alter the digestive process by reducing stomach acid secretion.

(These are important drugs when needed to treat gastritis, gastric reflux, or ulcers but are widely overused by physicians and the public.) With less stomach acid comes reduced pancreatic enzyme secretion, leading to poor digestion of proteins and absorption of substances triggering allergy. These drugs also contribute to nutritional deficiencies (B12, zinc, and other minerals) that affect the immune system as well.

Poor nutritional habits lead to greater food allergy incidence through continual exposure to the same foods, fast foods, sugars, and unhealthy oils and fats. The typical American diet, rich in omega-6 fats and simple sugars and lacking omega-3 fats and complex carbohydrates, impacts the digestive process by encouraging abnormal bacterial growth in the gut while not providing the nutrients needed for the health of the gut wall cells, the mucocytes. Poor nutrition can lead to greater likelihood of viral illness that can at times trigger a food allergy problem.

The change in food composition of the American diet also plays a role. The number of food additives has skyrocketed over the past fifty years, leading to recurrent exposure to chemicals in foods. Foods containing preservatives, conditioners, and artificial colorings and flavorings, and foods that are contaminated with antibiotics from animal feed and pesticides, add to the impact on the immune system in the digestive tract. Other behaviors such as early weaning and premature introduction of solid foods to infants and the repetitive nature of most diets have been suggested to increase food intolerances.

Not only do food allergies increase the allostatic load and cortisol burden, food allergies themselves are the result of long-term stress. Allostasis and high cortisol levels inhibit the normal immune response in the gut, leading to more infections. High cortisol also increases stomach acid production, leading to more use of acid-blocking drugs, and furthering malabsorption. Chronic stress and allostatic load will eventually change the immune response, leading to more allergies. Managing food allergies is a major part of the dietary control of cortisol and regaining adaptation.

Studies of the most common chronic symptoms associated with food allergies and food intolerance have led to many useful findings in designing a diet to improve adaptation and well-being. In a study of migraine patients reported by Ellen Grant in 1979, 85 percent became headache free after going on an elimination diet. The most common food triggers were as follows:

- Wheat—78 percent
- Orange—65 percent
- Eggs—45 percent
- Tea and coffee—40 percent each
- Chocolate and milk—37 percent each
- Beef—35 percent
- Corn, cane sugar, and yeast—33 percent each

In children with migraines, Egger and colleagues (1983) found that seventy-eight of eighty-eight children became symptom free during a strict elimination diet. When foods were reintroduced, the most common that triggered reactions were, in order of frequency: milk, eggs, chocolate, orange, wheat, benzoic acid (a food preservative), cheese, tomato, fish, pork, beef, corn, and soy. Many other studies have confirmed the importance of food allergy in migraine as well as tension headaches.

Headaches are easier to study than many other symptoms because they are episodic. However, digestive problems such as irritable bowel syndrome, inflammatory bowel disease, gallbladder symptoms, gastritis, and other problems have been shown definitively to have a link with food allergy. Irritable bowel syndrome (IBS) is a chronic condition with alternating diarrhea and constipation, cramps, and mucus in the stool. It is not progressive and involves no pathological changes in the gut wall, though many patients have symptoms that greatly impact their well-being. I have found food intolerance and food allergy to be a major component in many of my IBS patients. In a study with double-blind feeding challenges, two-thirds of the patients showed increased levels of prostaglandins in their stool, indicating an inflammatory reaction to the foods. The most common foods in order of reactivity for IBS patients were wheat, corn, dairy, coffee, tea, and oranges.

Other studies have shown that elimination diets help more than half the people with IBS. In a study of 189 patients by Nanda (1989), most reacted to between two and five foods, with the most common as follows: dairy 40 percent, onions 35 percent, wheat 29 percent, chocolate 27 percent, coffee 24 percent, eggs 23 percent, oranges 18 percent, tea 17 percent, and potatoes 15 percent. Of seventy-three patients who avoided their symptom-provoking foods, seventy-two remained well for longer than a year.

Children with attention-deficit/hyperactivity disorder (ADHD) often have food allergies as a trigger for their behavioral and cognitive symptoms. There is a great deal of controversy over the effect that diet and especially food colorings and additives have on these children. However, in a study by Boris and Mandel (1994), nineteen out of twenty-six children placed on an elimination diet improved. Children with allergy histories such as eczema or hay fever were more likely to be reactive to the food challenge. The most common provoking agents were corn, wheat, milk, soy, food color, and oranges. My experience confirms the importance of evaluating food allergies in these children, especially if they have a respiratory allergy history or a family history of allergies. Even in adults with ADD, food allergies play a major role.

Other areas where research has found food allergy to be a significant trigger for symptoms include bed-wetting in children, asthma, allergic rhinitis, hives, ear infections, and arthritis. Joint and muscle pain are symptoms that I have found to be commonly triggered by food allergy. My patients with poorly defined muscle and joint pain, often diagnosed with fibromyalgia, myofascial pain, seronegative arthritis, arthralgia, or myalgia, frequently improve by identifying and eliminating food allergies. Even in rheumatoid arthritis, food allergies can contribute to symptoms.

Conditions Found to Have a
Food Allergy Component

- Irritable bowel syndrome

- Gallbladder disease

- Inflammatory bowel disease

- Allergic rhinitis

- Asthma

- Eczema

- ADHD and ADD in children and adults

- Rheumatoid arthritis

- Fibromyalgia, myofascial pain

- Arthralgia and myalgia

- Bed-wetting in children

- Migraine and tension headaches

The bottom line is that any patient with chronic symptoms that are not easily treated with medical therapy and cannot be easily explained deserves to be evaluated for food allergies by a well-trained physician. Even if the problems are less serious but involve reduced quality of life and well-being, changes in diet and avoidance of food triggers as described in the Adaptation Diet will reduce allostatic load and improve adaptation.

Rotary Diversified Diet:
A Solution for Multiple Food Allergies

The rotation diet has been a core approach in managing food allergies. There are many benefits to the rotation diet, not the least of which is unmasking the symptoms caused by food allergy. The original idea of a four-day rotation comes from studying gut transit times, or how long a food takes to completely leave the body. While food remnants remain in the gut, it is possible that the immune system continues to react to the food through production of antibodies or cell-based immune responses. It appears that for most people with a typical fiber intake, four days is the time it takes to clear a food completely from the digestive tract.

Based on this information, the four-day rotation became the standard for managing food allergies. Additionally, because foods of the same family might cause similar allergic responses, rotating through food families is also recommended. Using chicken as an example, if this was part of Monday's food intake, it should not be eaten again until Friday. In addition, other foods of the same family, like eggs, should also be rotated on those days. The benefit beyond unmasking reactions to foods is to reduce the likelihood of creating additional allergic reactions to tolerated foods. The rotation diet supports the process of desensitization and tolerance, reducing allostatic load.

For most people, rotation of the whole diet is not needed unless food allergy is a major problem. Foods that are symptom triggers discovered through the challenge part of the Adaptation Diet require avoidance for three to four months. This usually brings back tolerance, but if symptoms still occur when reintroducing the food, then a four-day rotation diet makes sense. The bottom line is that the more variety in one's diet, the less likely one is to develop a food allergy.

For tens of thousands of generations, humans were hunter-gatherers, picking berries and other fruits and fishing and hunting game for food. There was no repetitive exposure to foods, since you ate what was available and then moved on to the next food source. Until the cultivation of grains and the rise of cities, this was the diet of *Homo sapiens*. Compare that to how we eat now. Most people eat the same limited number of foods every day. Seasonal availability is often overcome by transporting foods from other continents so that the same meals can be consumed regardless of season or time of year.

The repetitive nature of our diets is one of the causes of the epidemic of food allergy. The rotation diet, encouraging the maximum variety of food, can modulate this problem and prevent additional food allergies and food intolerance. Even incorporating just some of these concepts improves adaptation. For many people, a strict four-day rotation diet is not necessary. However, knowledge of food families as well as awareness of the need for variety will encourage greater adaptation, lower allostatic load, and improved cortisol control.

Appendix D contains lists of food families, examples of four-day rotation diets, and suggested rotations. This can be incorporated into the maintenance Adaptation Diet by rotating foods as possible. If the food challenge shows evidence of multiple food allergies and symptoms that point to other food allergies, the four-day rotation of the Adaptation Diet is critical. As with any chronic medical condition, the rotation diet should be supervised by a physician with training in environmental medicine. For those people who do not have any evidence of food allergy, simply trying to get the greatest variety possible in the diet will suffice.

5

Phase Three of the Adaptation Diet

*Control Inflammation
and Maintain Healthy
Cortisol Levels
throughout Life*

Maintaining adaptation in the diet is a major contributor to balanced cortisol levels and healthy aging. Completing Phase One of the Adaptation Diet improves the detoxification pathways and removes offending foods. Phase Two identifies food intolerance and food allergy. Phase Three builds on the benefits of detoxification and identification of food allergies to create a dietary program that controls cortisol, helps achieve normal body weight, and supports healthy aging.

The long-term goal of the Adaptation Diet is the reduction of allostatic load from poor dietary habits that trigger inflammation, allergies, insulin resistance, and hypoglycemia. The diet is rich in foods that normalize cortisol response—high-fiber beans, adequate amounts of low-fat protein, flaxseeds, omega-3 fats from fish and nuts, carotenoids and flavonoids from vegetables and fruit, and sulfides for detoxification from garlic, onions, and cruciferous vegetables.

The Adaptation Diet is a modern version of the Mediterranean diet, which has been proven to reduce overall mortality, especially from heart disease and cancer. The Adaptation Diet is not really a diet, but a lifelong pattern of consuming health-enhancing foods. At every meal, the goal is to seek out the foods that improve adaptation and promote healthy aging and avoid those that induce inflammation, blood-sugar problems, and allergic reactions. There is no doubt that healthy aging depends on eating correctly.

Fats and Adaptation

The typical American diet promotes inflammation through the use of a higher percentage of animal foods and processed foods containing omega-6 fats (linoleic acid) and trans fats. One hundred years ago (and currently in most traditional diets worldwide), the ratio of omega-6 to omega-3 fats was between 2:1 and 4:1. Today, in the average American diet, the ratio is closer to 25:1, dramatically increasing inflammation in every organ of the body. In addition, the poisonous trans fats introduced by the food industry over the past fifty years directly increase free-radical production, damaging cell membranes and triggering additional inflammation.

The fats that are so crucial to adaptation are more correctly termed essential fatty acids (EFAs). These nutrients are not made in the body; therefore, dietary sources or supplements are needed to obtain these critical substances. EFAs are incorporated into cell membranes throughout the body, especially in the brain and nervous system. They are needed for the transport of nutrients, chemical messengers, hormones, and neurotransmitters into cells, leading to normal cell function. The integrity of the cell membrane and organelles inside the cell is dependent on normal levels of fatty acids.

Essential fatty acids are important in energy production, oxygen transport, cell-to-cell communication, and the myelination of neurons in the central nervous system. They are the building blocks of the eicosanoid hormones and the prostaglandins, which are key regulators of inflammation in the body. Any change in the dietary intake of fats has a profound effect on cell membranes, cell function, and levels of inflammatory hormones. It's no wonder that so many studies have confirmed the importance of eating the right fats to maintain health.

One example of the impact of using unhealthy fats is a recent study on ulcerative colitis, a severe inflammatory bowel disease. Nearly a third of ulcerative colitis cases may be associated with high dietary levels of linoleic acid, according to a study by Tjonneland

and colleagues (2009). Linoleic acid is an omega-6 polyunsaturated fatty acid found in red meat and some cooking oils and margarine.

More than two hundred thousand subjects in five European countries submitted food-frequency questionnaires at the start of the study, and incident cases of ulcerative colitis were identified from disease registries, follow-up questionnaires, and hospital and pathology databases. After a median follow-up of four years, those with the highest quartile of linoleic acid intake showed a 2.5-fold increased risk for ulcerative colitis relative to the lowest quartile.

Several types of fatty acids are found in foods. Fats from animal products, including meat and dairy, contain saturated fats and arachidonic acid, an omega-6 fatty acid that increases levels of pro-inflammatory prostaglandin hormones. Monounsaturated fats (also called omega-9) are neutral and stable fats that are generally anti-inflammatory. Polyunsaturated fats include both omega-6 and omega-3 fatty acids. Most omega-6 fatty acids are pro-inflammatory, including those found in corn oil, safflower oil, soybean oil, peanut oil, and cottonseed oil. However, some omega-6 oils are beneficial and can be used as supplements, including those found in primrose, borage, and black currant seed oils. (They contain gamma linolenic acid, a healthy EFA.) Omega-3 fatty acids, found in cold-water fish and flaxseeds, support the anti-inflammatory prostaglandin hormones and are the most beneficial in controlling inflammation.

Trans fats, a synthetic chemical used to make liquid fats solid (as in margarine), are also called hydrogenated or partially hydrogenated oils. Trans is the mirror image of the normal fatty acid configuration, called cis. When these oils are incorporated into cell membranes, they become stiff and reduce their membrane transport function. This leads to cell dysfunction and has been associated with increased risk for heart disease and increased inflammation. Unfortunately, trans fats are found in many processed foods, including chips, cookies, soups, pastries, French fries, margarine, and fast foods. Recently, the food industry has finally accepted the decades-old research that proved these fats are dangerous and has begun removing them from a number of products.

The current (2010) USDA food recommendations (My Plate) finally have recognized the difference between healthy and unhealthy fats that previous guides such as the Food Pyramid did not. In the past, the USDA made no distinction between healthy fats like monounsaturated oils and unhealthy fats like saturated fats found mostly in red meats and tropical oils, and trans fats found mostly in margarines, snack foods, processed peanut butter, and commercial baked goods.

A major step in reducing inflammation and controlling cortisol is choosing the right fats: omega-3 fats from cold-water fish (wild salmon, sardines, herring, low-mercury tuna), as well as vegetable sources (flaxseeds, walnuts, pumpkin seeds, and dark green leafy vegetables). Monounsaturated fats from almonds, avocados, olive oil, grapeseed oil, and canola oil should be the main fats in the diet. In addition, strictly avoid trans fats. Also reduce the use of polyunsaturated omega-6 fats found in corn oil, safflower oil, soybean oil, and other partially hydrogenated oils. Reducing the intake of saturated fats from beef, whole dairy products, and egg yolks also decreases the inflammatory response.

The Mediterranean Experience

Just as important as avoidance of pro-inflammatory foods is the inclusion of foods that are anti-inflammatory. The Mediterranean diets found in Greece and Italy, shown to reduce markers of inflammation and thereby lead to less heart disease, cancer, diabetes, obesity, and other aging phenomena, are templates for the construction of the Adaptation Diet. The characteristics of these diets are the following:

- Low-glycemic-index carbohydrates such as whole grains, fruits, and vegetables in large amounts

- Minimal snacking between meals and no fast foods
- Moderate consumption of red wine (five ounces per day)
- Olive oil as the principal fat, with significant amounts of fish, nuts, and seeds and a balanced omega-6 to omega-3 ratio
- Significant intake of fish, especially salmon and small fish like sardines rich in EPA/DHA fatty acids
- Fat consumption is 25–35 percent of calories, with saturated fat (from butter, cream, full-fat dairy, or red meats) less than 8 percent
- Protein primarily as beans and lentils with moderate amounts of fish and poultry
- Dairy consumed as low-fat yogurt, kefir, or cheese
- Desserts are fruits, often fresh
- Use of local produce, fish, and poultry with minimal importation from distant sources
- Slow food approach, eating leisurely meals in a social setting with family and friends

In a study of cortisol levels and hypothalamic-pituitary-adrenal (HPA) activity in women in the Mediterranean area, García-Prieto and colleagues (2007) found disturbed HPA axis was associated with abdominal obesity and a higher content of fat and saturated fatty acids in the diet. Women who chose a dietary pattern closer to the Mediterranean diet, with high monounsaturated fatty acid intake, showed lower levels of HPA axis disturbance.

The Mediterranean diet protects against obesity and diabetes through reducing inflammation and cortisol elevation. It includes consumption of significant amounts of vegetables and fruits and using olive oil as the principal fat. Both epidemiological and interventional studies have revealed a protective effect of the Mediterranean diet against mild chronic inflammation and its metabolic complications. Mounting evidence suggests that Mediterranean diets could serve as an anti-inflammatory dietary pattern, which could help in fighting diseases that are related to chronic inflammation, including visceral obesity, heart disease, type 2 diabetes, and the metabolic syndrome. There is also a lower incidence of several types of cancer with these dietary practices.

Dietary patterns close to the Mediterranean diet, rich in fruit and vegetables and high in monounsaturated fats, are negatively associated with features of the metabolic syndrome. The metabolic syndrome, also called syndrome X, includes high blood pressure, insulin resistance, truncal obesity, high triglycerides and blood sugar, and low HDL cholesterol. It is a major risk factor for heart disease and diabetes. Some recent studies, including one done by Balbio (2009) in Spain, have demonstrated a 25 percent net reduction in the prevalence of metabolic syndrome following lifestyle changes mainly based on nutritional recommendations.

Olive oil is also an integral ingredient of the Mediterranean diet, and accumulating evidence suggests that it may have health benefits that include reduction of risk factors of coronary heart disease, prevention of several varieties of cancers, and modification of immune and inflammatory responses. Olive oil appears to be an example of a functional food, with varied components that may contribute to its overall therapeutic characteristics. Olive oil is known for its high levels of monounsaturated fatty acids and is also a good source of phytochemicals, including polyphenolic compounds, squalene, and alpha tocopherol (vitamin E). A unique characteristic of olive oil is its abundant oleuropein, a member of the secoiridoid family, which functions as a hydrophilic phenolic antioxidant.

Inhabitants of the Greek island of Crete are 20 percent less likely to die from coronary artery disease as, and have one-third the cancer rate of, Americans. A study comparing foods that are typically found in a Greek diet to what is often consumed in the United States shows the following:

- Greeks consume much less red meat and use many more plant-based foods, averaging nine servings a day of antioxidant-rich vegetables.

• Greeks ate cold-water fish several times a week—another heart-healthy investment because fish contain omega-3 oils that not only reduce heart disease risk but also boost immune system functioning.

The Greek diet contains little of the two kinds of fats known to raise blood cholesterol levels: saturated fat and trans fats.

Sugar, Carbohydrates, Metabolic Syndrome, and Adaptation

In the 1980s, under the leadership of the FDA and cardiologists nationwide, Americans were given an ultimatum: reduce your fat intake or die. All fats were bad, and little distinction was made between the various fatty acids as previously discussed. Unfortunately, this fat-avoidance craze has actually resulted in even more obesity, more heart disease, and more diabetes. Over the past thirty years as low-fat processed foods have flooded the grocery stores, Americans have reached the highest percentage of obesity ever seen. The reason is that in most processed foods that are low fat, refined sugar products have been used to replace the fat. Consuming an excess of refined sugar products leads to higher insulin levels and eventually insulin resistance. In fact, fat in food decreases overall caloric intake by leading to faster satiety and lower insulin response, leading to improved weight management. The reality is that research has shown that incorporating the right dietary fats will lead to better weight management and less inflammation.

If the makers of nutrition policy had paid attention to an event that occurred as a result of the Cold War, possibly the fat-avoidance craze would have never happened. In the 1950s, the Distant Early Warning radar system was built in the Arctic regions of the United States, Canada, Greenland, Iceland, and the Faroe Islands. Some of the construction was done in native Eskimo areas. At that time, there was essentially no heart disease or diabetes in these Native Americans, despite the fact that their diet had a huge percentage of calories from fat (from seal blubber and other animal fats). But they also ate no fast food and little sugar.

As "civilization" descended on these people and they adopted the sugar-rich, fast-food habits of most Americans, the incidence of heart disease, diabetes, and obesity skyrocketed. It wasn't the fats that caused these problems, but the sugar and processed carbohydrates that were to blame. This taught me and others who were knowledgeable about nutrition that the low-fat craze that started in the 1980s, ignoring the science such as the Eskimo studies, was bound to be a disaster.

These studies and many others have emphasized the need to restrict simple and refined sugars and starches to avoid blood-sugar problems, which can lead to insulin resistance and more inflammation. Insulin, a hormone made in the pancreas, brings sugar from the bloodstream into the cell for energy production. As noted earlier, in insulin resistance cell-membrane receptors become inefficient at responding to the signal from insulin to produce the changes needed to absorb glucose into the cell. This leads to higher and higher levels of insulin and blood sugar. Insulin resistance is often the result of decades of poor dietary habits leading to abdominal obesity. Insulin resistance affects up to one-third of the population and greatly increases the risk for diabetes, heart disease, cancer, and high blood pressure. Elevated insulin leads to more inflammation and higher cortisol levels.

Insulin receptors on the cell surface can be affected by hormones and chemical messengers made by adipocytes, the fat cells found in visceral or abdominal fat. Increased visceral fat increases inflammation through production of adipocytokines. They include TNF-alpha and IL-6, which prevent insulin receptors from working well, increasing the risk for metabolic syndrome, diabetes, inflammation, and elevated cortisol levels.

The sequence of this all-too-common cycle of events starts with increased abdominal fat from using simple sugars and refined carbohydrates. For example, in one study, consumption of soft drinks was measured in middle-aged adults over a four-year period. Consumption of more than one soft drink per day increased the odds of developing metabolic syndrome and insulin resistance. After a period of time, and with weight gain of as little as nine pounds of visceral fat, insulin resistance can occur. Elevated insulin further increases abdominal obesity through mobilization of free fatty acids and movement of glucose into fat cells to store as extra calories. As the abdominal girth grows, these changes accelerate and increase the inflammatory state, leading to more insulin resistance at the cell membranes.

Increased free fatty acids from inflammatory chemicals made by fat cells (adipocytokines), like TNF-alpha, increases triglycerides, insulin, and apolipoprotein B, leading to elevated cortisol and a marked increased risk of heart disease. Increased C-reactive protein and lower adiponectin, an anti-inflammatory adipocytokine that sensitizes cell-membrane insulin receptors, further worsens insulin resistance in obese people. Increased belly fat also leads to higher levels of resistin, a hormone that increases insulin resistance. These changes are the underlying events that lead to metabolic syndrome.

Metabolic syndrome is defined as having three of the following risk factors: increased waist girth—greater than forty inches in men, and greater than thirty-five inches in women; fasting blood sugar above 100 mg/dL; blood pressure above 130/85; triglycerides above 150 mg/dL. Here is where the story comes back to allostatic load and cortisol as a major component of these epidemic changes.

Many characteristics of metabolic syndrome are similar to those of Cushing's disease, a condition caused by either a pituitary or adrenal tumor secreting massive amounts of cortisol. The hallmark of Cushing's is visceral abdominal obesity, fatigue, mood changes, and marked increased risk for diabetes and heart disease. This similarity has led several researchers to propose that the key hormonal change in the development of metabolic syndrome is not just insulin resistance, but continued elevation of cortisol production.

In a study by Vogelzangs and colleagues (2009) of 1,200 depressed older persons, those with higher levels of free cortisol showed higher odds of developing metabolic syndrome. Especially in women, depressive symptoms were associated with elevated afternoon and evening cortisol levels. In a review of the research from the past twenty years, the authors concluded that metabolic syndrome is associated with a state of "functional hypercortisolism" leading to increased fat deposition around the abdominal organs. In addition, the adipose tissue itself creates a huge amount of cortisol through the 11-beta-HSD1 enzyme system, which converts inactive cortisone to active cortisol, contributing to metabolic syndrome. The amount of cortisol produced by visceral fat is actually greater than what the adrenal glands produce in obese individuals, contributing to the biochemical chaos of the overweight state. Once a person is obese, the normal feedback mechanism that shuts down cortisol production is impaired, contributing to this vicious cycle.

Signs of Metabolic Syndrome and Markers of Obesity

- Elevated blood pressure above 130/85
- Increased waist size: men, greater than forty inches; women, greater than thirty-five inches
- Blood glucose above 100 mg/dL fasting
- Triglycerides above 150 mg/dL
- HDL less than 40 in men and 50 in women
- Elevated waist/hip ratio: greater than 1 in men and 0.8 in women
- Triglyceride-to-HDL ratio greater than 3
- Body mass index over 30
- Elevated GGT liver enzyme

Elevated levels of insulin have also been associated with high blood pressure as well as increased growth-factor production, leading to a higher incidence of cancers. All of this further impacts the level of cortisol, which is produced to counterbalance many of the effects of insulin, leading to even more damage from allostatic load.

The key to reducing allostatic load and controlling cortisol excess and the risks for chronic disease is to reduce the amount of processed carbohydrates in the diet.

In addition, refined sugar and grains lead to a rapid spike in blood glucose and increased oxidant stress, leading to inflammation in just a few hours. The body's response is to produce more cortisol to reduce inflammation. Foods that cause a slower and more gradual and prolonged elevation of glucose do not cause the same inflammatory cascade and high cortisol levels. Several studies have shown that low-glycemic-index, carbohydrate-based diets are more effective than low-fat diets in treating obesity, metabolic syndrome, heart disease, and diabetes.

This is why the glycemic index is helpful in choosing what to eat. The glycemic index (GI) is a ranking of foods based on their potential to raise blood glucose. It compares the levels of blood-sugar elevation after eating a portion of food and ranks them relative to glucose levels after either straight glucose ingestion or white bread. Low-glycemic-index foods have a glycemic index below 55; high is above 70. For example, some candy bars have an index as high as 101, and cornflakes are 72, whereas an apple is 38, lentils are 29, and string beans are 32. In general, anything that is not whole and fresh probably has a high glycemic index.

However, some nutritious foods are listed as high GI although they really do not impact insulin production. For example, watermelon and carrots have high GI marks even though they do not create a negative impact on insulin sensitivity. The impact a food will have on blood-sugar levels depends on many other factors: ripeness of a food, cooking time, fiber and fat content, time of day, blood insulin levels, and recent activity. Therefore, this index is not to be used in isolation. The total amount of carbohydrate, amount and type of fat, fiber and salt content, as well as the caloric value of a food are also very important. Another set of data, the glycemic load, has been developed to take into account all of these factors. Appendix A contains a table identifying the glycemic index for some common foods. The internet has multiple sites to research glycemic load information.

Avoiding high-glycemic-index food will reduce the likelihood of insulin resistance and metabolic syndrome. Low-glycemic-index diets have many benefits, including fewer food cravings, fewer calories consumed, and decreasing weight gain. In addition, people on a low-glycemic-index diet have less hunger and lower serum triglycerides, lower blood pressure, higher beneficial HDL cholesterol, and less insulin resistance than those on high-glycemic-index diets.

The Adaptation Diet emphasizes the use of low-glycemic-index vegetables, fruits, grains, proteins, and fats. The percentage of

---

Examples of High-Glycemic-Index Carbohydrates

- Refined flour products, including white bread and bagels
- Frozen yogurt
- Orange juice
- Macaroni and cheese
- Crackers
- Candy
- Cookies and all other desserts
- Juice drinks with added sugar
- White potatoes
- Chips (corn and potato)
- Most breakfast cereals
- Sweetened soda

Selected Low-Glycemic-Index Carbohydrates

- All-bran cereal
- Peaches
- Plums
- Cherries
- Barley
- Grapefruit
- Legumes (lentils, beans, peanuts)
- Nuts (almonds, walnuts, soy nuts)
- Oatmeal (steel-cut, slow-cooking, and unsweetened)
- Green peas
- Tomatoes
- Unsweetened plain yogurt

---

calories from the three major food groups should be as follows: mostly low-glycemic-index carbohydrates, including predominately vegetables, legumes, and fruits and limited grains: 40–50 percent; protein from vegetarian and some animal sources: 30–40 percent; and fat from healthy oils, nuts, seeds, and fish: 20 percent. Carbohydrates including vegetables, legumes, and fruits are nature's powerhouse of adaptation containing thousands of beneficial phytonutrients, including flavonoids, carotenoids, vitamins, minerals, and fiber.

Phytonutrients protect cell membranes, prevent damage to the cell nucleus, are required for detoxification by the liver and other organs, and help with normal cell-to-cell communication. They are the premier antioxidants, preventing inflammation and allostatic load and reducing the need for cortisol every time they are eaten. Numerous studies comparing American diets to Asian or other diets where there are much lower rates of cancer and heart disease show that one of the main differences is the lower level of phytonutrients in the American diet.

Protein sources should be carefully chosen as well. The best sources of protein as described in the Mediterranean diet include a balance between vegetarian sources such as legumes (beans), nuts, and seeds and fresh organic animal sources including fish and fowl, and if tolerated, low-fat unsweetened dairy (best as cultured foods such as yogurts and kefir). Protein is needed for every cell and organ in the body to maintain healthy function. It is the basis of muscle, skin, connective tissue, hormones, and all body proteins essential for life. Inadequate intake of protein leads to a breaking down of muscles and other vital organs and tissues to compensate. Weight management and normalizing blood glucose and insulin are best accomplished by eating protein at every meal and snack.

When to Eat

Another important point is not just what is eaten but when. As every mother would say, breakfast is the most important meal. Here is the reason. The circadian rhythm for cortisol appears to be deeply set in every person's brain. Cortisol levels peak at 8 a.m., preparing one for the challenges of the day. Cortisol gradually comes down during the course of the day, until it reaches a low point at midnight. Production is gradually ramped up during sleep, again peaking at 8 a.m.

One of the major effects of cortisol is raising blood sugar for brain function. Glucose is the fuel that is used by brain neurons to produce energy. In the morning, cortisol induces gluconeogenesis by converting protein (specific amino acids) into glucose and releasing glycogen from stores in muscle and the liver. Breakdown of muscle protein to satisfy the brain's need for glucose is one aspect of catabolism, an important, though potentially destructive, function of cortisol. In addition, inadequate protein at breakfast followed by fewer and larger meals during the day does not effectively reduce the appetite-stimulating hormone ghrelin, leading to greater food consumption throughout the day.

To counteract the catabolic effects of cortisol, breakfast should contain high-quality protein to provide energy for the brain and stop the breakdown of muscle. The typical American breakfast of high-glycemic-index, low-protein cereals is exactly the opposite of what is needed at that time of day. Add a glass of orange juice, or worse, a juice drink that is loaded with added sugar, and a low-fiber bread or muffin, and you have the makings of a veritable cortisol festival leading to additional catabolic effects, including muscle loss and detrimental changes in body composition.

One other consequence of inadequate protein at breakfast is fluctuating blood glucose later in the day leading to hypoglycemia, another trigger for cortisol release. In my patients with hypoglycemia, protein at breakfast in addition to high-fiber foods such as steel-cut oats prevents hypoglycemia in the afternoon after lunch. A healthy lunch is just as important as a well-balanced breakfast to prevent cortisol dysregulation.

Many cultures, not influenced by the American food industry, eat a breakfast that satisfies what the body really needs. The Japanese often have fish products and sea vegetables, while Europeans have fish such as kippers or smoked salmon. Even the much-maligned English breakfast of a boiled egg, cooked tomatoes, and toast is better than a bowl of cornflakes. Here is another radical thought I often suggest, especially if eggs are not appropriate because of allergy or elevated cholesterol: eat dinner at breakfast. Make enough dinner for two meals and have leftovers if time is short in the morning.

Other ideas for breakfast include steel-cut oatmeal (slow-cooking) with walnuts, almonds, and flaxseed powder, or a serving of low-fat yogurt. Add berries and other fruits and a slice of whole-grain bread or brown rice cake with almond butter to round out the protein, complex carbohydrates, and essential fatty acids. Eggs, boiled, poached, or over easy, cooked without breaking the yolks (when the cholesterol in the yolk is directly exposed to high temperatures it becomes oxidized and is injurious to arterial walls), generally do not raise cholesterol. If concerned regarding cholesterol, use egg whites instead. Low-fat yogurt or goat-milk yogurt is a quick and easy protein source. Smoked salmon, herring, or tuna can all be used if the idea of kippers does not seem enticing. Well-designed protein powder, based in whey, soy, or rice, is another alternative source that works especially well with children and teenagers.

What about that cup of coffee that is part of breakfast for so many people? Studies have shown that caffeine raises cortisol and epinephrine levels, especially in people at higher risk for hypertension. Al'Absi and colleagues (1998) measured cortisol levels at rest and sixty minutes after continuous work on a mental stressor and a psychometric task. Findings showed an increased elevation in cortisol response when combining caffeine and the stressful task. This was true in both the controls and those at higher risk for hypertension, but even more exaggerated in the group at higher risk for hypertension. Caffeine also increases ACTH from the pituitary, leading to a greater cortisol response.

However, recent data has also demonstrated a beneficial effect of coffee consumption on preventing type 2 diabetes as well as reducing the risk of dementia. Researchers (Atanasov et al. 2006) found that the amount of caffeine typically found in a cup of espresso inhibited 11-beta-hydroxysteroid dehydrogenase type 1 (11-beta-HSD1) activity. This is the same enzyme found to have increased activity in obese patients, raising cortisol levels in fat cells. Whether it is the caffeine or a polyphenol in the coffee that has this effect is not clear. My suggestion is that one cup of coffee per day can be used by obese patients or those at low risk for activating the adrenal response or hypertension.

Another important eating pattern, especially if low blood sugar or the need for weight loss is an issue, is to have protein-rich snacks between meals. Eating every three hours will maintain normal blood sugar, prevent the breakdown of muscle protein, and keep insulin levels under control. In addition, smaller, frequent, protein-rich meals reduce levels of ghrelin, a key hormone released from the stomach that drives appetite and caloric consumption. Ghrelin also stimulates cortisol release independent of the HPA axis, further driving appetite and weight gain. Eating more frequently is one of the most potent ways to control ghrelin and therefore lose weight. Nut butters, seeds and nuts, yogurts, or other easily accessible foods are good choices for between-meal snacks.

As I discuss later in Chapter 9, "Beyond Adaptation: The Promise of Epigenetics," the new field of epigenetics has identified specific dietary components that protect gene expression and can reduce the risk for obesity, cancer, diabetes, heart disease, and other diseases of aging. These bioactive foods, an integral part of the Adaptation Diet, include broccoli, green tea, garlic, aged soy products such as tofu and tempeh, and the spice turmeric, which provides curcumin, a powerful anti-inflammatory agent. The outline of the Adaptation Diet below highlights the key dietary factors needed to improve adaptation, lose weight, protect the genome, and prevent chronic disease. These suggestions are at the core of the maintenance Adaptation Diet that will reduce cortisol and promote well-being.

The Adaptation Diet Outline

What to include:

- The largest portion of every meal should be vegetables (50 percent), with grains and animal protein in smaller amounts.
- Use one cup of cruciferous vegetables per day (broccoli, Brussels sprouts, kale, cauliflower, and cabbage), and liberally use onions, shallots, and garlic. Sulforaphane, a phytonutrient found in the highest amounts in broccoli, is a powerful protector of gene expression and has multiple anticancer properties.
- Have at least one vegetarian dinner every week.

- Use one cup of beans (kidney, navy, mung, or lima), lentils, or split peas five times a week–they are a great source of fiber, complex carbohydrates, and omega-3 fats.
- Eat organically grown foods whenever possible, especially protein, including free-range chicken and eggs.
- Avoid hypoglycemia and control ghrelin and appetite by eating a protein-rich breakfast and using only protein-rich snacks (for example, nuts and nut butters, low-fat yogurt, soy products) between meals. Consider eating five small meals per day and do not eat after 8 p.m.
- Drink juice made from organic green vegetables, including kale, Swiss chard, and spinach, mixed with carrots at least three days a week. It's best to use a machine that keeps the pulp with the juice rather than extracting the juice.
- Include anti-inflammatory and membrane-stabilizing fats–omega-3 fatty acids from walnuts, flaxseeds, pumpkin seeds, beans, salmon, herring, tuna, and sardines; and monounsaturated fats from olive oil, almonds, avocados, hazelnuts, and canola oil (cook only with olive, grapeseed, or canola oil).
- Have at least three portions of fish a week (wild salmon, anchovies, herring, mackerel, sardines, sturgeon, low-mercury tuna).
- Use two tablespoons a day of fresh ground organic flaxseed powder on salads or cereals (flax lignans reduce cortisol overproduction and detoxify hormones).
- Take a supplement with at least 1,000 milligrams of EPA/DHA fish oil on days when no fish is eaten, to control excess cortisol production (unless on blood-thinning medication).
- Incorporate colorful vegetables (carrots, squash, cabbage, tomatoes, etc.) and fruits (blueberries, pomegranate, and cherries, for example) rich in flavonoids and carotenoids into every meal, with at least seven portions per day.
- Eat eggs that come from free-range and organically fed chickens and are cooked without breaking the yolk (boiled, poached, fried over easy).

- Use herbs and spices that are anti-inflammatory and detoxifying: turmeric, cardamom, cilantro, ginger, onion, garlic, parsley. Curcumin in turmeric has great benefits in protecting gene expression, reducing inflammation, and protecting the brain against degenerative disease.

- Liberally use flavonoid-rich detoxifying vegetables, including shiitake and ganoderma mushrooms, broccoli, tomatoes, arugula, chard, kale, spinach, and other dark greens. Cooked tomato products protect against prostate disease in men.

- Consume a wide variety of foods rich in flavonoids (green tea, cherries, blueberries, red grapes, beets, legumes, asparagus, purple onions, sweet potatoes, and spices such as ginger, parsley, sage, and turmeric). Other potent members of the flavonoid group include rutin in buckwheat, hesperidin in citrus fruits, silymarin in milk thistle, genistein in soybeans, and apigenin in chamomile.

- Drink one-half (in ounces) of your body weight in filtered or bottled water every day. For example, if you weigh 130 pounds, drink 65 ounces of water. This will reduce aldosterone levels, help with weight loss, and normalize blood pressure.

- Choose green tea over black tea or coffee as a hot beverage. Green tea contains more catechins and the polyphenol epigallocatechin-3-gallate (EGCG). Green tea has been shown to protect gene expression and protect against cancer, hypertension, and diabetes.

- Use soy products rich in genistein and daidzein in the form of miso, tofu, edamame, and tempeh to detoxify hormones and to protect cell membranes and gene expression.

- Maintain a healthy weight to reduce inflammation and leptin resistance (even the loss of 5-10 percent of body weight changes cortisol and leptin levels).

- Supplement with probiotics (beneficial bacteria, including lactobacillus and bifidobacter), especially after antibiotic use. Probiotics can assist in weight loss and prevention of diabetes.

- Snack on protein-rich foods and never with high-glycemic-index carbohydrates as they will trigger more hypoglycemia. Nut butters, nuts, seeds, and low-fat yogurts are a few ideas for good snacks. Adding protein between meals can help with weight management and maintenance of good muscle mass.

- Strive for at least 25 grams of fiber per day from beans, whole grains, vegetables, flaxseed powder, chia seeds, or supplemental products such as psyllium seeds to reduce harmful bacteria in the gut and promote healthy bacteria that reduce inflammation, remove toxins from the body, and produce fatty acids like butyrate that regulate gene expression.

What to avoid:

- Avoid foods identified as allergy triggers (as documented in Phase Two) for at least three months. (If unclear about which foods to eliminate, avoid for one month the following trigger foods: wheat, sugar, eggs, dairy products, corn, beef, tomatoes, soy, chocolate, coffee, and alcohol. These can be reintroduced one per day after avoidance, observing for reactions.)

- Avoid hypoglycemia by eating a protein-rich breakfast and eating only protein-rich snacks between meals.

- Limit pro-inflammatory saturated fats (red meat, pork, lamb, poultry skin, whole dairy products, and tropical oils) and omega-6 vegetable oils (corn, soy, sunflower, safflower, cottonseed, and peanut).

- Eliminate all trans fats (hydrogenated and partially hydrogenated vegetable oils).

- Eliminate gluten grains (wheat, barley, and rye), especially in breads and baked goods, for three months and use in limited quan-tities after that (most people can use steel-cut oats as a cereal, which is a good source of fiber, and brown rice as their primary grain).

- Limit high-glycemic-index foods, especially sodas and candies sweetened with high-fructose corn syrup, which increase obesity and liver dysfunction (see Appendix A), and emphasize fiber-rich carbohydrates such as beans and root vegetables.

- Reduce caffeine intake to one cup of coffee or black tea per day to reduce inflammation and cortisol levels and prevent elevated cholesterol and homocysteine. Avoid all soft drinks. Use green tea as the primary hot beverage.
- Consume alcohol in moderation—no more than one drink every other day for women and one drink per day for men, preferably red wine or beer that contains polyphenols such as resveratrol, which reduces inflammation.

Following is a sample menu that puts into practice the key points of the Adaptation Diet to optimize weight and improve adaptation.

Breakfast

2 organic poached eggs or 1 cup organic low-fat yogurt

1 cup quinoa with 2 tablespoons ground flaxseed powder

1 cup blueberries

1 cup green tea

Mid-morning snack

1 tablespoon almond butter with celery sticks

Lunch

Salmon salad with romaine or kale with jicama and pecans

1 cup steamed broccoli florets

1 cup green tea

Mid-afternoon snack

Black lentils, brown rice, and salsa mixed together and served in a lettuce wrap

Dinner

Black Bean Soup (see recipe on page 286)

Roasted cauliflower with red pepper flakes

Green salad (spinach, kale, chard, arugula, or other
dark greens)

Evening snack

⅛ cup walnuts with ½ cup snow peas

This sample menu controls cortisol and assists in weight loss in the
following ways:

- Low-glycemic-index carbohydrates and protein snacks
  normalize blood sugar and control insulin production.
- Essential fatty acids from salmon and flaxseed and
  antioxidant-rich fruits and vegetables reduce inflammation,
  lowering cortisol secretion.
- Green tea, flaxseed, and EPA/DHA from the salmon
  improve the feedback in the midbrain to control cortisol.
- Fiber-rich complex carbohydrates from legumes (black
  beans, lentils) improve gut bacterial balance and
  detoxification.
- Adequate dietary protein protects against muscle breakdown from excess cortisol.
- In addition, as discussed in Chapter 9, broccoli, green tea,
  and other foods protect the normal gene expression that
  controls inflammation and cortisol levels.

Appendix C contains a wide variety of recipes to put the Adaptation Diet into action.

The Adaptation Diet emphasizes the use of inflammation-
controlling foods. Avoiding pro-inflammatory foods and emphasizing those that control inflammation can prevent many of today's
major epidemic degenerative diseases. Diet is the single most important factor in reducing inflammation and normalizing cortisol levels.
Below are lists of foods to avoid and foods to include to accomplish
the goal of reduced inflammation.

Pro-inflammatory Villains to Avoid

- Cold cuts, bacon, hot dogs, canned meats, sausages
- Pork, beef (organically fed and free range is better), eggs (except organic and free range; no more than four per week, preferably just egg whites)
- All trans fats in baked goods, chips, cake mixes, crackers, fried foods, shortenings, hydrogenated and partially hydrogenated vegetable oils
- All deep-fried foods
- Whole dairy products except from organically fed cows (low or moderate amounts of cultured dairy such as yogurt and kefir are acceptable)
- Polyunsaturated oils (peanut, safflower, sunflower, soy, corn) and lard
- White flour and white sugar products, including cookies, baked goods, candy, ice creams, ketchup, and other condiments
- Caffeinated coffee, soft drinks, sweetened fruit drinks, black teas

Anti-inflammatory Good Guys

- Vegetables: asparagus, beets, broccoli, Brussels sprouts, cabbage, carrots, cauliflower, celery, chard, bean sprouts, kale, spinach, lettuces (not iceberg), red onions, garlic, avocados (actually a fruit), cooked tomatoes (also a fruit), red and yellow peppers, squash, zucchini, sweet potatoes, yams
- Legumes: soybeans (best as edamame, tempeh, tofu, miso soup), green beans, navy beans, mung beans, lentils, split peas, white beans, black beans (never refried beans)
- Fruits: red grapes, blackberries, cranberries, red currants, blueberries, cherries, apples, pears, plums, pineapple, mangoes, tangerines, grapefruit, oranges

- Herbs: turmeric, parsley, sage, rosemary, thyme, basil, mint, ginger
- Protein: wild salmon, anchovies, herring, sardines, tuna (low mercury), mackerel, tilapia, cod, red snapper, organically raised poultry
- Nuts and seeds (best raw and unsalted; can be used as nut butters): almonds, flaxseeds (best if ground), shelled pumpkin seeds, walnuts, pepitas, sunflower seeds, sesame seeds (tahini)
- Grains: buckwheat, brown rice, millet, quinoa, steel-cut oats, smaller amounts of corn, whole wheat, rye
- Beverages: green tea, red wine (limit to one glass per day), herbal teas

In addition to the effects of phytonutrients in foods—such as flavonoids, other polyphenols, and carotenoids on reducing inflammation and controlling cortisol—vitamin C, vitamin E, zinc, copper, selenium, and other minerals and vitamins play a major role in normalizing cortisol and enhancing adaptation. Consider the use of a multivitamin/multimineral that provides adequate amounts of these nutrients.

Choosing Organically Raised Foods

For decades I have been a strong proponent of eating organically grown foods. After spending many years studying and becoming board certified in environmental medicine, I found alarming evidence of the sheer volume of man-made chemicals allowed in the food chain. Pesticides, herbicides, and fungicides are a major source of premature aging. All of these chemicals have a toxic effect and require the body's concerted effort to detoxify itself. This leads to greater oxidant stress and increases the need for cortisol to reduce the subsequent inflammation, triggering the aging effect of elevated cortisol levels. In addition, chemicals termed persistent organic pollutants (PCBs, bisphenol A, phthalates) are widespread in soils and foods and increase inflammation as well as alter gene expression. (See Chapter 9 for more on the POPs.)

I have recently discovered another major link between pesticide use, cancer risk, and premature aging: the health-protecting properties of foods like broccoli and berries are severely diminished through the plants' contact with pesticides. In broccoli, for example, the active phytonutrient (the glucosinolate glucoraphanin, which becomes sulforaphane when broccoli is chewed), a proven anticancer agent, exists as a natural pesticide to protect the broccoli plant from insects. However, this health-protecting nutrient is deactivated when the plant is exposed to man-made pesticides. Unfortunately, the same effect of pesticides is found in other foods rich in anti-aging nutrients, including berries, grapes, chard, kale, and spinach. This process is repeated throughout the vegetable kingdom, reducing the anti-aging benefits associated with the use of flavonoid- and carotenoid-rich vegetables and fruits. The exception is organically raised produce.

Luckily, organic produce is now widely available. Taking it one step further, freshly harvested produce has the highest content of polyphenols and flavonoids. To ensure the most nutritious vegetables and fruits, I suggest to my patients that they buy their organically grown produce at a local farmer's market when possible. Otherwise, health-oriented supermarkets have a wide variety of organic produce.

I also suggest the use of organically produced dairy products, fowl, pork, red meat, and eggs when possible. As I mentioned earlier, the essential fatty acid content of eggs is dramatically better in free-range and organically fed chickens. If red meat is to be used, look for grass-fed free-range cattle, which have lower levels of harmful fatty acids like arachidonic acid. Especially with beef, but also with chicken, organically raised animals will not have the extra burden of antibiotics, growth hormones, pesticide residues, and other harmful chemicals that have made their way to the dinner table via the typical industrial farming techniques.

6

The Stars of the
Adaptation Diet

The maintenance of allostasis and adaptation depends on making good choices at the dinner table. Understanding the science of adaptation makes it easier to employ the Adaptation Diet and create eating habits that fit each person's lifestyle. This chapter contains details about the beneficial effects of foods rich in phytonutrients that decrease inflammation, prevent free-radical damage, protect cell membranes, and decrease the impact of toxins. All of these foods and phytonutrients protect the midbrain and brain from damage and reduce allostatic load and the need for cortisol production. These foods form the basis of the Adaptation Diet. The major groups of these adaptive superstars are carotenoids, flavonoids, polyphenols, and isoflavones.

Carotenoids

I remember bringing my children to an exhibit at Epcot Center in Disney World and seeing a kitchen come to life with dancing and singing by the different food groups as well as the appliances. (Sadly, this is no longer one of the shows at Epcot.) The line that caught my attention was "Remember, vegetables are your friends." It certainly is true that the vegetable world is packed full of life-protecting and detoxifying nutrients, including the carotenoids. These critical antioxidants are found in yellow, orange, red, and green vegetables as well as tomatoes, sweet potatoes, sea vegetables such as kelp, and squash.

There are more than six hundred carotenoids in the food chain, with new compounds being isolated seemingly every month. They all protect cell membranes against free-radical damage from toxins, protecting the heart, prostate, breasts, liver, and other vital organs. For example, lycopene, a potent antioxidant that gives tomatoes their red color, is effective in scavenging free radicals in cell membranes, preventing oxidation of lipoproteins (the proteins that carry fat such as cholesterol through the blood), and reducing the incidence of prostate cancer, breast cancer, and heart disease. Lutein and zeaxanthin, carotenoids found in dark green leafy vegetables such as spinach and kale, are the chief constituents of the macular pigment in the eye and protect against adult macular degeneration, the leading cause of blindness in older Americans. These carotenoids might also protect against heart disease and other vascular problems.

Beta-carotene, the most thoroughly studied carotenoid, a precursor of vitamin A and an important antioxidant in its own right, is found in the greatest amounts in yellow and orange vegetables such as carrots, squash, sweet potatoes, and yams. Beta-carotene appears to accumulate in arterial plaque and might protect against heart disease. However, in human studies (Goralczyk 2009), supplementation of beta-carotene alone (with no other antioxidants given) in cigarette smokers demonstrated a slight increase in the incidence of smoking-related cancers. The most likely reason was the lack of other antioxidants provided to these patients. Beta-carotene, vitamin E, vitamin C, and other nutrients work as a team to detoxify free radicals and protect DNA and cellular membranes. Excessive use of any antioxidant causes a relative deficiency in the others. In addition, beta-carotene needs to be combined with the other carotenoids to be protective.

The average daily intake of carotenoids for adult women in the United States has been estimated to total 6 milligrams. However, optimum intake of beta-carotene itself is estimated to be 9–12 milligrams per day, while the typical average intake is only 1.8 milligrams. The following list is a guide to foods rich in carotenoids and estimates how much is currently used on average in a typical American diet. These are all inadequate amounts to ensure detoxification and cell protection. The Adaptation Diet calls for much greater intake every day of all these foods.

Carotenoid Intake in a Typical American Diet

Total carotenoids = 6.0 mg/day

	Category Intake (mg)	Dietary Sources
Beta-carotene	1.8	Carrots, cantaloupe, broccoli, tomatoes, apricots, green peppers, leafy greens, spinach, squash, and sweet potatoes
Alpha-carotene	0.4	Carrots, tomatoes, apples, corn, green bell peppers, leafy greens, peaches, potatoes, squash, and watermelon
Lycopene	2.6	Tomato products, watermelon, apricots, carrots, green peppers, and pink grapefruit
Lutein/ zeaxanthin	1.3	Spinach, green leafy vegetables, and broccoli
Beta- cryptoxanthin	0.03	Oranges, tangerines, apples, apricots, corn, green bell peppers, lemons, papayas, and persimmons

---

Flavonoids

Another major group of important phytonutrients and antioxidants is the flavonoids. There are more than four thousand flavonoids in the diet, mostly found in fruits and vegetables, herbs and spices. The flavonoids provide the dark color to the skin of vegetables and fruits, such as the color of red onions. Americans consume about one-fifth the amount of flavonoids as Asians, explaining in part the lower incidence of cancer and heart disease in people with traditional Asian diets compared to Americans. Total flavonoid intake is inversely related to the incidence of heart disease.

The flavonoids include catechins from green tea; polyphenols from red grape skin found in wine, which protect against heart disease; and quercetin, a potent antioxidant in grapefruits that helps regenerate vitamin C. Foods richest in flavonoids include legumes, green tea, cherries, blueberries, raspberries, red grapes, beets, asparagus, onions, sweet potatoes, and spices such as ginger, parsley, sage, and turmeric as well as many Chinese and Ayurvedic herbal remedies. Other potent members of the flavonoid group include rutin in buckwheat, hesperidin in citrus fruits, silymarin in milk thistle, genistein in soybeans, apigenin in chamomile, and resveratrol in red grapes and wine.

A superstar of the flavonoids is green tea, produced by lightly steaming the leaves of the tea plant *(Camellia sinensis)*. Polyphenols, the biologically active compounds in teas, are partially deactivated when tea is oxidized, as in black tea. The polyphenols in green tea include catechin, proanthocyanadins, and epigallocatechin, considered the most active flavonoid in tea.

Green tea polyphenols have shown higher antioxidant activity than vitamin C and vitamin E. Green tea can also increase the activity of detoxifying enzymes, including glutathione and catalase, active in the liver, lungs, and small intestine. Green tea activates both Phase I and Phase II detoxification.

Green tea consumption has been linked to the reduced incidence of many cancers, including stomach, small intestine, bladder, prostate, skin, pancreas, colon, breast, and lung. The lower incidence of cancer in Japan might be explained at least in part by green tea consumption. One of the effects of green tea is to normalize gene expression, reducing cancerous cellular changes. (See Chapter 9 for more information on the epigenetic effect of green tea.) Green tea appears to inhibit estrogen's stimulation of breast receptors in estrogen-sensitive cancers. Additionally, green tea suppresses the activation of carcinogens, detoxifies carcinogens, and inhibits nitrosamine production from foods such as bacon, hot dogs, ham, and other processed meat.

In most studies, green tea consumption was four to ten cups per day. Each cup contains an average of 80–120 milligrams of polyphenols. Green tea extracts can be used that contain 300 to 600 milligrams of polyphenols standardized to contain 80 percent polyphenols and 55 percent epigallocatechin. To reach the possible benefit found in population studies, a minimum of 300 milligrams should be taken as a supplement.

Studies have shown remarkable properties in another under-utilized food, wild blueberries. In animal studies, Papandreou and colleagues (2009) found that rats fed wild blueberries had better memory for spatial tasks and improved coordination. During World War II, British pilots ate wild blueberries to improve their night vision and coordination. Blueberries contain high amounts of polyphenols that give the berries their blue color and tartness. These chemicals have been shown to be strong antioxidants that are cardioprotective, improve circulation, inhibit certain cancers, and protect against age-related cognitive dysfunction and motor deficits. It appears that the more tart wild blueberry has a higher concentration of these polyphenols than those commercially produced. In either case, these studies show the benefit of eating a wide variety of fruits and vegetables, especially those with intense coloration, including pomegranate, raspberries, blackberries, and red grapes.

Quercetin, found in a wide range of foods, including red onions, grape skins, green tea, and tomatoes, is one of the most potent flavonoids and has been shown to protect against the development of diabetic complications such as diabetic cataracts, neuropathy, and retinopathy. Quercetin can possibly lower cardiovascular risk, lower cholesterol, and improve endothelial function. In a study by Kleemann and colleagues (2011), quercetin was found to lower arterial inflammation and an important marker of heart disease risk, C-reactive protein (CRP). Quercetin also appears to have potent antiviral properties, as do most of the flavonoids, with inhibition of viral infections, including herpes type 1, parainfluenza, polio, and respiratory syncytial virus. Quercetin might also have some benefit in treating the common cold. The recommended daily dosage as a supplement is 200–400 milligrams taken twenty minutes before a meal. It is also helpful to take bromelain, a digestive enzyme from pineapple, with the quercetin to enhance its anti-inflammatory effect.

Proanthocyanadins, which are found in grape seeds, red wine, and commercial extracts from maritime pine bark, have potent antioxidant and anti-inflammatory effects. They prevent damage to collagen, the protein that constitutes much of the connective tissue, tendons, and ligaments. These potent antioxidants have fifty times the effect of vitamin C in protecting connective tissue and can reduce symptoms from arthritis and allergies, lower cholesterol, strengthen capillaries, and promote healthy skin.

Soybeans and Isoflavones

Soy protects against heart disease and stroke, lowers cholesterol, and protects against hormonally influenced cancers such as breast and prostate. Soy products, including tofu, soybeans (edamame), miso, soy milk, tempeh, and soy nuts, contain the isoflavones genistein, equol, daidzein, and others that are critical in the detoxification process and reduce the effect of hormones on receptors. They lower inflammation by reducing levels of inflammatory mediators, C-reactive protein, TNF-alpha, and interleukin-6. They also enhance detoxification of estrogen and testosterone, one reason for the very low incidence in Asia of breast cancer and menopausal symptoms. Genistein and the other soy isoflavones influence the synthesis of tumor proteins, slow the growth of malignant cells, block procancer enzymes, and inhibit the growth of blood vessels that nourish tumors.

In women who are low in estrogen, such as during menopause, soy isoflavone stimulation of estrogen receptors can reduce symptoms of menopause significantly. Many of my patients can reduce hot flashes by using miso, tempeh, and tofu products. The fermented soy products are higher in genistein and might provide greater detoxification and protection against hormonally induced disease. I recommend consuming one serving of soy per day if needed. That's about three ounces of tofu or one-half cup of tempeh or miso. I don't recommend primarily using soy milk as a source of these isoflavones because it is not a food that was part of traditional Asian diets and has never been studied long term. There has been much controversy over the negative effects of excess soy products on breast health and thyroid function. Using only fermented traditional sources of soy reduces these risks and is an appropriate food choice.

Other foods that contain smaller amounts of these isoflavones are the other legumes, alfalfa, clover, licorice root, and kudzu root. Kudzu root has been used in supplements in place of soy in soy allergic patients.

Legumes

If there is one group of foods that most Americans underutilize, it is legumes. These nutritional powerhouses are a perfect blend of soluble and insoluble fiber, essential fatty acids, protein, and complex carbohydrates. They contain phytohormones, lignans, and isoflavonoids, which provide cancer protection, lower LDL cholesterol, and act to detoxify hormones and toxins. Because of their fiber properties, they stabilize blood-sugar levels, preventing obesity and type 2 diabetes. The legumes include soybeans, kidney beans, lentils, adzuki beans, black beans, brown beans, chickpeas, mung beans, navy beans, pinto beans, red beans, and split peas. One cup of cooked beans per day is a worthy goal.

Cruciferous Vegetables

Your mother was right when she told you to eat your broccoli. Broccoli is one of the cruciferous (*Brassica* family) vegetables, an essential food group for detoxification and healthy aging. Other crucifers include cauliflower, Brussels sprouts, cabbage, bok choy, kale, mustard greens, rutabaga, turnips, and watercress. They induce several enzyme systems, including glutathione S-transferase and glutathione peroxidase, that are potent cell-membrane protectors. The compounds in these foods include aryl isothiocyanates and indole-3-carbinol, which detoxifies estrogen, protecting against breast and prostate cancer. Animals fed cruciferous vegetables and then exposed to the deadly carcinogen aflatoxin had a 90 percent reduction in the incidence of cancer. Smokers who chewed two ounces of watercress at each meal had a significant increase in the detoxification of nicotine compared to controls. Because indoles are easily destroyed during cooking, either steam your crucifers or eat them raw.

Cruciferous vegetables are rich in glucosinolates that enhance glutathione levels, protect the genome, and increase detoxification. Glutathione is a key antioxidant that protects cell membranes from oxidative damage. An overload of toxins from poor diet, alcohol, cigarettes, or over-the-counter medication can deplete glutathione and pose risks for cancer and inflammatory processes.

Turmeric

A good example of the potency of spices and herbs is turmeric, used in Indian cooking for centuries. It contains curcumin, a potent antioxidant that influences cell signaling pathways. Turmeric inhibits the inflammatory process and reduces the need for cortisol production, lowers total cholesterol, raises HDL, and prevents abnormal clotting. Turmeric reduces lipid peroxides, a measure of oxidant stress, and protects lipids from oxidation. This spice is found in yellow curry, prepared mustard, and as a supplement. (See Chapter 9 for additional discussion of the powerful effects of this ancient food.)

Methionine and Cysteine

Amino acids, the building blocks of protein, are used in the detoxification process. The most important of these are the sulfur-containing amino acids, cysteine and methionine, which lead to the manufacture of glutathione, a compound that detoxifies and acts as a powerful antioxidant. Glutathione levels can be increased through the use of meats, nuts, asparagus, and avocados. However, glutathione is easily destroyed by the use of alcohol, acetaminophen, and other drugs. Vitamin C at 500 milligrams can protect glutathione from degradation. N-acetylcysteine, available as a supplement, increases glutathione levels and can treat toxicity from drugs such as acetaminophen as well as from environmental toxins.

Foods that are rich in the sulfur amino acids methionine and cysteine include eggs, fish, dairy products, poultry, beans, nuts, and seeds. The more environmental stress from toxins and drugs, the higher the need for these foods to provide the sulfur as a building block for detoxification. The sulfur amino acids also are the key factors in sulfation, which converts many toxic intermediaries into harmless substances.

Garlic

Garlic has been used for five thousand years as a medicinal food. Pasteur noted that garlic was an antiseptic. It has long been used as an antiparasitic in many cultures throughout the world. Garlic has immune-system-stimulating properties as well, activating natural killer cells against tumor cells (Ishikawa et al. 2006). Stomach cancer rates are lessened significantly in people with high levels of garlic intake (Zhou et al. 2011).

A clove of garlic is a gold mine of phytonutrients with more than thirty different active compounds that detoxify and protect against free-radical damage. (Chives, leeks, onions, and shallots also contain many of these nutrients.) These active compounds include the sulfur-containing phytonutrients allylic sulfides (thiols), allicin, ajoene, saponins, and phenolics. These substances have been shown to lower cholesterol; reduce the stickiness of blood platelets; act as natural antibiotics against viruses, bacteria, fungi, and parasites; and block tumor growth.

Garlic (as well as onions) also contains flavonoid compounds, including quercetin, which have anticarcinogenic effects. These are potent antioxidants associated with reduced risk of skin cancer, leukemia, and experimentally induced cancers in rodents.

Phytochemicals That Improve Detoxification and Protect Cell Integrity

Compound	Source
Isothiocyanates	cruciferous vegetables (broccoli, cabbage, kale)
Glucosinolates	cruciferous vegetables
Organosulfurs	garlic, onions
Curcumin	turmeric
Flavonoids	numerous fruits and vegetables
Monoterpenes	citrus peel

Mushrooms

The medicinal use of mushrooms such as maitake, reishi *(Ganoderma lucidum)*, enoki, and shiitake *(Lentinula edodes)* is highly developed in Asia. These mushrooms have strong effects on enhancing immune function, including natural killer-cell activity and inhibiting tumor growth. The oral extract of maitake, which contains beta-glucan, a polysaccharide, has been shown by Shomori (2009) to have potential antitumor effects in gastric cancer-cell lines.

The dose needed to stimulate the immune response is 900 milligrams per day. Shiitake is available in many food stores and can readily be added to meals. I have my patients use an alcohol tincture of a mixture of ganoderma, shiitake, and *Ophiocordyceps sinensis* for acute viral illness. For people who need immune enhancement because of a chronic illness, these mushrooms can be used in capsule form. A typical combination includes cordyceps, ganoderma, *Coriolus versicolor,* shiitake, and *Grifola frondosa.*

Yogurt and Beneficial Bacteria

Although yogurt is often overlooked as an adaptogenic food, it can have a significant impact on the level of systemic inflammation and weight, and therefore cortisol production. Yogurt as well as kefir (a liquid cultured dairy product), and to a lesser degree buttermilk, are a great source of easily utilized protein and, most importantly, beneficial bacteria for the digestive system.

Yogurt and kefir are fermented dairy products that contain active cultures of lactobacillus and bifidobacter bacteria (probiotics). (Check the label, because not all commercially available yogurts have live cultures.) There are trillions of bacteria in the digestive tract, many of which are essential to human health. Until recently, medicine has focused on unhealthy bacteria in the gut as a source of illness; however, it is now clear that ensuring adequate levels of beneficial bacteria is required for overall health. The intestinal world of bacteria, called the microbiota, can be dramatically altered by the use of antibiotics, anti-inflammatory medications, acid-blocking and proton pump inhibitor (PPI) medications, alcohol, poor diet (especially high-glycemic-index foods and low fiber intake), toxins, and stress. Reduced levels of healthy gut bacteria have been implicated in chronic inflammation of the digestive tract, lower immunity against infection, and an increased risk of diabetes. The most effective way to ensure good microbiota populations is to minimize the damaging medications, consume foods rich in probiotics, maintain a high fiber intake, and, if needed, supplement with probiotic capsules.

Probiotics also play a major role in regulating allergic reactions to foods and reducing inflammation through suppressing growth of abnormal bacteria and yeasts. These beneficial bacteria aid in the detoxification of hormones and other chemicals and prevent reabsorption of antigens and chemicals that trigger inflammation. They inhibit the formation of carcinogens from dietary sources and enhance immune function. In addition, they produce vitamins B and K, which are necessary for normal clotting and nervous system function. Probiotics are also needed for weight control, as demonstrated in a large population study of dietary habits where the only food associated with weight loss was yogurt.

Yogurt with live cultures shows beneficial immune system effects, including tripling of interferon production, raising the activity of natural killer cells (cells that destroy potential cancer cells), and blocking the effect of carcinogenic agents in the colon on the development of colon cancer. In a study of women with breast cancer (van't Veer et al. 1989), there was an inverse relationship between the amount of yogurt consumed and the incidence of breast cancer, most likely because of the beneficial effects of the probiotics. (It is essential that all dairy products used are organic, due to the increasing levels of persistent organic pollutants [such as PCBs and bisphenol A] found in dairy.) Yogurt is best used without added sweeteners, especially aspartame. Blended fruit yogurts with high amounts of fructose should also be avoided. In addition to dairy products, other food sources of probiotics (though not as potent) include kimchee (fermented cabbage), tempeh and miso (fermented soy), sauerkraut, and kombucha.

Recent evidence (Muccioli et al. 2010) further links the bacterial pattern in the gut with both obesity and diabetes. It appears that certain unhealthy strains of bacteria affect gut wall permeability, leading to greater absorption of lipopolysaccharides (LPS), a component of bacterial cell walls, that markedly increases the inflammatory response. Increased gut permeability leads to heightened immune response in the gut wall as well as higher levels of systemic inflammatory hormones. Increased LPS levels directly impact the fat cells and increase their size and activity, leading to more visceral fat and a vicious cycle of inflammation and more fat deposition. All of these changes lead to more cortisol production to suppress inflammation, as well as higher cortisol secretion from adipocytes (fat cells). As we have seen, elevated cortisol increases blood sugar, impairs insulin receptors, and leads to more visceral fat. Diabetes appears to also be closely linked to this sequence, possibly from the increased inflammatory state induced by gut bacteria. The gut microbiota has been found to differ in both obese and diabetic individuals compared to nonobese, nondiabetic individuals. This then leads to the vicious cycle of gut wall dysfunction, inflammation, and obesity.

Targeting the gut bacterial population can be a potent avenue to weight loss and reduced risk of metabolic syndrome and diabetes. Finnish scientists have shown that *Bifidobacterium* numbers were much higher during infancy in children who had normal weight later in childhood, compared to obese children. Weight loss induced by diet and exercise has been associated with increased levels of lactobacillus. Lactobacillus supplementation has also been associated with weight loss and improved glucose metabolism, probably through downregulation of LPS-mediated inflammation. Even supplementing women in pregnancy with *Lactobacillus rhamnosus* prior to delivery and for the first six months of breast-feeding showed a clear trend of reduced weight in the child's first four years of life compared to placebo.

To ensure adequate beneficial microbiota in the digestive tract requires a diet rich in soluble fiber containing prebiotics that promote the growth of good bacteria. These foods include the bean family (legumes), whole grains (especially oatmeal), onions, leeks, flaxseed, greens, and berries. Using well-designed probiotics and prebiotics (soluble fiber like inulin from chicory) as supplements can further reduce the systemic levels of LPS, improve intestinal permeability, and reduce inflammation and cortisol levels. In addition, inulin fructans have been shown to improve blood-sugar response to meals and to lower insulin levels.

To increase healthy adaptation, effectively lose weight, and improve glucose metabolism, I suggest that my patients supplement with probiotics, prebiotics, and, if needed for immunity, colostrum extracts. (Colostrum is a form of milk from both human breast milk and cow sources that is rich in immune proteins and antibodies.) Several strains of lactobacillus that have been studied are especially effective against abnormal gut organisms, reducing LPS levels and helping with gut permeability. These include *Lactobacillus rhamnosus* GG, *Lactobacillus rhamnosus,* and *Lactobacillus acidophilus* NCFM. Strains of bifidobacter, also needed to regulate the health of the small intestine, reduce inflammation, and control weight, should be included in any supplement program. It is important that the manufacturer guarantees the potency of the strain to contain at least ten billion live organisms per capsule. Most need to be refrigerated to maintain potency. There is little doubt that the science now supports the importance of normalizing the gut microbiota.

Berberine: Normalizing the Gut Microbiota, Blood Sugar, and Weight

A remarkable botanical that might become a core part of the management of obesity through the microbiota/inflammation connection is berberine, an alkaloid originally isolated from traditional Chinese herbs that has been used in Chinese and Ayurvedic medicine for more than 2,500 years. For many years I have used berberine as a way of reducing abnormal gut bacteria and treating dysbiosis, or unhealthy bacterial patterns in the gut. (As noted above, this is now termed alterations in the gut microbiota.) Recent studies have shown that this is just one of several beneficial effects of berberine.

In a study by Hu and colleagues (2012), obese subjects were given 500 milligrams of berberine orally three times per day. The result was a modest weight loss of five pounds but a much greater improvement in blood lipids, including a 23 percent decrease in triglycerides and a 12.2 percent decrease in cholesterol. (These results were replicated in animal studies.) In addition, vitamin D (calcitriol) levels increased by 59 percent, leading the authors to suggest that berberine might also be useful in the prevention of osteoporosis. Berberine can contribute to significant weight loss, in addition to reduction in fat mass and improvements in blood-sugar levels and insulin resistance.

Berberine has been used in China for many years to treat type 2 diabetes. Compared to medications often used in the United States like metformin, berberine has broader benefits, including lowering blood sugar by up to 25 percent, triglycerides by 17 percent, and insulin by 28 percent in a study of 50 patients with diabetes. Berberine has also been found to improve insulin sensitivity in rodents fed a high-fat diet through improved mitochondrial regenesis. (The mitochondria are intracellular organelles critical for cellular energy and burning of fats.) One study (Han et al. 2011) showed that some of these changes stemmed from berberine's antibacterial effect on the gut microbiota, leading to less absorption of lipid polysaccharides and reduced inflammation. These findings are in line with the current concept that diabetes and obesity are triggered by inflammation from the gut microbiota.

A study by Chang and colleagues in 2012 showed that berberine also reduces homocysteine (a metabolite associated with increased risks for heart disease and strokes) in rats fed a high-fat diet. In addition, significant weight loss, improved triglyceride levels, and lower LDL cholesterol were seen. Another study (Zhang et al. 2012) showed that berberine actually prevented the development of obesity and insulin resistance in rats fed a high-fat diet. Zhang and colleagues also felt that these effects were from modulation of the gut micro-biota, leading to lower levels of inflammation and weight loss.

Berberine has become a significant tool in the battle to improve the gut microbiota, reduce inflammation, lose weight, improve insulin sensitivity, prevent diabetes, and improve cholesterol and triglyceride levels. There are no pharmaceutical agents that have such a sweeping effect on weight loss, reduction of inflammation, and normalizing blood sugar. Another mechanism of action, in addition to changes in the gut microbiota, is the inhibition of visceral fat activation of cortisol, a major contributor to the excess cortisol seen in obesity. Berberine also affects the gene expression that promotes increased burning of fats and carbohydrates, leading to weight loss. Berberine can have significant effects on cholesterol levels equivalent in many cases to the effects of statin drugs. Experts are now recommending berberine as a first-line treatment for type 2 diabetes, high cholesterol, metabolic syndrome, and obesity. Berberine has also been found to improve endothelial function, thought to be the key factor in the development of heart disease. All of berberine's broad-based benefits make it a powerful ally in lowering cortisol through reduction in inflammation, blood sugar, and harmful fats. The daily dose of berberine needed for these benefits is about 1,000 milligrams.

Protecting the Amygdala and Hippocampus through Nutritional Supplements and the Adaptogenic Diet

When all is said and done, one of the most important goals of proper dietary habits is to protect the brain from damage induced by elevated cortisol and oxidant stress. Food-based nutrients are the cornerstone of preserving cell-membrane health. However, with the stress patterns that I see in my patients as well as the pollutants from the environment and the food chain, using nutritional supplementation targeted at protecting the neurons of the midbrain is often required.

Cortisol and epinephrine increase lipid peroxidation and cause damage to cell membranes from free radicals, including singlet oxygen, super oxide, and hydrogen peroxide. Injury can be to the cell membrane, the DNA, or the mitochondria, the energy-producing organelles inside the cell. Protecting against this damage are antioxidant molecules that are either made in the body or derived from food and supplements.

Stress, poor adaptation, and elevated cortisol age the brain. Aging itself increases cortisol and its damaging effect on the cerebral cortex and the hippocampus, which is intimately involved with memory and mood. Damage to the hippocampus alters the feedback control of cortisol production, making the situation even worse. This leads to early memory loss, depression, anxiety, and fatigue.

Protecting the brain from damage should be everyone's number-one priority. The Adaptation Diet, stress reduction through meditation and relaxation techniques, exercise, and changes in attitude and

Effects of Elevated Cortisol on Brain Aging

- Increases inflammatory hormone gene expression (5-lipoxygenase)
- Increases nerve sensitivity to toxins and poor blood flow
- Inhibits sex- and growth-hormone secretion
- Affects mood and behavior
- Permanently downregulates hippocampal cell receptors
- Alters neurotransmitter function
- Disrupts memory recall and cognition
- Increases insulin resistance
- Affects neuronal cell atrophy, injury, and death
- Promotes failure of the mitochondrial mechanism and neurotoxicity

behavior are all needed to improve adaptation. In addition, several nutrients have been shown to be neuroprotective through specific membrane-sparing effects, preventing free-radical damage to the brain from allostatic load. One of these nutrients is alpha lipoic acid, which improves healthy glucose transport and metabolism and promotes proper function of the mitochondria, the cellular energy factory. Lipoic acid is a potent antioxidant and helps regenerate vitamin C and vitamin E, particularly in the nervous system tissue.

Alpha lipoic acid improves energy production through adenosine triphosphate (ATP) synthesis. It is a strong antioxidant and acts as a chelator of heavy metals. It increases the synthesis of glutathione, the most important antioxidant found in brain tissue, and scavenges reactive oxygen species (its antioxidant effect). It works both inside and outside the cells of the nervous system. It improves the removal of glucose from the bloodstream, increasing insulin receptor sensitivity. In patients with diabetic neuropathy, 800–1200 milligrams per day of alpha lipoic acid has been used with positive results. For nondiabetic individuals, a time-released preparation of 400–800 milligrams per day is suggested.

The brain has its own immune cells, the microglia, which can become upregulated, triggering inflammation leading to neurodegenerative processes including Parkinson's disease, Alzheimer's disease, and other forms of dementia. Reducing the overall inflammatory state with the Adaptation Diet is the first step in preventing these changes. In addition, nutrients that target the Nrf2 transcription factor can increase antioxidant protection and downregulate the brain's inflammatory state. These include curcumin from turmeric (yellow curry spice), green tea, sulforaphane from broccoli and other cruciferous vegetables, and resveratrol from red grapes and red wine. (This is the same group of bioactive foods that have been found to be powerful regulators of gene expression as discussed in Chapter 9.) Emphasizing the foods that contain these critical nutrients is important, while specific supplements of these can be used if there is concern regarding risk for neurodegenerative disease.

Other key brain nutrients include acetyl-L-carnitine; N-acetyl-cysteine; carotenoids, including lutein; the B vitamins, especially B6, B12, and folic acid (critical for methylation to detoxify toxins); coenzyme Q_{10} for mitochondrial function and antioxidant effect; *Ginkgo biloba* for improved blood flow and antioxidant protection; EPA/DHA (cold-water fish oils, especially from salmon and tuna) for support of the membranes of the brain cells (a higher concentration of DHA in supplements would be preferred for protecting the brain and nervous system); and vitamin E, including both alpha and gamma tocopherol.

Acetyl-L-carnitine is a nonessential amino acid derivative that improves mitochondrial energy production. It has been shown to improve cognitive function and delay the onset of dementia. It also increases the production of acetylcholine, a critical neurotransmitter. Carnitine can also clear abnormal deposition of fatty acids and has been shown to decrease triglyceride levels. Acetyl-L-carnitine is more active in the brain than carnitine itself. Doses used in the studies of dementia ranged from 1.5 to 3 grams per day.

Magnesium is needed for normal mitochondrial function in the production of energy. It is depleted when glucose is elevated from increased cortisol levels. Elevated intakes of dietary fats and calcium also deplete magnesium stores. Magnesium is needed for normal muscle tone and is useful in the treatment of asthma, migraine, anxiety, and muscle spasm. In patients with chronic pain, magnesium levels are often depleted and cause additional lack of stress resistance. The best form of magnesium is citrate with a dose of 300–500 milligrams per day.

Coenzyme Q_{10} is protective of brain and heart cells through its antioxidant effect and improvement of mitochondrial function. CoQ_{10} has a sparing effect on vitamin E, while vitamin E allows CoQ_{10} to be more effective when it is taken as a supplement. A dose of 150 milligrams was shown to improve brain function in Parkinson's patients. CoQ_{10} also showed significant effects in improving cardiac function in patients with cardiomyopathy. (One-third of the heart weight is composed of mitochondria, which are dependent upon adequate CoQ_{10} levels.) Doses should be at least 100 milligrams daily of a crystalline-free oil-based preparation.

CoQ_{10} Facts

- Protects against cholesterol oxidation
- Found in organ meats
- Decreases after age forty
- Decreased mitochondrial function occurs with aging.
- Useful in atrial fibrillation, congestive heart failure, mitral valve prolapse, hypertension
- Decreases angina and ST depression
- Improves exercise tolerance, reduces LDL oxidation
- All patients on statin drugs should supplement with at least 100 milligrams per day of CoQ_{10}.

N-acetylcysteine (NAC) has a potent antioxidant effect through increasing levels of glutathione, the key cellular antioxidant. Glutathione also increases disposal of peroxides and protects cell membranes and the nucleus. NAC has been shown to increase electron transport in the mitochondria and activates enzymes to increase energy production from the mitochondria. There is also evidence of reduction of cell death or apoptosis with the use of NAC. Doses of NAC should range from 500 to 1,000 milligrams per day.

Vitamin E is the primary fat-soluble antioxidant found in all tissues. Low levels lead to higher risk for degenerative diseases of the brain such as Alzheimer's and Parkinson's. It is protective against the oxidative stress effects of elevated cortisol levels. High doses of vitamin E up to 2,000 IU per day have been shown to slow the onset of progression of Alzheimer's by up to two years. Mixed tocopherols including both the gamma and alpha forms are more consistent with what is found in food and should be the only form of vitamin E used as a supplement. Blood levels of vitamin E are also predictive of heart disease, with the lowest levels showing an increased risk of developing coronary artery disease. In fact, vitamin E levels are a more important predictor of heart disease than are cholesterol levels. For brain protection, 200–800 milligrams of mixed tocopherols are suggested. Using high doses of one antioxidant such as vitamin E without corresponding doses of other antioxidants such as vitamin C can be harmful. I always recommend a mixed antioxidant supplement that contains adequate amounts of mixed tocopherols, vitamin C, and carotenoids.

Food Sources of Vitamin E

- Almonds
- Asparagus
- Avocados
- Olive oil
- Wheat germ
- Soybeans

Niacinamide (vitamin B3) helps maintain normal blood-sugar levels in people prone to hypoglycemic reactions. Niacinamide is a potent inhibitor of inflammation in the brain caused by enzymes such as nitric oxide synthetase and poly (ADP-ribose) polymerase (PARP). It has antioxidant effects as well as protects mitochondrial function in the brain. Recommended dosages of niacinamide are 100–500 milligrams per day.

Folate (folic acid), vitamin B6, and vitamin B12 are important in detoxifying homocysteine, a product of protein metabolism that can cause vascular disease of the brain and heart. These three vitamins are needed for methylation reactions that detoxify homocysteine and protect the brain and blood vessels. Cognitive dysfunction is seen in deficiencies of these vitamins, with symptoms of memory loss, forgetfulness, confusion, depression, mood changes, and dementia. Changes in stress levels and elevated cortisol can increase the requirement for these vitamins. Daily intake should be at least 1 milligram folic acid (as tetrahydrofolate), 25 milligrams B6, and 1,000 micrograms of B12, preferably as methyl B12.

Essential fatty acids are incorporated into the tissue membranes of nerves. There is less inflammatory activity in these membranes if EPA and DHA are substituted for arachidonic acid (from red meat, dairy, and eggs) in the membranes of the brain. These fatty acids are found in high amounts in cold-water fish such as salmon, cod, and mackerel as well as in walnuts and other nuts. The dose per day should be a minimum of 400 milligrams for prevention and up to 3 grams for treatment of chronic inflammation. Capsules of EPA/DHA are readily available. It is important to make sure the fish were caught in nonpolluted waters, because of possible contamination with toxins from the ocean.

Resveratrol is a polyphenol found in the skins of red grapes and other plants. It is the only nutrient shown to enhance mitochondrial regeneration. In animals fed high doses of resveratrol, aging was slowed and longevity increased. Resveratrol also reduces inflammation through inhibition of COX-1, COX-2, and 5-LOX pathways. (This is the same effect as many of the common anti-inflammatory medications such as ibuprofen, aspirin, and prescription anti-inflammatory medications.) It also is a strong antioxidant and protects lipid membranes, inhibits platelet aggregation, and improves liver detoxification. Resveratrol activates the sirtuin gene, which protects the cell against damage and slows cell death. The only other activator of this gene is reduced caloric intake. Resveratrol in the diet could explain the so-called French paradox—that despite high-fat diets and large amounts of red wine, there is little heart disease in France.

Suggested Daily Dosages for Brain Protection

- Alpha lipoic acid 400–800 mg
- Acetyl-L-carnitine 500 mg
- Coenzyme Q_{10} 100 mg
- N-acetylcysteine 500–1,000 mg
- Vitamin E 200–800 IU of mixed tocopherols
- Vitamin C 500–1,000 mg ascorbates with flavonoids
- Niacinamide 100–500 mg
- Folic acid (as tetrahydrofolate) 1 mg (if no cancer risk)
- Vitamin B6 25–50 mg
- Vitamin B12 500–1,000 mcg of methyl B12
- EPA/DHA 400–3,000 mg

This is not meant to be an exhaustive list of supplements that might impact brain health. I suggest a good multivitamin/multimineral complex in addition to some of the above nutrients. Remember that taking supplements is not a replacement for the benefits from the Adaptation Diet, good eating habits, and appropriate self-care. Use of these supplements should be under the supervision of a health care professional.

7

Cortisol Tamers

My experience observing the wide-ranging impact of diet on my patients' ability to adapt has helped me identify several factors that directly reduce elevated cortisol levels. These include foods, herbs, vitamins, and minerals that constitute a group of substances called adaptogens. They are instrumental in managing allostasis and ensuring adaptation.

Controlling cortisol should start early in life. However, for some people childhood already presents a challenge in terms of allostatic load. Several studies (Reynolds et al. 2007, Herrick et al. 2003) have shown that maternal diet can influence the cortisol levels of children. For example, Herrick and colleagues (2003) looked at the children of women who had a diet containing excessive animal protein (greater than seventeen portions of meat or fish per week) and minimal amounts of carbohydrate-rich foods in the second half of pregnancy. These children had up to 46 percent higher levels of salivary cortisol in response to the Trier Social Stress Test (a standardized psychological stress test). Children of women who consumed a more balanced diet using complex carbohydrates and less protein (less than thirteen portions of meat or fish per week) had significantly lower cortisol levels. In addition, there is evidence that low birth weight might also increase cortisol production and stress responsiveness later in life. Despite what may have happened in utero, there are still many things that can be done to alter cortisol levels. Following are dietary and lifestyle factors that I have found to have a significant impact on regaining adaptation.

Lose Weight and Cut Calories

Obesity itself increases cortisol levels, leading to an increased risk of metabolic syndrome, diabetes, and heart disease. The pro-aging impact of obesity is enormous in Western society, where one of every two adults is overweight and 40 percent of children are obese or overweight. A striking example of this childhood epidemic was pointed out to me on a recent ski trip. Several of the ski instructors told me that half of the young children they teach are so overweight and out of shape that they can barely get up if they fall during ski lessons! The instructors had seen a dramatic change in the number of obese children in their classes over the previous five years.

Obesity stems from a combination of genetic susceptibility, diet, and lack of exercise. Diet is the number-one reason for this epidemic. Perhaps the biggest culprit is the use of high-glycemic-index foods, including refined sugars and other carbohydrates, which stimulate increased appetite and craving for additional carbohydrates, greatly increasing caloric intake. Eating these foods causes an initial spike in blood sugar, followed by elevated insulin levels that then lead to lower blood sugar, increased hunger, and more food intake in an attempt to restore energy balance. Studies in both humans and animals consistently confirm these findings as underlying much of the obesity epidemic.

In obese children the amount of daily food intake was measured after the ingestion of a high-glycemic-index food (instant oatmeal) compared to a low-glycemic-index meal (steel-cut oats). Food consumption throughout the day after a breakfast and lunch of the two types of oatmeal was 53 percent higher with the high-glycemic-index food. A study in the UK by Warren and colleagues (2003) measured food intake at lunch following either a high- or low-glycemic-index breakfast and found that the low-glycemic-index meal reduced caloric intake later in the day in both normal and overweight children. Another study, by Ebbeling and colleagues (2005), found that children who were allowed to eat as much low-glycemic-index food as they desired lost significantly more weight than those children on a diet that was low calorie and fat restricted. The bottom line is that eating high-glycemic-index foods markedly increases appetite and leads to a greater intake of calories throughout the day.

Certainly there are other factors contributing to the obesity epidemic, including lack of exercise, high fat intake, the use of fast foods, enormous portion sizes and excess caloric intake ("super-sized"), a lack of nutrient-rich foods like legumes and cruciferous vegetables, and exposure to chemicals such as bisphenol A and phthalates (called persistent organic pollutants), which are known to be obesogens and contribute to weight gain. However, the most potent pro-obesity dietary factor in the United States is the use of high-glycemic-index carbohydrates.

Once obesity occurs, a vicious cycle ensues of inflammation, insulin resistance, and more obesity. A person with abdominal obesity (a waist size greater than forty inches in men and greater than thirty-five inches in women) is at much greater risk for heart disease, diabetes, and metabolic syndrome. Metabolic syndrome includes insulin resistance as the key metabolic derangement as well as hypertension, elevated triglyceride levels, and lower levels of high-density cholesterol. Twenty-five percent of obese people and 50 percent of hypertensives are insulin resistant. It is estimated that 25 percent of the U.S. population may be insulin resistant and have metabolic syndrome.

The cortisol connection appears here as well. Obese women, after eating a high-carbohydrate meal, have a marked elevation in cortisol production compared to normal-weight women. This increase in cortisol often includes elevated norepinephrine levels as well and creates a maladapted response and additional allostatic load. On the other hand, a high-protein and low-carbohydrate meal did not elevate cortisol in the obese women studied.

Obesity and excess abdominal girth themselves increase cortisol levels and interfere with adaptation. One of the most dangerous and discouraging aspects of being overweight is that once established, it is self-perpetuating. Cortisol appears to be one reason that obese people do not slim down easily. It has been shown that in the obese individual, there is a greater release of cortisol from the adrenal glands when stimulated with corticotropin-releasing hormone (CRH) from the hypothalamus and midbrain. This implies that stress from any source will cause a greater secretion of cortisol in obese people, further complicating the connection between excess weight and stress hormones and the risk for metabolic syndrome, diabetes, and heart disease.

As noted earlier, the adipocytes (fat cells, especially those in visceral fat in the abdominal cavity surrounding the internal organs) increase conversion of inactive cortisone to active cortisol through the enzyme 11-beta-HSD1, resulting in elevated cortisol systemically. Amazingly, it appears that the amount of cortisol produced by this mechanism is equivalent to the amount manufactured by the adrenal system. Obesity itself increases this enzyme activity in the fat cells, leading to more circulating cortisol, elevated cortisol in visceral fat, and additional risk for metabolic syndrome. This makes weight loss even more challenging. In addition, the hypothalamic-pituitary-adrenal axis is activated more in obese individuals, further increasing cortisol production.

Research by Schinner and colleagues (2007) has shown remarkably that adipocytes secrete a signaling molecule (Wnt-signaling) that directly stimulates the adrenal glands (through StAR transcription) to produce higher levels of cortisol and aldosterone, the hormone that raises blood pressure. The greater the abdominal fat, the higher the cortisol and the faster that premature aging, high blood pressure, heart disease, and diabetes occur. Obesity and increased abdominal fat also contribute to insulin resistance and a cluster of metabolic abnormalities, including type 2 diabetes, hypertension, and abnormal levels of blood fats, including cholesterol and triglycerides.

If a person is overweight, there are also lower levels of the binding protein, corticosteroid-binding globulin (CBG), that prevents cortisol from stimulating receptor sites. This makes cortisol more available, amplifying its damaging impact. The reason the body is so intent on increasing cortisol in obesity is to attempt to reduce the chronic low level of inflammation seen in most overweight people, especially if they are eating a typical American inflammatory diet. In a study done in Spain with two hundred subjects (Fernandez-Real et al. 2002), the greater the waist/height ratio (a simple measure of obesity), the lower the CBG levels, leading to elevated free (active) cortisol. In a study in England by Steptoe and Kunz-Ebrecht (2004), men with abdominal obesity had morning cortisol levels that were higher than those in men with normal weight. Elevated morning cortisol is typically seen in high levels when stress is a major factor. It appears that simply being overweight is enough to cause malad-aptation and premature aging.

Visceral abdominal fat, especially when greater than normal, functions as an endocrine organ. This startling finding flies in the face of all previous ideas about hormones and how they are pro-duced from endocrine glands. In addition to making cortisol, fat cells make leptin, a hormone that signals the brain to reduce appe-tite. In many cases of obesity, leptin levels become elevated because the signal is disrupted, probably from inflammatory foods, prompt-ing more leptin production. Similar to insulin resistance, leptin resis-tance is associated with a chronic inflammatory state caused by dietary habits. The leptin no longer effectively shuts down appetite. Excess simple carbohydrates, the wrong fats, and too many calories all contribute to leptin resistance. The Adaptation Diet, as well as appropriate nutritional supplementation, can reduce inflammation and overcome both insulin and leptin resistance.

Visceral fat can directly increase endothelial dysfunction, a major risk factor for heart disease. (Endothelial function is a marker of the ability of blood vessels to dilate and prevent inflammatory changes leading to atherosclerosis.) It has been shown that as little as a nine-pound weight gain of visceral fat is associated with significant endothelial dysfunction and elevated cortisol levels. Researchers at the Mayo Clinic (Corral et al. 2007) studied forty-three lean people, put thirty-five of them on a weight-gaining diet, and compared them to the others who did not gain weight. The researchers measured endothelial function through blood-flow parameters both after the thirty-five people gained the weight and again after they subsequently lost weight. They found impaired function of the endothelium from this modest weight gain even if blood pressure and other markers were normal, implying that even a small amount of increased visceral fat can start the process of metabolic syndrome and heart disease.

The bottom line is that even mild obesity causes inflammation leading to greater cortisol response. Obese individuals show higher IL-6, NFK alpha, CRP, leptin, and insulin, all markers of inflammation. Besides releasing free fatty acids, adipocytes secrete substances that contribute to insulin resistance, including resistin. Increased turnover of free fatty acids interferes with intracellular metabolism of glucose in the muscle, and exerts a lipotoxic effect on pancreatic beta cells. The pre-receptor metabolism of cortisol is enhanced in visceral adipose tissue by the activation of 11-beta-hydroxysteroid dehydrogenase type 1. As noted, adipose tissue itself is the source of many of these inflammatory hormones and signaling molecules. All these changes indirectly stimulate cortisol release to reduce inflammation.

The vicious cycle of too much abdominal fat leading to elevated cortisol, which makes insulin resistance worse, leading to more weight gain, has to be broken to regain adaptation. Luckily, it does not take massive weight loss to regain appropriate cortisol balance. Losing as little as 5 percent of total body weight can stop the cycle of increased cortisol release and lead to adaptation. For some people 10 percent is needed, but even that is possible to accomplish with appropriate dietary changes. The majority of my patients who stay with the Adaptation Diet for at least three months, emphasizing frequent protein meals and low-glycemic-index carbohydrates, while eliminating food allergens as well as glutens, sugars, and all processed foods, will lose enough weight to accomplish the goal of cortisol control. For those patients who need extra help to lose the 5 percent, supplementation with acetyl-L-carnitine, alpha lipoic acid, irvingia, and green tea can jump-start the process.

Of course, calorie control is also a key in weight management. Cutting calories has been proven to be the most effective anti-aging strategy ever researched. In the 1990s, evidence for the efficacy of caloric restriction did appear in a most unlikely setting. Biosphere 2 was an experiment of living in a completely self-contained closed environment in the desert outside Tucson, Arizona. A self-sustaining ecological system was developed to show that humans could thrive in this setting. However, because of an unanticipated decrease in food availability, the eight men and women who lived in Biosphere 2 were forced to consume 22 percent fewer calories, while still sustaining high levels of physical activity over an eighteen-month period.

The result was a 17 percent decrease in body weight and a marked reduction in metabolic risk factors for heart disease in the Biosphere 2 inhabitants. They had lower blood pressure, cholesterol, and glucose levels. Most interestingly, they showed lower cortisol levels and markers of inflammation such as CRP. They had higher DHEA levels, lower thyroid hormone levels, lower core temperature, improved insulin sensitivity, and reduced markers of oxidative stress.

Caloric restriction also leads to a reduction in inflammation, the key to aging well. Long-term human studies have not yet been done, so many scientists hesitate to tout caloric restriction as an anti-aging miracle. However, it is clear that losing weight and cutting calories, regardless of initial weight, will reduce inflammation and cortisol levels, leading to much-improved adaptation and lower allostatic loads.

Flaxseed Powder

Surprisingly, one of the most powerful regulators of cortisol production is flaxseed powder. In a study done by Spence and Thornton

(2003), volunteers were fed diets containing flaxseed supplementation with differing concentrations of lignans and alpha linolenic acid. They were then given a stressful and frustrating task to perform, after which the researchers measured their levels of plasma cortisol, fibrinogen, and peripheral resistance (a marker for the elasticity of arteries). The flaxseed highest in lignans had the most significant effect in reducing plasma cortisol.

Flaxseed has been called nature's perfect food, because it contains soluble fiber, omega-3 essential fatty acids, and lignans, a potent phytohormone. The omega-3 essential fatty acid is anti-inflammatory, decreasing the need for cortisol and reducing the risk for heart disease and diabetes. Lignans in flaxseeds are phytoestrogens (plant-based substances that attach to estrogen receptors, reducing stimulation from circulating hormones) and have been shown to reduce the incidence of breast and prostate cancer. In postmenopausal women with breast cancer, Canadian researchers (Thompson and Chen et al. 2005) found that dietary flaxseed increased cancer-cell apoptosis (cell death) and reduced tumor growth rate.

In a study by Prasad (2005), lignans from flaxseed reduced atherosclerosis plaques in rabbits fed a high-fat diet. The protective mechanisms of the flaxseeds included decreased oxidative stress, lower total cholesterol and LDL, and higher HDL. Lignans from flaxseeds also improved glucose control and reduced both insulin levels and insulin resistance in human volunteers.

I recommend two tablespoons of ground organic flaxseed daily, sprinkled on salads, cereals, or other foods. It is best to grind the seeds in a coffee grinder and use them right away to prevent rancidity. If you are not able to grind your own, purchase organic flaxseed powder that has vitamin E in it to prevent rancidity. Flaxseed oil capsules generally do not have the same effect unless they have added lignans.

Fish Oil and Supplements of EPA/DHA

Researchers in France (Delarue et al. 2003) did one of the most important studies regarding the connection between omega-3 fatty acids and stress. They measured the stress response to mental arithmetic and other stressors before and after feeding human volunteers 7.2 grams of fish oil a day as supplements for three weeks. The measurements included plasma cortisol, catecholamine (epinephrine and norepinephrine), and non-esterified fatty acid. The response to stress, including elevations of cortisol, epinephrine, and fats, was dramatically reduced by supplementation with omega-3 fatty acids. They concluded that adrenal activation could be inhibited by adequate intake of omega-3 fatty acids. The site of action is in the central nervous system. Furthermore, it was postulated that essential fatty acid supplementation might reduce the injury to the hippocampus from cortisol and slow the subsequent development of Alzheimer's disease and other manifestations of premature aging.

Low dietary intake of omega-3 fats from fish has been associated with promoting anger, aggression, and depression in some people. Taking EPA/DHA supplements (EPA and DHA are the two key fatty acids in fish) can reduce this effect. A study done at the New York Veterans Administration hospital by Buydens-Branchey and colleagues (2000) found that in male outpatients who had aggressive behavior and substance abuse, 3 grams of fish-oil supplements daily (containing 2,250 milligrams of EPA and 500 milligrams of DHA) reduced anger scores significantly compared to placebo. Because anger and aggression equate to high cortisol levels, this study confirms the benefits of omega-3 supplementation in reducing cortisol elevation.

Researchers in Japan (Hamazaki and Itomura 2000) showed a decreased norepinephrine concentration (31 percent less) in students given 1.5 grams of DHA during exam week. They also showed a marked reduction in measures of hostility (72 percent less) in students on EPA supplementation compared to controls, when faced with the stress from final exams. (Norepinephrine, the acute stress hormone of the autonomic nervous system and the midbrain, will eventually lead to higher cortisol levels when chronically elevated.)

In 2010, Noreen and colleagues showed that EPA/DHA can blunt the increase in cortisol found after intense exercise. They studied forty-four men and women, who were put on either 4 grams of EPA/DHA providing 1,660 milligrams of EPA and 800 milligrams of DHA, or 4 grams of safflower oil. After six weeks of treatment there was a significant decrease in cortisol and fat mass and an increase in fat-free mass in the group on EPA/DHA. This study showed the benefit of lowering cortisol in terms of reducing fat mass and losing weight. The proposed mechanism of lowering cortisol is through reduction of the inflammatory cytokine IL-6, which can stimulate the hypothalamic-pituitary-adrenal axis independent of CRH. Controlling inflammation is a critical goal in managing weight and reducing excess cortisol.

All these studies have the same conclusion: if enough of the right fats are eaten, the brain will not respond excessively to stress. The fats in the diet matter in terms of brain health and adaptation because they are incorporated right into the brain itself. This was also the opinion of other researchers, including Lanfranco and colleagues (2004), who found that essential fatty acid administration inhibits cortisol production through a mechanism in the brain itself, not in the pituitary or the adrenal glands. In mice who have brain lesions similar to those of Alzheimer's disease, use of essential fatty acids reduced damage to the hippocampus during stress and prevented the development of additional Alzheimer's-like brain lesions.

Another major connection between EPA/DHA and reduction of cortisol is the impact these fatty acids have on inflammation. As I discussed earlier, EPA and DHA are building blocks for the anti-inflammatory eicosanoid hormones. The use of foods rich in EPA/DHA tips the balance of eicosanoid hormones toward the anti-inflammatory cytokines helping to resolve inflammation. In addition, recent findings by Calder (March 2012) reveal another target of these valuable fats. Substances called pro-resolution molecules, including lipoxins, resolvins, and protectins, are used by the body to turn off chronic inflammation. EPA/DHA has a major influence on enhancing production of these molecules, reducing chronic inflammation and therefore cortisol levels.

In addition to eating fatty fish such as wild salmon, to control cortisol levels it is helpful to supplement with EPA/DHA capsules on days when fish is not consumed. A reasonable dose for cortisol balance and adaptation is 1,000–1,200 milligrams of EPA and at least half as much DHA. Most supplements have between 160 and 320 milligrams of EPA per capsule. If you have any bleeding problems or use anticoagulants, fish-oil use needs to be supervised by a physician. Some people cannot tolerate fish oils without digestive upset. To prevent oxidative stress from high-dose fish-oil supplements, it is important to use a good antioxidant supplement.

Linolenic Acid Supplementation

A study by Bruder and colleagues (2006) found a connection between gamma linolenic acid (in primrose, borage, and black currant seed oils) and reduction of cortisol production. An oxidized derivative of linoleic acid (EKODE) reduced cortisol production by 25 percent in adrenal cells. It also increased production of DHEA, the other main adrenal hormone that reduces the destructive effect of cortisol by promoting tissue repair. It is thought that these fatty acids are oxidized in the liver and form compounds that modulate adrenal steroidogenesis, changing the amounts of cortisol and DHEA the adrenal glands produce.

Supplementing the diet with one of these oils is the easiest way to obtain the key omega-6 fatty acid, DGLA. Although this study looked at a synthetic derivative of these oils, I have observed improvement in my patients with symptoms such as premenstrual tension and anxiety with the use of evening primrose, borage, and black currant seed oils. A typical dose of gamma linolenic acid in borage oil is one to two 240-milligram capsules per day.

Phosphatidylserine

Phosphatidylserine (PS) is a major component of cell membranes and may restore sensitivity to cortisol receptors in the midbrain, hypothalamus, and pituitary to improve the feedback loop when cortisol levels are elevated. This is particularly important because long-term elevation of cortisol can damage the cells in the hippocampus that regulate cortisol secretion, disrupting the normal feedback control over production of this hormone.

I have used phosphatidylserine with my patients to help dampen excess cortisol production, improve memory, and treat depression. I often have them use it at night if there are symptoms of insomnia, anxiety, and memory loss. If tests reveal elevated cortisol at other times of the day, the PS is used at those times. Elevated nighttime cortisol occurs with breakdown of the feedback to the midbrain and is strongly associated with depression, anxiety, and insomnia.

Phosphatidylserine was first isolated in 1943 and has been extensively studied in more than three thousand papers. It contains both fatty acids like DHA, an omega-3 essential fatty acid, and amino acids. It is vital to the function of brain cells and other cells throughout the body. Dietary sources of PS are organ meats, chicken skin, fatty fish, and red meat. The average daily intake in Western diets is 130 milligrams; however, a low-fat diet provides even less. In the 1980s, the average intake was 250 milligrams. Modern food production of fats and oils decreases all the natural phospholipids in our diets, including phosphatidylserine. Phosphatidylserine (like phosphatidylcholine found in lecithin) is a phospholipid that is incorporated into cell membranes, especially in the brain. PS has been shown to reduce cortisol response to both psychological and physical stress. In a 2008 study by Starks and colleagues, short-term supplementation of phosphatidylserine was able to blunt increases of cortisol after exercise by 39 percent compared to placebo. Ten healthy males were given 600 milligrams of phosphatidylserine or placebo for ten days and their cortisol levels measured after moderate exercise. The authors concluded that phosphatidylserine is effective in combating exercise-induced cortisol secretion and could prevent the physiological deterioration caused by elevated cortisol while improving the overall hormonal state. Similar to psychological stress, strenuous exercise can also induce an unwanted increase in cortisol and add to allostatic load.

Phosphatidylserine improves communication between cells in the brain by increasing the number of membrane receptor sites for receiving messages. Phosphatidylserine modulates the fluidity of cell membranes, essential to the brain cells' ability to send and receive chemical communication.

Stress increases the demand for phosphatidylserine. Supplementing with PS has been shown to reduce exercise-induced stress by blunting the increase of cortisol after intense exercise. PS can improve mood and relaxation in stressful situations and increase dopamine production, helping with depression. It enhances metabolism of glucose in the brain, improving neurotransmitter function. It increases the synthesis of acetylcholine, needed for memory, leading the FDA to state that phosphatidylserine may reduce the risk of cognitive dysfunction in the elderly. PS has also been recommended for treating ADD and ADHD in children and adults. (Many of the studies with the strongest results for treating cognitive decline, even in Alzheimer's disease, were based on animal-derived PS from bovine brain tissue, which is no longer in use because of mad cow disease. The jury is still out on soy-based PS for these severe problems.)

The adaptogen effect of phosphatidylserine appears to be multifocal, including enhanced neurotransmitter release, which can moderate cortisol levels. By blunting the excess release of cortisol and sensitizing the feedback loop to the midbrain, there is less risk for allostatic load. Most supplements of phosphatidylserine are soy derived with a typical dose of 100 milligrams up to three times per day. If insomnia is an issue, one of the doses should be one hour before sleep.

Vitamin D

Vitamin D has emerged recently as a nutritional superstar. Among its many proven benefits are improving bone density and preventing osteoporosis, reducing the risk for prostate, colon, and breast cancer, improving immunity to viral infections, reducing the risk of heart disease and diabetes, and reducing the incidence of autoimmune diseases, including multiple sclerosis and systemic lupus erythematosus. It is this last finding regarding reduction of autoimmune processes that makes vitamin D important in the world of adaptogens.

A telling study by Alele and Kamen (2010) on vitamin D and inflammation looked at sixty-nine healthy women and measured vitamin D—25(OH)D3—levels in the blood. The women with the highest level of vitamin D had the lowest markers of inflammation, including TNF-alpha, a key lymphokine indicating immune activation. Women with regular UVB sun exposure had serum 25(OH)D3 concentrations that were significantly higher and parathyroid hormone concentrations that were significantly lower than those in women without regular UVB exposure.

Vitamin D deficiency affects between 30 and 50 percent of the general population. This epidemic is a result of many factors. Vitamin D gets activated from sunlight and UVB rays. As people age, the skin is less adept at converting precursors into vitamin D. In addition, the use of sunscreen and the presence of air pollution block vitamin D activation. Especially in children, reduction in outdoor time has contributed to this alarming increase in vitamin D deficiency. Vitamin D is formed in the skin from 7-dehydrocholesterol and then converted in the liver and kidneys to the active form. Adequate sunlight would theoretically provide 90 percent of the needed amount of about 10,000 IU per day. However, in my practice even my patients who are surfers show that is clearly not happening. Possibly another factor in this epidemic of low vitamin D levels is the overuse of statin drugs, which lower cholesterol, the precursor of vitamin D in the skin.

Low vitamin D levels appear to be a major risk factor for cardiovascular disease. Low levels lead to high renin levels and hypertension, inflammation, insulin resistance, and increased risk of diabetes. Low vitamin D has also been linked to unexplained muscle pain, fatigue, poor resistance to infections, and a variety of autoimmune conditions. Vitamin D supplementation, which achieves ideal blood levels, could lead to lower cortisol requirements by reducing inflammation and immune system problems. Normal blood levels of 25(OH)D3 are from 30 to 100 ng/mL (nanograms per milliliter), with ideal levels between 40 and 80 ng/mL. Many of my patients are at the lower end of normal or even below 30 ng/mL, despite living in one of the sunniest climates in the United States.

In the past, normal vitamin D blood levels were thought to be lower. However, after studying groups in tropical areas, like Central American natives, it was realized that blood levels should be significantly higher and might reduce the incidence of multiple sclerosis, a disease with a greater incidence the farther north one lives. It was also noted that vitamin D is needed to reduce the number of inflammatory cells in the brain of MS patients. In a study by Munger and colleagues (2004) of 180,000 women, those who took 400 IU of vitamin D daily were 40 percent less likely to develop multiple sclerosis. These findings led researchers to suggest that maintaining higher levels of vitamin D could influence the occurrence of MS and other autoimmune conditions.

Lupus is another example of how low vitamin D possibly contributes to autoimmunity and inflammation. Inadequate levels of vitamin D are frequently found in lupus patients, contributing to this inflammatory condition. In obese patients, vitamin D supplementation significantly improved markers of inflammation, reducing the risk of cardiovascular disease.

In the past, the recommended doses of vitamin D supplementation were too low and not based on good science, because there was a lack of understanding of the crucial nature of this vitamin. It was assumed that sunlight would be enough and if any extra vitamin D was needed, a teaspoon of cod liver oil (with about 400 IU) was adequate. Current research supports using doses of up to 5,000 IU daily to achieve a blood level of 40 ng/mL, the minimum found to reduce inflammation and help prevent heart disease, cancer, hypertension, and other major disease.

If signs of deficiency exist, I recommend at least 2,000 IU of vitamin D3 in an oil-based form daily, though many patients need quite a bit more to achieve ideal blood levels. Higher doses require monitoring with blood tests to prevent toxicity, because vitamin D is fat soluble and excess buildup of vitamin D can cause problems with calcium metabolism and parathyroid secretion while increasing the risk of kidney stones. It should be used cautiously in anyone with high blood calcium levels or a history of kidney stones. In addition, high doses of vitamin D should be accompanied with vitamin K and possibly vitamin A to prevent abnormal arterial calcification and vitamin A deficiency.

Botanical Adaptogens

Adaptogens, a term first proposed by Soviet researchers in the 1950s, are a group of natural substances, including herbs and vitamins, that improve responsiveness to stress and prevent allostatic load. The original research from the Soviets was focused on surviving extreme physical stress. However, my experience with patients under emotional stress as well as physical stress who become maladapted has demonstrated that these botanicals are helpful not only in the Gulags of Siberia, but in daily life.

Most adaptogens work through modification of cortisol production, leading to enhanced immune function, better stress responsiveness, and the ability to recover from physical and emotional challenges. Though the exact mechanism of action for these herbs has not been identified, it is thought that they restore hypothalamic and midbrain sensitivity to modify cortisol secretion. Research has also shown that adaptogens affect tolerance for stress through their phytonutrient (flavonoids, lignans, carotenoids) content, acting as antioxidants and membrane stabilizers. They have demonstrated immune-regulatory and blood-sugar-stabilizing effects, further leading to reduced cortisol response.

Adaptogens reduce an excessive immediate fight-or-flight response and elevated epinephrine and norepinephrine levels, as well as reduce allostatic load and adrenal exhaustion. They reduce symptoms of fatigue by making cellular energy production more efficient and reducing lactic acid buildup (from inefficient anaerobic metabolism). Adaptogens also improve the homeostatic mechanism, overcoming allostatic load and reestablishing allostasis.

Another benefit described for adaptogens is a normalization effect. For example, if one person has elevated blood pressure as a result of stress, while another experiences blood pressure drops when stressed, adaptogens—through improvement of the midbrain and the hypothalamic-pituitary-adrenal axis—normalize blood pressure response, either raising or lowering it as required. Adaptogens can reduce excessive host defense reactions, decreasing the damaging effect of allostatic load, while at the same time allowing for an appropriate response to stress.

Breakdown of the cortisol feedback control mechanism during long-term stress occurs because of neuropotentiation of the amygdala, decreased sensitivity in the hippocampus, and increased locus coeruleus production of epinephrine from CRH stimulation. The hypothalamus is affected by all these changes. In some cases this will lead to a lack of responsiveness in the midbrain to appropriately stimulate cortisol release when in stressful situations. This is the "adrenal exhaustion" phase mistakenly thought by many to be a problem with the adrenal glands themselves. Because part of the effect of adaptogens is thought to occur at the hypothalamic level, it is possible that their impact can also be on the midbrain, resetting its control over cortisol production. The botanical adaptogens that I use the most in my practice include Siberian ginseng, Chinese (Panax) ginseng, ashwagandha, *Rhodiola rosea, Ginkgo biloba,* and *Ophiocordyceps sinensis.*

It is imperative that these botanicals be used with medical supervision if there is any concern about a medical condition or if any blood-thinning medications are used. Each of these herbs might affect any one individual in a negative manner if the person's current state of the HPA axis does not call for the specific effect of the adaptogen. These are powerful herbs with multiple effects and should be treated with respect.

Siberian Ginseng

One of the most widely studied adaptogens is Siberian ginseng *(Eleutherococcus senticosus).* In the 1950s, Russian scientists discovered that this herb, distinct from Chinese or Korean ginseng (Panax ginseng), had powerful adaptogenic properties. Siberian ginseng used as a supplement showed an increased ability to adapt to adverse physical conditions as well as improved mental performance and enhanced quality of work under stressful conditions. It has shown strong antioxidant effects and the ability to protect nerve and heart cells from damage.

Siberian ginseng has six compounds that are antioxidants, four with anticancer activity, three that lower cholesterol, two that stimulate the immune system, and one that modulates insulin levels. Studies on Siberian ginseng (more than a thousand have been done, most of them in Russia and other countries previously in the Soviet bloc) showed improved adaptation in several areas.

Soviet studies on Siberian ginseng and its effects on adaptation showed:

- Improved stamina and recovery in Soviet Olympic athletes
- A 40 percent decrease in high blood pressure and a 30 percent decrease in total reported symptoms in auto factory workers

- A 30 percent reduction in the incidence of influenza in long-distance truck drivers
- A 50 percent decrease in immune suppression from chemo-therapy in patients with gastric cancer
- Increased endurance in Soviet cosmonauts during long-duration space flights

Siberian ginseng appears to improve hypothalamic receptor sensitivity, leading to normalized cortisol production, less immune suppression, lower blood pressure, and improved glucose metabolism. It acted as a true adaptogen, demonstrating increased cortisol output below a stress threshold and decreased cortisol output above a stress threshold, enhancing the physiologic response to mild stress and modulating the response to extreme stress. It prevents some of the immune suppression seen with elevated cortisol. Siberian ginseng can normalize blood sugar through stimulating the release of glycogen stored in muscles for immediate energy, reducing long-term elevation of glucose and insulin resistance, and reducing catabolic (muscle-wasting) effects on muscle and endurance.

I generally recommend the use of a combination of adaptogens to improve adaptation. The dose of Siberian ginseng in most formulations is 200 milligrams, containing 0.8 percent eleutherosides E and B. The active compounds for most adaptogens have been identified and are usually listed as a percentage of total ingredients. For example, the eleutherosides are the active compounds in Siberian ginseng and should constitute at least 0.8 percent of total compounds.

Panax Ginseng

The other ginseng often used, Asian (also called Korean) or Panax ginseng, has different active compounds (ginsenosides) than Siberian ginseng. Panax ginseng has a long history of use in Chinese medicine, employed as a tonic to improve energy and adaptation. It appears to improve the feedback loop of the hypothalamic-pituitary-adrenal axis. In one study reported by Le Gal and colleagues (1996), the use of 80 milligrams of Panax ginseng per day in addition to a multivitamin/multimineral was associated with a significant improvement in energy levels in most participants in the study.

Panax ginseng has a variety of actions on the adrenal glands and HPA axis. In animals, it has been shown to increase the size of adrenal cells, enhancing activity. It can increase HPA sensitivity to cortisol through effects on the hypothalamus. Certain ginsenosides have shown a buffering ability to reduce an exaggerated adrenal stress response. In the brain, ginseng stimulates ACTH and the cortisol response to acute stress but also demonstrates improved negative feedback and greater sensitivity of the brain to circulating levels of cortisol, reducing allostatic load. It can upregulate the HPA axis, reducing fatigue, and is especially useful in the later stages of HPA axis underfunctioning. Typical doses range from 200 to 400 milligrams with 8 percent ginsenosides.

Ashwagandha

Ashwagandha *(Withania somnifera)* is another invaluable adaptogen. It has been used for centuries in Indian Ayurvedic medicine to improve adaptation to both physical and emotional stress. Animals pretreated with this adaptogen and exposed to stressful conditions did not have as much adrenal hypertrophy, blood-sugar elevation, or cortisol depletion as untreated animals. Ashwagandha also has anabolic activity (increasing androgens, such as DHEA, needed for tissue repair), and normalizes inflammatory prostaglandins. It also reduces catecholamine (epinephrine) production and normalizes blood-sugar and cholesterol levels.

People treated with ashwagandha report feeling less anxious in stressful situations. It appears to enhance GABA levels and in animal models has a neurorestorative effect in Parkinson's and Alzheimer's disease. In addition, it demonstrates significant immune-enhancing effects as well as anti-inflammatory properties. Other stress-modifying effects include reduction of the incidence of peptic ulcers and improvement of thyroid function. A typical dosage of ashwagandha is 200 milligrams containing 5 percent withanolides.

Rhodiola Rosea

Rhodiola rosea (also called Arctic root) is native to high mountainous areas of Asia and Eastern Europe. It is another herb that the Soviets studied extensively, finding that it enhanced work performance and resistance to stress. I have found it is one of the most clinically useful adaptogens, especially when combined with phosphatidylserine, which improves the midbrain's response to stress.

Rhodiola appears to affect neurotransmitters, including dopamine, serotonin, catecholamines, and beta-endorphins. It is also cardioprotective, maintaining higher levels of cAMP (an energy-producing enzyme) in the heart muscle. It reduces catecholamine stimulation of cardiac tissue, leading to less arrhythmia. It is often useful in the person who is easily overstimulated and is wired and tired. Rhodiola also stimulates immune function while reducing stress-induced beta-endorphin production. (Beta-endorphin and ACTH are both produced in the pituitary as a response to stress.) Rhodiola has been studied extensively for more than thirty-five years. In a study by Darbinyan and colleagues (2000) of work-fatigued physicians, rhodiola produced an improvement in cognitive function and performance. The dose is about 200 milligrams containing at least 1 percent salidrosides.

Ginkgo Biloba

Ginkgo biloba is a well-researched herb that has strong adaptogenic properties. It reduces elevated cortisol levels and can increase ACTH levels. Ginkgo has been shown to reduce stress-induced learning impairment in rats and potentially to reduce stress-induced cognitive dysfunction in humans. It increases acetylcholine synthesis and the turnover of norepinephrine.

Ginkgo has been shown to reverse age-related losses of adrenergic receptors in the neocortical area of the brain. It increases uptake of choline in the hippocampus and could have an anticonvulsant effect. Studies on the effects of ginkgo on dementia have shown both beneficial effects in some results and little impact in others. However, a recent study in Germany by Herrschaft and colleagues (2012) showed that ginkgo extract improved cognitive function in mild to moderate dementia.

Ginkgo protects mitochondria from oxidative damage and has potent antioxidant effects that are protective of brain tissue. Ginkgo has been shown to increase blood flow in the central nervous system. It has a mild anticoagulant effect, inhibiting platelet aggregation, which improves the general circulation. Ginkgo can improve cognitive function and possibly slow degenerative disease of the brain. Supplements should contain at least 120 milligrams with 24 percent of the active ingredient, ginkgo flavonglycosides. Caution should be used if surgery is imminent or if blood-thinning medications are combined with ginkgo.

Cordyceps

Another potent adaptogen, especially useful with "adrenal fatigue," is *Ophiocordyceps sinensis,* a medicinal mushroom that is one of the most valued therapies in Chinese medicine. Wild cordyceps is a rare, blade-shaped fungus found at high altitudes in China and Tibet. Chinese scientists have been able to produce a water-soluble extract of the mycelial component of the fungus that contains the active ingredients cordycepic acid and adenosine.

Cordyceps has been used in traditional Chinese medicine to support vitality, improve kidney and lung function, and enhance libido. It has been shown to have beneficial effects on immune function as well as normalizing glucose metabolism. As an adaptogen, cordyceps has been shown to have substantial effects on adrenal function.

The hot-water extract of cordyceps improves endurance of mice in response to physical stress, inhibits cholesterol elevation, and inhibits enlargement of the adrenal glands. (The size of the adrenal glands is often used as a measure of stress effects, because chronic allostatic load typically increases the size of the adrenal glands as the body attempts to react to the stressful situation.) Rats increased their ability to secrete cortisol when stimulated with cordyceps in a manner differing from stimulation by ACTH.

Cordyceps is most useful when fatigue and anxiety are significant symptoms. In human studies, Zhu and colleagues (1998) found that cordyceps improved fatigue, cold intolerance, and cognitive function in elderly people. It has been shown to improve stress tolerance and endurance. Cordyceps has also demonstrated an ability to improve respiratory function in patients with COPD (emphysema) and increase energy levels in patients with heart failure. It has many effects on the immune system, increasing T-cell activity, promoting natural killer-cell function, protecting against the side effects of radiation therapy, and reducing inflammation in autoimmune states. Like other medicinal mushrooms, cordyceps has shown apoptotic (cell death) effects in cancer-cell lines including leukemia and colon and liver cancer. A typical adaptogenic dose to help with cortisol control is 400 milligrams of the hot-water extract standardized to contain 8 percent cordycepic acid and 0.25 percent adenosine, taken twice daily.

Licorice

Another approach to controlling cortisol production is the use of licorice extracts (carbenoxolone) to inhibit the conversion of cortisone to cortisol by adipocytes. These extracts can block the 11-beta-HSD1 enzymes needed to convert inactive cortisone to cortisol in fat cells. It is possible that using small amounts of licorice-root extracts (not Red Vines or other licorice candies) can slow down the production of cortisol.

One other effect of licorice is mimicking the physiologic effects of aldosterone to raise blood pressure. This can be most helpful in people who are fatigued and have low blood pressure but can be a problem in hypertensives. Careful monitoring and change in dose as needed can be required with the use of licorice extracts. Licorice can

---

Typical Adaptogen Dosages

- Siberian ginseng 200 mg containing 0.8 percent eleutherosides E and B
- Panax ginseng 200 to 400 mg with 8 percent ginsenosides
- Ashwagandha 200 mg containing 5 percent withanolides
- *Rhodiola rosea* 200 mg containing at least 1 percent salidrosides
- *Ginkgo biloba* 120 mg with 24 percent ginkgo flavonglycosides
- Cordyceps 400 mg of hot-water extract containing 8 percent cordycepic acid and 0.25 percent adenosine, taken twice daily
- Licorice 300-600 mg with 25 percent glycyrrhizic acid

---

be used in a daily dose of 300–600 milligrams with 25 percent glycyrrhizic acid if there are no concerns regarding high blood pressure.

Nutrient Adaptogens

I'm using the term "nutrient adaptogens" to describe vitamins, minerals, fatty acids, and sterols that have been shown to improve allostasis and the body's response to stress. Before the availability in my practice of many of the botanicals listed above, I relied on vitamins such as pantothenic acid (B5) and vitamin C to modify cortisol function. Following are the most useful of these nutritional adaptogens.

Most of the research on vitamin C has been to evaluate the antioxidant, immune-enhancing, and tissue-repairing properties of this critical vitamin. However, it also has a strong effect on cortisol production. I have found in my practice that high-dose vitamin C mimics the effect of cortisol, reducing inflammation and allergies and thereby reducing the need for cortisol production. For example, in marathon runners who took 1,500 milligrams of vitamin C a day for one week before a race, significantly lower post-race cortisol levels were found than those given 500 milligrams or a placebo.

A study by Brody and colleagues (2002) on the effect of vitamin C on cortisol levels from elevated psychological stress (Trier Social Stress Test, which measures the response to mental arithmetic and mock job interviews) demonstrated lower subjective stress levels, cortisol levels, and blood pressure in individuals who took 3,000 milligrams of vitamin C compared to placebo. The minimum dose of vitamin C needed for an adaptogenic response is 1,000 milligrams per day, preferably in the form of a buffered ascorbate, not ascorbic acid.

Another old standby in my practice is pantothenic acid, or vitamin B5. It is found in many foods, including eggs, yeast, red meat, poultry, and whole grains, yet despite its widespread availability, many of my patients respond to supplementation. Deficiency of B5 compromises adrenal function, whereas supplementing with B5 can downregulate hypersecretion of cortisol secondary to high-stress conditions. Fatigue and intolerance to stress can be a sign of B5 deficiency. A dose of 100 to 500 milligrams a day of vitamin B5 is recommended.

B vitamins have long been known to help with stress. The most research has been done on pyridoxine or vitamin B6. Deficiency of B6 leads to increased sympathetic nervous system outflow and even hypertension. Supplementing with B6 can reduce the levels of epinephrine as well as blunt the cortisol response. Deficiency of B6 also leads to reduced production of GABA and serotonin, neurotransmitters that reduce anxiety and depression.

In a study of bereavement-induced psychological stress, low B6 levels worsened the maladapted state. Twenty-five years ago, pyridoxine was called the "anti-stress factor," because it was shown to prevent increased tissue sensitivity to cortisol. It appears that B6 decreases glucocorticoid-mediated protein induction, downregulating the tissue response to cortisol, while severe pyridoxine deficiency strongly upregulates the cellular response to cortisol.

Supplementing with high-dose B6 (up to 200 milligrams per day under a physician's direction only) could be required to see a marked reduction in stress-hormone responsiveness. The active form of B6, pyridoxal-5-phosphate, is now available, and doses of 50–100 milligrams daily might be enough to achieve the same effect. It is thought that B6 affects depression and stress reactions through diminishing sympathetic nervous system overactivity and decreasing cortisol production evoked by stress.

A word of caution on the use of high-dose B vitamins is warranted. They should be used under the supervision of an experienced physician, because high-dose B6 has been associated with peripheral nerve problems when used without other B vitamins. I always have patients use 1,000 micrograms of B12 as well as 1 milligram of folic acid and a well-balanced B complex when taking B6 above 50 milligrams a day. B12 and folic acid have their own adaptogenic effects and should be part of a well-rounded nutritional approach to maladaptation.

Adaptogenic Nutrients

- Vitamin B6 up to 200 mg per day (only under supervision by a physician at this dose) or P-5P at 50-100 mg per day

- Vitamin B5 (pantothenic acid) 100-500 mg per day

- Vitamin B complex 50 mg per day

- Vitamin B12 1,000 mcg per day in a sublingual tablet

- Vitamin C 1,000 mg per day

- Phosphatidylserine 200-300 mg per day

- Multivitamin/multimineral supplement (preferably from a reputable vitamin company) that has more than the RDA minimums

8

The Curious Cases of Gluten and Candida

Beginning to cultivate wheat and other grains was a watershed moment in human evolution, providing a stable and nutritious food source and moving our early ancestors from hunter-gatherers to a society able to develop cities and commerce. Wheat is believed to have originated in southwestern Asia; some of the earliest remains of the crop have been found in Syria, Jordan, and Turkey. Primitive relatives of present-day wheat have been discovered in excavations in eastern Iraq dating back nine thousand years. Other archaeological findings show that wheat was grown in the Nile valley about 5000 BC, as well as in India, China, and even England at about the same time. Despite this illustrious history, wheat and other grains are a common trigger of maladaptation and allostatic load, linked to conditions such as celiac disease, osteoporosis, headaches, joint pain, and digestive inflammation.

When I was growing up in New York, one of my family jobs was to go to the neighborhood bakery to buy a loaf of freshly baked rye bread before dinner. By the time I got home, I had consumed four or five slices, cutting into my appetite, much to the chagrin of my mother. That same degree of craving is not uncommon in my adult patients, as wheat is one of the most addictive of all foods. Wheat uniquely contains exorphins, a substance similar to endorphins, the pain-relieving and mood-elevating chemicals made by the brain. After digestion of a slice of bread or serving of pasta, the exorphins from wheat go to the same brain receptors as endorphins, explaining the addictive nature of this food.

It doesn't make much sense that a food that was integral to human evolution has caused so many people health problems. However, like many things in life, too much of a good thing has become a problem for some people. Sensitivity to gluten (the protein in wheat) is widespread in the United States, especially in people of northern European extraction (Scandinavian, English, Irish, and German).

Gluten is found in wheat, barley, rye, malt, triticale, spelt, and kamut. It is found in the greatest amount in wheat and rye. There is some controversy about whether the protein in oats triggers the same response as glutens, because it is a different branch of the grass family of foods (more information on food families is found in Appendix D) and contains avenin protein, not gluten protein. However, some of the oats commercially available can be contaminated with wheat and other grains and generally should be avoided. If pure oats can be obtained, 98 percent of celiac patients can use them without triggering inflammation. Hidden sources of gluten include many processed foods such as cold cuts and deli meats, frozen vegetables, soups, salad dressings, and soy sauce. Gluten is composed of gliadin and glutenin proteins.

Individuals vary in their response to gluten proteins. On one end of the continuum is simple gluten intolerance (also called non-celiac gluten intolerance) with symptoms of fatigue, headaches, digestive bloating, flatulence, diarrhea, weight gain, skin problems, depression, and joint or muscle pain. It is estimated that one in ten Americans could have gluten intolerance or wheat allergy. On the other end of the continuum is the more serious celiac disease, a less common problem with an incidence of 1 in every 133 Americans. The University of Chicago Celiac Disease Center estimates that 1 percent of healthy Americans could have celiac disease, affecting three million people, 97 percent of whom are undiagnosed.

Incidence of Gluten Intolerance and Celiac Disease

- 1 in 133 asymptomatic healthy Americans have celiac disease
- 1 in 22 have a family member with celiac disease
- 1 in 30 adults with digestive complaints have celiac disease
- 1 in 8 people of northern European heritage have celiac disease
- 30 million Americans have gluten sensitivity
- 3 million Americans have been diagnosed with celiac disease
- 19 out of 20 cases go undetected

In celiac disease, gluten protein causes the destruction of the intestinal villi (fingerlike protrusions that provide most of the surface area for nutrient absorption) in the small intestine from exposure to the gluten protein in grains. It takes less than 1 gram per day of gliadin (less than 2 percent of an ounce) to cause an inflammatory response. This leads to malabsorption, weight loss, and severe fatigue and is associated with osteoporosis, autoimmunity, arthritis, and other systemic problems. One quarter of patients with celiac disease have a chronic skin condition known as dermatitis herpetiformis, which can involve intense itching and blisters. Other conditions seen in celiac disease are listed below.

The diagnosis of celiac disease is best made through an intestinal biopsy that demonstrates changes in the wall of the intestine, including inflammation and atrophy. The only treatment for celiac disease is lifelong avoidance of all gluten sources. It can be lifesaving to make this diagnosis. Non-celiac gluten intolerance does not involve any organ damage.

A minority of patients with celiac disease will have obvious symptoms: weight loss, diarrhea, cramping, and appearing ill. The more common presentation involves symptoms outside the gastrointestinal tract: neurological, endocrine, psychiatric, and

Conditions Associated with Celiac Disease

- Diabetes
- Obesity
- Depression
- Neuropathy
- Osteoporosis
- Thyroid disease
- Sjögren's syndrome
- Rheumatoid arthritis
- Autoimmune liver disease

rheumatologic. Malabsorption can lead to deficiencies in fat-soluble vitamins, including vitamin A needed for vision, skin, and reproductive function; vitamin D needed for bones, prevention of breast, ovarian, and prostate cancer, and normal immune function; vitamin E needed for heart health, antioxidant function, and detoxification; and vitamin K needed for blood clotting and strong bones. In addition, minerals such as calcium and iron can be deficient in celiac disease. This can lead to osteoporosis and anemia.

Fatigue and depression are common problems in both celiac disease and non-celiac gluten intolerance. Fatigue can be caused by a combination of malabsorption of nutrients, especially B vitamins, inflammation in the gut, iron deficiency, and anemia and autoimmunity affecting thyroid function. Depression is most likely a result of deficiency of fatty acids, such as EPA/DHA, which are needed for brain function, and lack of B12 and other B vitamins. Many times I have seen patients with gluten problems who were treated with antidepressants when they simply needed to change their diets.

Symptoms found with gluten intolerance are also often mistakenly attributed to other conditions. In addition to depression and

---

Nutrient Malabsorption in Celiac Disease

- Essential fatty acids, omega-3 and omega-6
- Iron, zinc, calcium, and magnesium
- Selenium
- Water-soluble vitamins: B1, B6, B12, folic acid
- Fat-soluble vitamins: A, D, E, K

---

fatigue, obesity, food cravings, diarrhea, constipation, lethargy and lack of interest in life, poor concentration, back pain, muscle cramps, and joint pain are commonly seen. It is not hard to imagine each of these complaints being treated with medications rather than identifying their underlying cause. Even in my practice, I have been fooled several times into thinking gluten intolerance was not the trigger for certain symptoms (see below). However, by keeping an open mind regarding the varied presentations of gluten problems, eventually a diagnosis can be made. It has been estimated that on average it can take as long as nine years between the onset of symptoms and proper diagnosis of celiac disease or gluten intolerance.

I have also found that in wheat allergy even without gluten intolerance, depression, fatigue, and anxiety are common symptoms. Many times while skin testing patients for food allergies with the provocative-neutralization technique, I have seen mood changes and problems with concentration, which resolve once this food is removed from the diet. The most common food that contributes to depression and cognitive issues is wheat. Avoidance and challenge as described in Chapter 4 is the best method to confirm a wheat allergy if appropriate skin testing is not available.

Diagnosis of these conditions can be difficult. Genetic markers found on cell surfaces through blood tests (HLA-DQ2 and HLA-DQ8) can be useful but often are not conclusive. Blood antibody tests for celiac disease (antigliadin antibodies, including IgA

Common Symptoms of Gluten Intolerance

- Abdominal cramps, bloating, gas
- Diarrhea or constipation
- Poor concentration, brain fog
- Irritability and unpredictable moods
- Weight gain, obesity
- Long-standing fatigue
- Food craving, especially for starches and sweets
- Depression
- Lethargy, lack of interest and motivation
- Joint pain, muscle cramps, muscle pain, back or neck pain
- Unexplained elevation of liver enzymes on blood tests

endomysial antibodies, IgA tissue transglutaminase antibodies, and IgG tissue transglutaminase antibodies) are positive only in celiac disease and are often negative in gluten intolerance. Salivary IgA antigliadin antibodies can be a good screen but still present false negatives and false positives. The best way to identify gluten intolerance is avoidance of these foods for several months. If gluten is a significant trigger for allostatic load, many symptoms will improve within three months, though some problems might take as long as six months to resolve. If you are concerned that celiac disease is present, you should consult a gastroenterologist immediately for biopsy of the small intestine, a test that is more accurate while still ingesting gluten foods.

European physicians are much more aware of the problems that gluten can trigger than most physicians in the United States. We were on vacation in Ireland several years ago, and I was amazed to find that at a restaurant run by the national park service in

Killarney Lakes National Park, there was a gluten-free section in the cafeteria. The Irish are particularly susceptible to this problem and have made great strides in making gluten-free foods available. Fortunately, gluten-free grains and foods have recently become much more available in the United States.

Wheat allergy and gluten intolerance (also called idiopathic gluten sensitivity) are different, though overlapping, conditions. Strictly speaking, wheat allergy is a reaction to one of several storage proteins in wheat and is not the same as gluten intolerance. Skin testing or blood-antibody tests can identify wheat allergy, with different testing needed for gluten intolerance. Even in cases without the intestinal pathology of celiac disease (also called non-tropical sprue), gluten intolerance causes some inflammation in the gut wall, while food allergy to wheat might not involve the digestive tract. This is a confusing area for my patients who had negative skin tests to wheat but still benefit greatly from gluten avoidance. Whether gluten intolerant, wheat allergic, or suffering from celiac disease, the result of eating wheat and other gluten grains is a dramatic increase in cortisol production to counteract the inflammatory changes induced by these conditions. To regain adaptation, it is critical to identify these problems and make the appropriate dietary changes to reduce cortisol and allostatic load.

Wheat-Less/Weigh-Less Diet

In the early 1990s I started an experiment to see if my patients could lose weight simply by eliminating gluten-containing foods. They stopped eating all breads, muffins, baked goods, and pizza as well as cereals with wheat, rye, barley, and oats but did not cut their caloric content in other ways. We devised recipes for nongluten grains, though there were few good alternatives available then as compared to now. (When looking to see if a food is wheat free, remember that wheat can be listed as durum, enriched, wheat germ, bulgur, couscous, triticale, orzo, or semolina.)

Gluten-Containing Foods: A Short List

- Beverages: coffee substitutes, malted drinks, beer, ale
- Baked goods: whole wheat, graham crackers, pretzels, rolls, muffins, doughnuts, sweet rolls, pancakes, waffles, crackers, prepared bake mixes, ice cream cones, pies, pastries
- Pastas: spaghetti, noodles, macaroni, dumplings (unless gluten free)
- Cereals: wheat, barley, rye, some oats, kamut, spelt
- Animal protein: possible in deli meats, packaged cold cuts, frankfurters, chili con carne, croquettes, fish or meat patties and loaves, any breaded meat
- Thick liquids, condiments, and sauces: malt products, soups, chowders, soy sauce, bisques thickened with wheat, puddings, cheese spreads

---

Almost every patient lost weight effortlessly if they stayed on strict gluten avoidance. They also noted improved energy, less muscle and joint pain, fewer headaches, better digestive function, and, most surprisingly, better moods and less anxiety. They reduced markers of inflammation and allostatic load and maladaptation. Many of them brought their cortisol levels back to an adapted state.

Alternatives to gluten are widely available. Though gluten is the material that causes grain to be sticky, yielding breads and baked products that are so satisfying, the new gluten-free products such as brown rice pastas can be quite good. Products made from rice, millet, buckwheat, amaranth, quinoa, potato, tapioca, and arrowroot provide a rich alternative to wheat and other gluten grains. For example, tapioca bagels are available through several internet sources. Grain-free starches that are excellent sources of fiber and nutrients include yams, sweet potatoes, parsnips, winter squash, and other root vegetables.

Even if good alternatives to gluten exist, it is still wise to remember that refined grains should not be a large part of the diet. Eating refined grains, including oats and wheat, early in the day will increase caloric intake of other foods. In a study of obese children at Children's Hospital in Boston, Ludwig and colleagues (1999) found that after a meal of instant oatmeal as compared to a vegetable omelet and fruit, children consumed 81 percent more calories throughout the day. In a study of overweight adults performed in Italy by Vicennati (2002), a high-carbohydrate meal activated the HPA axis and cortisol production to a much greater degree than a high-protein meal.

Combining gluten avoidance with the other aspects of the Adaptation Diet, including limiting total grain intake, especially refined grains, makes weight loss even easier. For those people who are gluten intolerant, it is essential that these foods be removed from the diet to ensure reduction in stress and allostatic load. For anyone who wants to shed pounds and improve their tolerance for stress, a time-out for wheat and baked goods will pay off. At least three months is needed to have the desired effects. If gluten is not a major issue, it can be reintroduced at that time using a rotation diet. (See Appendix E for gluten-free recipes.)

Some Alternatives to Gluten

- Baked goods: breads made from rice, oats, soybean, tapioca, garbanzo beans, corn, buckwheat

- Cereals: oatmeal, oats, buckwheat (check label, as many buckwheat products contain wheat), millet, amaranth, corn, rice, cream of rice, quinoa flakes

- Sauces and deserts: meringues, rice pudding, tapioca pudding, gelatin, all fruits

The Candida Connection

One of the most powerful regulators of adaptation is a healthy intestinal tract. Since the early 1980s when William Crook identified a common syndrome of yeast overgrowth in the digestive tract and the resulting increased inflammation, food allergies, and poor well-being, a controversy has raged about a lowly inhabitant of the gut, a yeastlike organism, *Candida albicans*. Despite tremendous resistance from traditional medicine in recognizing this problem, my patients have benefited to an enormous degree from treating candida overgrowth syndrome. Let me explain why this is so controversial.

Within the first year of life, essentially all human digestive tracts are colonized with *Candida albicans*. Unlike beneficial inhabitants of the gut such as lactobacillus and bifidobacter, candida provides no benefit to the host. Because it is found in everyone, academic medicine has scoffed at the idea that it contributes to any problems other than yeast vaginitis in women, penile rashes in men, and thrush in the mouth. It is known to be a problem in the colonization of internal organs in immunosuppressed patients with AIDS or patients on medications that suppress the immune response. Except in those extreme circumstances, candida is not found in body cavities except in the digestive tract and the vaginal area in women.

However, even in patients who are not severely ill, candida can contribute to allostatic load. The digestive tract has the ability to be tolerant to candida if it is found in small amounts or if the immune system in the gut is operating in a normal fashion. Unfortunately, through the use of medications and poor diet, tolerance to candida can be lost. This frequently occurs from the excessive use of antibiotics for infections, acne, or other reasons. These medications reduce the amount of beneficial bacteria in the gut that produce lactic acid, which controls the proliferation of candida and other unwanted inhabitants of the gastrointestinal tract. Candida then overgrows, adhering to the wall in the large intestine, creating an excessive immune response to this fungal organism, sensitizing the body to other allergens.

Overgrowth of candida can even result from ingestion of the antibiotics found in meats and poultry. Any use of prescription cortisone (Prednisone), some birth control pills, or, most importantly, diets with excessive sweets and other simple carbohydrates help candida prosper. Candida in the gut, like nutritional yeast in bread or wine, thrives in a high-sugar environment. White flour products, including breads and other baked goods, processed sugars of any type, and even the natural sugars found in fruit juice or dried fruit can lead to more growth. Alcohol is an especially important trigger for yeast growth.

Candida is a constant irritant to the immune system, causing increased production of inflammatory cytokines, leading to bowel symptoms of bloating and gas, fatigue, aches and pains, and other markers of allostatic load. It appears to upregulate the immune system so that there are greater sensitivities to molds, foods, and chemical substances. In addition, there is an increase in food allergy problems and worsening of the leaky-gut syndrome. In some women there will be an increased frequency of yeast vaginitis.

Testing for candida overgrowth is not straightforward, because there is always some growth in the gut, and a normal immune system should react to candida skin testing. In my practice I use a quantitative stool culture to assess excess colonization. I skin test patients and look for a heightened skin wheal response. However, often the most useful diagnostic information is a history of antibiotic use leading to symptoms of yeast overgrowth. As in many other aspects of medicine, the ultimate diagnosis of candida overgrowth is the response to treatment.

Symptoms of candida overgrowth include fatigue, stamina problems, frequent infections, mood swings, allergies, and poor stress tolerance. I have listed below the key signs and symptoms for this problem.

Signs and Symptoms of Candida Overgrowth

- Bloating of the abdomen, flatulence, poor digestive function
- Fatigue and stamina issues
- Mood swings, depression, irritability
- PMS, menstrual irregularity
- Recurrent yeast vaginitis, especially from use of antibiotics
- Frequent colds and flu
- Allergies to molds, foods
- Acute sense of smell and adverse reactions to chemicals such as paints, varnishes, car exhaust, gasoline, cleaning detergents
- Frequent or persistent antibiotic use
- Multiple pregnancies or high-dose birth control pills
- Use of steroid medications

Many times a vicious cycle of poor diet leading to more frequent infections and more prescriptions for antibiotics results in candida overgrowth. This then leads to more allergies, poor immune function, fatigue, and more infections. Another significant contributor to this cycle is elevated cortisol from other maladaptive causes. High cortisol and elevated blood sugar induce candida overgrowth. For example, it is well known that diabetics are much more prone to yeast infections and problems from candida. The consequence of overgrowth of candida is increased biochemical stress that then triggers even more cortisol production, and the cycle continues.

Though this seems like a dreadful situation, there are effective means to reduce candida overgrowth and bring tolerance back to the immune system. The first step is dietary. I have used the anti-yeast diet (see Appendix F) in my practice for the past twenty-five years to reduce the stimulus for candida overgrowth. It is essentially the Adaptation Diet with a few minor changes. Simple carbohydrates, alcohol, and concentrated fruit sugars are the most important foods to avoid. Yeast growth is directly stimulated by these foods. The second concern is the total amount of carbohydrate consumed. I instruct my patients to avoid all gluten grains, starchy vegetables like white potatoes, and fruit juice, and to reduce their overall intake of fruits for the first two months.

The third group of foods to avoid are those that contain molds and yeast. The concern with these foods is a cross-sensitivity to food molds as well as to the candida overgrowth in the gut. Foods in this group include any hard cheese, aged cheese like blue cheese, vinegar, mushrooms, dried fruit, fruits such as melons, and the skins of peaches and apricots. Yeast-containing foods such as bread and baked goods are to be strictly eliminated. Following the guidelines of the Adaptation Diet and making these few additional changes will help to control the yeast overgrowth. Usually three months on an anti-yeast diet will make a big difference in allostatic load.

In addition to diet, good self-care is critical in managing candida overgrowth. Exercise, rest, and managing stress effectively will assist the immune system in increasing tolerance. Most important is the avoidance of antibiotics whenever possible. For most viral respiratory infections, antibiotics are not needed, though they are often prescribed. As an alternative, if there are no signs of a bacterial infection, botanical therapies could be employed, including high-dose vitamin C, echinacea, astragalus, maitake extracts, and lactoferrin, as well as a variety of homeopathic compounds.

Probiotic therapy is very important in controlling yeast overgrowth, including high-potency lactobacillus and bifidobacter combinations. Specific botanical therapies are also useful, including plant tannins, uva ursi, gentian, caprylic acid, oregano oil, berberine, colloidal silver, and undecylenic acid. In some cases antifungal medications such as Nystatin, Diflucan, or Sporanox are needed. All these therapies have to be used under the direction of an experienced health care provider.

Highlights of the Anti-Yeast Diet

- The Adaptation Diet is the core diet.
- Focus on vegetables, proteins, legumes.
- Avoid all simple sugars, including cane sugar, corn sweeteners, honey, molasses, fructose, and milk sugar in milk products.
- No alcohol.
- Condiments like ketchup and mustard have sugar added and should be avoided.
- Avoid malt in cereals and other foods.
- Processed and canned foods often contain sugar products.
- Avoid all gluten grains (wheat, rye, barley); use only whole nongluten grains.
- Reduce the overall carbohydrate load.
- Avoid breads and all yeast-containing foods.
- No aged or moldy foods, including brick and aged cheeses, vinegar, mushrooms, dried fruits, melons.
- Avoid leftovers if there is any chance of mold contamination.

Many of my patients have experienced profound improvements in their health after reducing candida overgrowth. Roberta, a mother of three children, was thirty-seven years old when she consulted me for a long list of problems, including fatigue, digestive bloating, muscle and joint pains, and, most bothersome to her family, mood swings and severe premenstrual syndrome (PMS). She had allergies as a child and had received many courses of antibiotics for respiratory infections.

Roberta suffered from frequent yeast vaginitis, often after taking antibiotics for her recurrent respiratory infections. In addition, her allergies were returning after a hiatus of fifteen years, and she became sensitive to perfumes and cleaning materials. In addition to fatigue, she had problems with her memory and mental focus.

Roberta had intense cravings for sweets, breads, and other starches. Her candida testing revealed a very high level of growth in her digestive tract. I prescribed the anti-yeast diet (see Appendix F), antifungal medications, probiotics, and antifungal botanicals.

Within a month Roberta was a new person. Although she struggled to stop eating desserts and breads, her bloating and aches and pains diminished. Her energy returned and even the PMS was greatly reduced. What amazed her the most was her mental clarity. Roberta felt she had emerged from a fog. As she was able to control her sugar cravings and maintained the anti-yeast diet over the next three months, Roberta's allergies greatly improved as well.

Though the diet needed to suppress candida overgrowth is restrictive, there are still many options, even on a restaurant menu. Order carefully, skip the cocktail and wine and the breads and desserts, and the rest is relatively easy. Order entrées without sauces, grilled, broiled, or baked; and eat all the salads (skip the dressing) and vegetables you want. This diet is similar to the detoxification phase of the Adaptation Diet. For some of my patients, reducing yeast overgrowth was the most significant way to reduce their allostatic load and regain adaptation. If there is suspicion of candida overgrowth and it does not resolve from careful dietary management, consult with a physician familiar with this problem to determine what else should be done.

9

Beyond Adaptation

The Promise of Epigenetics

Can we influence our biological destiny? Our ultimate adaptation would be the ability to alter the genetic expression that determines the function of every cell and organ. It now appears that many of the choices we make in terms of diet and lifestyle actually do change how genetic information is expressed and passed from one generation of cells to the next. Research in epigenetics, the science that explores how genes are expressed, has shown how genetic control of essentially every cell in the body is influenced by diet and environment. One example of the adaptive power of diet is found in cells that have become abnormal, such as cancerous cells, which can be returned to a normal state through the influence on the epigenome of a group of powerful phytonutrients described by researchers as bioactive foods.

Throughout this book I have presented a program to protect health by improving adaptation and controlling cortisol levels through diet. Cortisol levels and all other biochemical functions are ultimately determined by the expression of genes. The next step in adaptation and healthy aging is to learn what controls gene expression in daily life and what we can do to impact it through changes in diet and exercise, while reducing toxic exposures from our environment.

Epigenetics refers to heritable (inherited) changes in gene expression, without changes in DNA sequence, that can be passed on through generations of cells in all organs. Unlike previous ideas about the fixed and unchangeable state of the genetic code that is carried in the DNA of every cell, epigenetics describes changes in the structure around the genes influenced by diet and environmental factors. This information, called epigenetic marks, can also potentially be passed from mother (and father) to child and even through several generations of offspring. Even cortisol levels in children can be altered through epigenetic mechanisms, as described in a 2012 study by Jiang and colleagues of pregnant women who were given high levels of the essential nutrient choline (found in eggs, fish, milk, red meat, and soy) during their pregnancy. The researchers found that genes that control cortisol levels in the offspring were downregulated through epigenetic marks from the use of choline during pregnancy. Possibly these epigenetic effects can lead to a less stressed and better adapted life in these children.

In addition, research has shown that not only diet, but also stress during adulthood, can alter epigenetic markers. For example, rats under restraint stress (an experimental procedure where an animal is stopped from moving, causing a strong stress response) demonstrate a rapid change in the proteins that surround the DNA (histones), leading to altered gene expression. Epigenetic alterations have been linked to obesity and diabetes, as well as cancer, cognitive dysfunction, and respiratory, cardiovascular, reproductive, autoimmune, and neurobehavioral conditions.

I observed the power of diet and the environment in shaping the expression of inheritance on a recent trip to Costa Rica. I had the pleasure of staying at a magnificent rain forest lodge in the Osa Peninsula of southwest Costa Rica. On our second day there we walked through the rain forest with the resident naturalist, Philip. As we approached an enormous mound of dirt, sticks, and mud, he pointed out that this was a colony of leaf-cutter ants. The colony consisted of millions of ants, each one of which had a specific job. There was the queen who literally created the colony, soldiers, leaf cutters, those who digested the leaf, those who moved the material to different parts of the nest, as well as many others. The differences in all these ants, which had common DNA and were part of what is called a superorganism, were their environment and diet as they developed. Differing temperatures inside the nest and differing food sources caused the ants to take on different job descriptions. They manifested who they were through the influence of their diet and environment on their genetics without any change to their underlying DNA, an example of the power of epigenetics.

In humans, the link between diet, environment, and epigenetics was first noted by Heijmans and colleagues (2008) when it was found that pregnant women in the Netherlands who were living under starvation conditions during World War II gave birth to relatively small babies, not unexpected considering their limited diet while pregnant. Surprisingly, when the Dutch mothers' female children who lived in relative prosperity with decent diets in terms of calories and macronutrients got pregnant, their children were unexpectedly small. The researchers felt that the effect of poor nutrition during World War II was carried through to the grandchildren of the Dutch mothers.

The explanation for this transgenerational transmission lies in the alteration of epigenetic markers on the DNA from a deficiency of key nutrients in the grandmothers. It is thought that lack of methylation (transferring a methyl group onto part of a gene), stemming from inadequate levels of methyl donors (choline, methionine, betaine, folic acid, B12) and zinc, altered gene expression and was passed on through the generations. The process of methylation switches off or represses genes, and prevents them from transcribing certain proteins that control cell function, which has wide-ranging effects on health and disease. The surprising part of this story is that changes in the grandmothers' epigenome were passed on through at least three generations without any changes in the underlying DNA.

In prenatal exposures, several studies, including one by Perera and Herbstman (2011), point to significant effects of not only diet but many different pollutants in altering epigenetic programming and disease risk through several generations. These toxicants include arsenic, tobacco smoke, air pollutants, and endocrine-disrupting chemicals. In 2005, Anway and colleagues reported that a brief exposure of pregnant rats to an insecticide (methoxychlor) and a fungicide (vinclozolin) resulted in changes in DNA methylation of two genes in male pups, causing decreased sperm counts and infertility. More alarmingly, these adverse effects lasted through four generations of male rats without any additional exposure, implying the epigenetic markers continued through several generations.

Epigenetic changes can occur throughout the life cycle; however, the most vulnerable time is in utero and during early childhood. For example, low birth weight from maternal malnutrition is associated with abdominal obesity in adult men and increased risk of cardiovascular disease, osteoporosis, type 2 diabetes, depressive disorders, and even certain cancers. The epigenetic adaptive response in the fetus to reduced calories persisted throughout life, leading to obesity from these epigenetic changes and increased disease risk.

In an important study that directly relates to adaptation and cortisol levels, Bagot and Meaney (2010) found that newborns of mothers who had symptoms of depression during pregnancy had increased methylation of the glucocorticoid receptor gene in umbilical cord blood cells, and at three months of age the infants had elevated salivary cortisol concentrations. This epigenetic remodeling in response to maternal environmental events appears to increase the risk for cortisol-related emotional problems early in childhood and later in life.

Dietary choices can have an enormous influence not only through the generations, as seen in the Dutch mothers, but on a person's health as they age. The research at this time points to key phytonutrients in the diet as having a major influence on epigenetic marks, leading to resistance to cancer, diabetes, and other chronic disease. These include sulforaphane from broccoli, genistein from soy, curcumin found in turmeric, and EGCG from green tea. In addition, green leafy vegetables and other sources of folic acid are essential for normal epigenetic function.

Dietary intake of these bioactive foods can go a long way toward improving adaptation and preventing cancer, heart disease, and premature aging. All these foods have been discussed earlier in the book in regards to antioxidant effects and improved cortisol management. Epigenetic research has taken this a step further and identified how these foods can literally change who we are on a cellular level. In addition to including bioactive foods in the diet to protect the epigenome, individuals should make every effort to reduce exposure to toxic chemicals and heavy metals by using only organic meats, dairy, and vegetables, avoiding farm-raised salmon, and giving up the plastic water bottles and food storage containers that contain chemicals like bisphenol A that alter the epigenome in significant ways.

The Science of Epigenetics

Genotype and phenotype are the scientific terms that describe how inherited genetic material determines a person's unique characteristics. The genotype is the inherited material coded in the DNA of genes, fixed and unchangeable. Genes code for many specific attributes like eye color and height. The phenotype is the manifestation of this inherited code, like having blue eyes and being six feet tall. However, over the past twenty years as the Human Genome Project unraveled the genetic basis of life, the field of epigenetics, researching how gene expression occurs, has become increasingly important.

In a 2008 article written by Andrew Feinberg, MD, director of the Center for Epigenetics, Johns Hopkins University School of Medicine, the importance of epigenetics was reflected in the title: "Epigenetics at the Epicenter of Modern Medicine." In fact, more than sixteen thousand scientific articles on epigenetics are published each year in medical journals. A major part of the focus of epigenetic research is on the effect food and the environment have on the health of the epigenome.

According to Feinberg, epigenetics is defined as modifications of the DNA or associated proteins in the cell nucleus other than DNA sequence variation that carry information content during cell division. Epigenetics is further defined as a heritable modification to the DNA that regulates chromosome architecture and modulates gene expression without changes in the underlying base pair sequence, ultimately determining phenotype from genotype. The way each cell and organism determines its path through life, leading to health or disease, is not only encoded in the genome and DNA but also in the epigenome, which defines whether a gene will be active or silent. Epigenetic phenomena, unlike the gene sequence, are a changing and dynamic system that ultimately can be impacted by personal choices.

For example, disordered gene expression that controls cell proliferation and differentiation can lead to a cell becoming cancerous. Gene expression is greatly influenced by epigenetic factors, with genes that protect the cell against cancerous changes (tumor suppressor genes) turned on or off based on diet and toxin exposures. Genes that regulate normal cell growth can also be influenced by diet. Through nutritional modification, disordered gene expression can potentially be reversed, moving an abnormal cell back toward a normal state of function. Though epigenetic phenomena are inherited from one generation of cells to the next, they can be modified at any time through the use of bioactive foods that alter the epigenome.

Compared to normal cells, the abnormal patterns of DNA methylation and histone modification in cancer cells are more easily influenced by bioactive foods. Normal cells are less affected by dietary intake of these potent and therapeutic foods. As cells first mutate, it appears that their vulnerability to these foods is greatest, preventing cancers and other chronic degenerative disease from taking hold. However, over time, with poor diet and inadequate self-care, these life-changing diseases can advance, leaving little that diet and the bioactive foods can change.

Every human cell has a nucleus that contains forty-six chromosomes. All the instructions needed to direct cellular activity reside in the DNA on the chromosomes. DNA for all living organisms is made of the same chemical and physical components. The DNA sequence is arranged in double strands that wind around each other, called the double helix, and is composed of nucleotides that spell out the exact instructions to create each unique trait. The DNA sequence is the specific side-by-side arrangement of bases along the DNA strand (ATCCGGA, etc.). The genome is an organism's complete set of DNA.

Each chromosome contains many genes, made up of DNA base pairs, the functional unit of heredity. Genes are specific sequences of bases that encode instructions to make proteins (which are the basis of all cell functions), translated through messenger RNA. Genes constitute about 2 percent of the genome, with about thirty thousand genes containing 3.2 billion nucleotides. Other sections of the chromosome contain noncoding regions that provide structural integrity and regulate protein quantities.

The double-strand DNA is coiled around proteins called histones; this combination is called chromatin. Chromatin is tightly bundled to fit into the cell nucleus. Methylation is a critical part of the structure of chromatin and occurs when a methyl group (CH_3, one carbon and three hydrogen atoms) is attached to a specific part of the DNA, determining if the gene at these sites will be activated or repressed.

DNA methylation is typically associated with gene repression and silencing; if aberrant, it can lead to disease and aging. The source of the methyl group, methionine, is an essential amino acid that depends on adequate dietary levels of folic acid, B12, and other nutrients to function in the methylation pathway. DNA methylation essentially causes DNA to stick to the histones, effectively silencing the gene, which is especially important with cancer-causing oncogenes.

The configuration of the histones around certain genes also determines if the gene can be accessed and create proteins. Histones can be modified by a host of dietary and environmental factors as well. If the histones are condensed and tightly folded, they are essentially closing off access to the gene; if they are more open, then the gene can transcribe its protein. Histone proteins may be tagged with methyl or acetyl groups, which modify their behavior and influence the way genes are expressed. Bioactive foods and environmental toxins greatly influence histone configuration as well, generally leading to increased expression of genes by relaxing the condensed histones through acetylation.

Epigenetic markers are copied from one cell generation to the next and may alter gene expression in the daughter cells. This mechanism explains how dietary or toxic exposures can have consequences years or decades later even with no change to the DNA sequence. The plasticity of the epigenome and its responsiveness to dietary factors allow for improved adaptation and changes driven by self-directed dietary and lifestyle behaviors. To maintain the correct pattern of methylation through cell divisions, new methyl groups are placed on the newly copied DNA strands in the nucleus of cells, a process that requires the presence of methyl donors.

Though much of the research I discuss in this chapter relates to the prevention and treatment of cancer, this information is applicable in preventing obesity and many other chronic illnesses and improved adaptation throughout life. It appears that the interaction between genes and the environment plays a crucial role in resistance to stress and maintaining the ability to adapt effectively to life's challenges. Disruption of normal phenotypic plasticity is the unifying theme of epigenetic disease. This is the ultimate loss of adaptability, as the gene expression is unable to operate in a normal fashion. Loss of responsiveness to stress exacerbates the effects of underlying disease and can lead to more rapid aging and the onset of heart disease, cancer, diabetes, and dementias. This loss of responsiveness is caused in part by inadequate dietary factors, because DNA methylation depends on dietary methionine and folate.

The pattern of epigenetic marks is extremely complex, with some parts of some cells' genome needing methylation, with other areas needing no methylation. Multiple modifications in histones—from

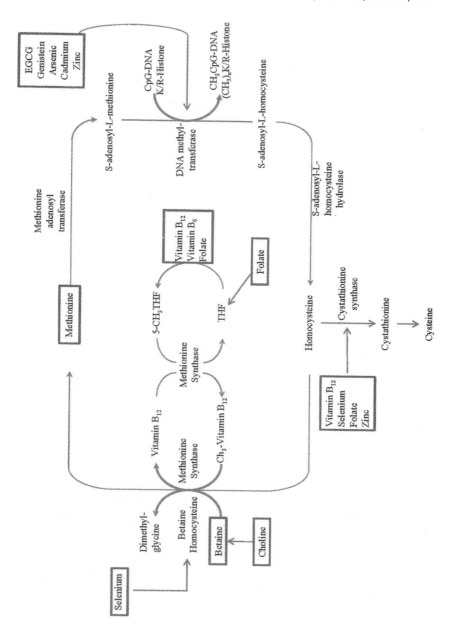

Figure 1: Nutritional and Toxic Influences on Epigenetic Methylation Pathways (from Su et al. *Frontiers in Genetics*. Jan 9, 2012)

chromosome to chromosome, cell to cell, organ to organ—present a mind-numbing number of variables. However, through all of these possibilities the wisdom of the body understands how to maintain healthy genomic and epigenomic function. It is only when an individual's diet is inappropriate, adaptation to stress is inadequate, or chemical exposure is too great, that it all goes awry.

Diet, Environment, and the Epigenome

A striking example of the effect of diet on genetic expression comes from the world of bees. Despite having the same genetics, honeybees grow up to be either workers or queen bees based on whether they are fed royal jelly or beebread as larvae. Studies of honeybees have shown that the key effect of the different foods is in methylation of the DNA, which controls the activity of multiple genes.

In humans, epigenetic effects also include methylation and histone modification, which impact gene expression and tremendously influence the risk for cancer, diabetes, obesity, heart disease, and neurodegenerative disorders, as well as affect the health and function of the brain and other vital organs. In situations where dietary deficiency or toxic exposures have led to global hypomethylation (too few methyl groups throughout the genome), there is a marked increase in cancerous cells. Hypomethylation often results from inadequate methylators in the diet, including folic acid, B12, betaine, and methionine, leading to excess activity of genes like oncogenes, increasing cancerous changes and abnormal cell function. On the other hand, triggers for hypermethylation, including toxins like arsenic and PCBs, alcohol, aging, or maternal protein deficiency, also increase risk for cancer and other diseases.

The Agouti gene in a strain of mice has been used to identify the impact of diet and toxins on epigenetic effects in pregnancy and their impact on future generations. These mice have multiple genes that control the color of the coat in the offspring. One of the genes, the Agouti gene, has several versions leading to different coats, ranging from brown to yellow. One version of the gene, called Avy, will express a yellow coat in the offspring if there is inadequate methylation. In addition to the mouse pup having a yellow coat, there is a greater risk for obesity, diabetes, and cancer and a shortened life span. If the Avy gene is switched off through adequate methylation, the mouse is brown or black in color and has fewer health problems.

Even though the DNA sequence of the Agouti gene does not change, the health and color of the mice are remarkably different based on how much methylation occurs at this gene location, providing researchers with a tremendous tool in assessing the impact of diet and toxins on the epigenome. What determines methylation in these animals and in general is primarily diet and environment. Diets rich in methylating nutrients, such as folic acid, betaine, choline, and B12, or with added genistein, a phytoestrogen from soy, will influence the color of the offspring dramatically, leading to more pure Agouti (brown) and healthier offspring.

On the other hand, exposure of a pregnant mouse to bisphenol A (BPA), an estrogen-like contaminant in food and water (used to make polycarbonate plastics found in water bottles, plastic containers, and tin cans), will increase the yellow coat frequency in the mouse's offspring. (Bisphenol A is one of several chemicals termed endocrine disruptors because of their hormone-like effect. It is found in great quantities in water, foods, and soils.)

Though no change occurs in the DNA sequence, the effect on the methylation status of the Agouti and other genes from exposure in utero to BPA (reduced methylation) can be found many generations later, showing that epigenetic changes can be heritable. However, in mice exposed to BPA and fed a diet supplemented with methyl donors, the damaging effect of BPA was greatly reduced.

Epigenetic effects not only occur in utero but continue throughout life. In a study of identical twins (identical genome and DNA), Esteller (2005) reported the underlying epigenetic reason why twins become less alike as they age. He evaluated forty pairs of identical twins ranging in age from three to seventy-four. The younger the twins, the more alike their DNA methylation and histone acetylation patterns appeared. Older twins, especially if they had differing diets and lifestyles, had much different patterns in several cell lines from a variety of organs, including white blood cells, fat cells, muscle cells, and epithelial (skin) cells.

He compared three-year-old twins and fifty-year-old twins and found four times as many differently expressed genes (including DNA hypomethylation and histone hyperacetylation, leading to overexpressed genes) in the fifty-year-old twins. Despite having identical DNA, the influence of their diet and environment changed the gene expression as they grew older and more dissimilar, supporting the notion that who we become is greatly determined by not just our genes, but by the epigenetic effects of diet and environment.

A study from King's College in London on twins (Bell et al. 2012) identified when epigenetic changes occur in genes that impact aging, cholesterol, and lung function. Looking at as many as 490 age-specific epigenetic changes, the researchers concluded that many epigenetic marks occur earlier in life (before age twenty-two) and continue to impact the aging process throughout life. Though these findings were significant, the researchers, recognizing the limitations in current technology that can look at only a small sample of epigenetic marks, emphasized the importance of more research into the effect of epigenetics on aging.

The first example of human disease with an epigenetic mechanism, colon cancer, was identified in 1983. By comparing normal cells to colon cancer cells from the same patient, the researchers identified hypomethylation in the cancer cells, associated with genetic instability and chromosomal rearrangements. Other cancer studies showed hypermethylation of tumor suppressor genes that prevented these genes—whose job it is to repair the early cellular changes that can lead to cancer (or cause the abnormal cells to self-destruct, called apoptosis, if repair is not possible)—from activating and transcribing proteins.

In addition to cancer, epigenetic changes are associated with aging in general, with progressive increases in DNA methylation and gene silencing noted in aging tissues, including the colon, stomach, liver, kidneys, bladder, and esophagus. There is evidence that heart disease and atherosclerosis are partially linked to hypermethylation. There are also some hints that psychiatric illness, including bipolar disorder and schizophrenia, has an epigenetic component. Disruption of epigenetic mechanisms can result in oxidative stress, obesity, insulin resistance, diabetes, and vascular dysfunction.

Though much of the current research on epigenetics is focused on dietary and toxic environmental triggers, behavioral patterns also play a role in how genes are expressed. Research by Szyf and colleagues (2004) found that in rats, healthy maternal behaviors such as grooming, licking, and nursing affected the amount of DNA methylation and histone acetylation in the genes associated with cortisol receptors in the pups' hippocampus, the area of the midbrain that controls cortisol levels and the stress response. The changes in behavior and epigenetic marks were heritable, with the nurtured pups nurturing their own offspring, leading to similar epigenetic changes in the next generation. These epigenetic heritable effects might explain the connection between early parenting and the way people deal with stress throughout their lives. Szyf (2012) described the epigenetic genomic adaptation mechanism (including methylation) as "the molecular links between nature and nurture," especially with changing social and physical environments in early life. Lifelong traits and adaptability to stress might be coded in these epigenetic changes that occur in early childhood.

Additional findings in human studies also point to an epigenetic component in psychological health. Gene expression has been shown to be altered in depressed and socially isolated subjects compared to normal individuals, while other studies have shown altered gene expression in highly stressed medical students before exams. In a study by Creswell and colleagues (2012), older individuals who were taught to meditate were found to be less lonely and to have downregulated the gene expression that controls inflammation. He looked at forty healthy but lonely adults and found that after eight weeks of a Mindfulness-Based Stress Reduction program and daily meditation at home, those who followed the meditation program, compared to controls, had lower levels of pro-inflammatory gene expression in their immune cells and lower levels of C-reactive protein, an important risk factor for heart disease. These findings are suggestive of the profound impact epigenetic changes have on adaptation and resistance to stress and how behavioral changes can influence epigenetic expression, change biochemistry, and protect against chronic disease.

Nutritional Epigenetics: Eating for Your Epigenome

As the science is beginning to show, it is possible to influence gene expression over a lifetime and affect your cortisol levels and the incidence of cancer, heart disease, obesity, diabetes, premature aging, and even your psychological state through proper nutrition. Many different nutrients have been found to impact the epigenome. These include nutrients involved in DNA methylation: folate, vitamin B12, vitamin B6, riboflavin, zinc, methionine, choline, and betaine, as well as bioactive food components such as resveratrol (grapes and red wine), curcumin (turmeric), sulforaphane (broccoli and other cruciferous vegetables), and tea polyphenols (green tea) that can modulate epigenetic patterns by altering the levels of S-adenosylmethionine and S-adenosylhomocysteine (the key methyl donors) or directing the enzymes that catalyze DNA methylation and histone modifications. Other bioactive food components that regulate the epigenome include genistein (soybean), silymarin (milk thistle), diallyl disulfide (garlic), lycopene (tomatoes), rosmarinic acid (rosemary), apigenin (celery, parsley), and gingerol (ginger). The bioactive food components isothiocyanates (cruciferous vegetables), resveratrol (grapes), and organosulfur compounds (garlic) affect histone proteins, leading to increased self-destruction of abnormal cells and a reduction in inflammation. (See Figure 1.)

As more is learned about epigenetics and risks for cancer, obesity, and other diseases, the more complicated it can seem. However, the majority of current studies lead to the conclusion that key nutrients and bioactive foods are powerful regulators of the epigenome. For example, sulforaphane from broccoli and curcumin from turmeric both modify histone acetylation, leading to de-repression (turning on) of tumor suppressor genes and apoptosis in cancer cells. In a study of patients with stomach cancer, Yuasa and colleagues (2009) found that intake of green tea and cruciferous vegetables has been linked to the methylation status of a key gene, reducing the incidence of this disease. These types of studies help us take the next step in understanding how deeply influential dietary habits are and that we truly become what we eat. Later in this chapter I will present greater detail on these epigenetic superstars.

There is evidence that in utero, levels of key nutrients such as folic acid can also affect the development of disease in the offspring in later life. In 2011, Sie and colleagues found that the offspring of mice given supplemental folic acid during pregnancy had a reduced risk of colon cancer as they aged. The effect might be from global DNA hypermethylation repressing (turning off) oncogenes that trigger colon cancer. In a very important study that might provide a way to protect against the epigenetic damage from environmental chemicals during pregnancy, Bernal and Jirtle found that genistein (from soy) intake during pregnancy reduced the effect of bisphenol A on methylation defects.

Looking after your epigenome doesn't have to be complicated. In addition to the foods mentioned, include in the diet the building blocks for methylation: get your folic acid from green leafy vegetables, peas, beans, sunflower seeds, and liver; get choline from eggs, beef, liver (organic only), peanuts, and cauliflower; increase methionine with tofu, Brazil nuts, spinach, garlic, fish, chicken, and beef; and get B12 from turkey, liver, shellfish, red meat, dairy, and fish. And don't forget a glass of red wine (no more than one per day for men and one-half for women) as a source of resveratrol, which can increase epigenomic protection.

The great nemesis of the American diet, excessive intake of simple carbohydrates, which leads to elevated blood sugar and insulin resistance, can also impact epigenetic mechanisms. It appears that histone methylation is affected by excess blood sugar, which induces vascular inflammation, increasing the risk for degenerative diseases. In addition, oxidized LDL cholesterol from unhealthy dietary fats (trans fats, excess omega-6 fats) alters the epigenome and leads to the activation of inflammation-related genes, while a maternal diet high in fat can lead to liver histone modifications affecting cholesterol metabolism. (The fetal origin of adult diseases, including obesity, diabetes, and cardiovascular disease, is an area of intense research at this time and all the answers are certainly not in.)

In addition to dietary choices, evidence is mounting that exposure to several environmental toxins can lead to hypermethylation and gene suppression, a major cancer risk. The culprits include bisphenol A, PCBs, arsenic and other heavy metals, and pesticide residues in foods. Protect yourself and your children by limiting the use of plastics for food storage, use only organically produced foods (especially animal protein, which can be highly contaminated with fat-soluble toxins), and filter your water. Improving your detoxification pathways (as described in Chapter 3) is vital.

Dietary exposures to toxins, as well as inadequate intake of key bioactive foods, can have health consequences years or decades later, even on future generations. Epigenetic memory is part of the mechanism by which dietary and environmental toxic exposures are "remembered." However, it is also becoming clear that the memory from these epigenetic marks can be altered through appropriate changes in dietary habits.

Key Concepts of Epigenetics

- Epigenetic changes can occur from dietary habits and environmental exposures to toxins.
- Unlike the genome, which is fixed, epigenetic changes can occur either in utero or during the life span.
- Epigenetic marks can be heritable through cell lines and be maintained over many generations of cells.
- Epigenetic marks can be passed down through several generations of individuals.
- Increased methylation of DNA sequence usually leads to repression of gene activity.
- Nutrients like folic acid and B12 contribute methyl groups to support methylation. If these key nutrients are inadequate in the diet, global hypomethylation can occur, leading to abnormal gene expression.
- Toxic chemicals can cause excess methylation, especially at tumor suppressor gene sites, turning off these genes.
- Bioactive foods, including genistein (soy), curcumin (turmeric), sulforaphane (broccoli), EGCG (green tea), and others, generally inhibit methylation and affect histone acetylation, turning on needed gene expression (such as tumor suppressor genes).
- Good dietary and lifestyle practices can have an enormous impact on the epigenome and determine the state of health.

Epigenetics and Obesity

The same epigenetic mechanisms that put us at greater risk for cancer and heart disease appear to increase the risk of weight gain and obesity. Researchers have been scouring the human genome to find the genetic connection to obesity. To date, there have been more than forty genetic variants associated with obesity. However, this explains only a small piece of the obesity epidemic, because over the time that there has been an explosion of worldwide obesity, there has been negligible change in the actual genetic sequence of the population. A larger factor might be the epigenetic marks influenced by diet and environmental toxicants, especially the endocrine-disrupting chemicals.

Heritability of obesity is found in 40 to 70 percent of individuals. This was determined through twin studies that measured body mass index, waist/hip ratios, and other obesity markers. In a 2011 study, Zhang and colleagues found that obese women tend to have obese children, with this outcome possibly modified by maternal weight loss during pregnancy. It is thought that epigenetic mechanisms in early development, heritable from the mother, determine much of the risk for obesity.

One epigenetic aspect found in obesity is the lack of methylating dietary factors in the maternal diet, leading to lifelong obesity in the offspring. This is a similar finding to the increased risks of cancer in the offspring of mothers with low folate in their diet. In 2007, Sinclair and colleagues reported on the effects of restricting folate and B12 in the diet of pregnant sheep. They found that the offspring of these sheep were heavier and fatter as adults as a result of epigenetic changes in methylation status from the maternal low-folate diet. The effects of exposure in utero to lack of methylating factors lasted throughout the life of the offspring. It is possible that one cause of the obesity epidemic is epigenetic programming as a fetus or early in life. To reduce this risk, it is prudent for prospective parents to consume folate-rich foods such as green leafy vegetables, eggs (a source of choline and methionine), tofu, and organic meats to possibly normalize epigenetic mechanisms and reduce the heritable patterns of obesity. As with cancer and other epigenetic-related diseases, histone modifications are also linked with obesity.

The silencing of the genes that control hormones like leptin (a hormone produced by fat cells that suppresses appetite by communicating energy reserve information to the central nervous system and other organs) is one of many potential links between epigenetics and obesity. It is felt that both maternal undernutrition (the children of the Dutch women who suffered a famine in 1944 had impaired glucose tolerance and insulin secretion in adulthood) and overnutrition, so common in the Western diet today, induce epigenetic changes leading to obesity in the offspring as adults. Ong and Muhlhausler (2011) have shown that perinatal exposure to high-fat and high-sugar diets resulted in permanent changes in the central reward system of the offspring, leading to increased preference for fat and overconsumption of calories, resulting in obesity. They studied rats and found that, after exposure to what they called a junk-food diet during pregnancy, the offspring ate excessive junk food throughout their lives.

Another aspect of the obesity epidemic is our exposure to obesogens, the same persistent organic pollutant chemicals that are putting us at greater risk for cancer and other maladies. BPA and other chemicals (persistent organic pollutants, POPs) found in fat cells can greatly impact the risk of diabetes and obesity. In fact, when comparing groups of obese patients, those with higher levels of POPs were more likely to develop diabetes even if they were less obese. Lang and colleagues (2008) found that higher BPA concentrations measured in urine were associated with both diabetes and cardiovascular disease.

Phthalates, another common plasticizer, have been linked to an increased incidence of abdominal obesity and diabetes, possibly through deregulation of metabolic pathways. A study of U.S. males (Stahlhut et al. 2007) showed that urine concentrations of four phthalate metabolites correlated with waist size and insulin resistance, a forerunner of diabetes. Other toxins linked to an increased risk of obesity and diabetes include PCBs and arsenic. It appears that the epigenetic mechanism of the POPs on weight gain is the same as it is for other conditions such as cancer: excess methylation of genes, leading to abnormal gene expression. The difference with obesity compared to cancer is the genes affected: those related to diabetes, abnormal metabolism, and obesity; or those involved with abnormal cell proliferation.

Only a small part of the puzzle connecting epigenetics and obesity has been solved, but it is clear that following the prescription to use bioactive foods, methyl donors, and a wide variety of plant-based nutrients would assist in protecting yourself and your offspring from the epidemic of obesity. Emphasizing green tea, broccoli, fermented soy, turmeric, and garlic, along with the information presented earlier in the book and the recipes in the appendixes, will further empower weight loss while reducing the risk for chronic disease. In addition, curcumin from turmeric has been shown to actually reduce the production of fat cells by inhibiting transformation of pre-adipocytes to adipocytes. The epigenetic model implies that the early years of life have greater plasticity to reverse abnormal epigenetic marks, leading to a reduction of obesity and chronic disease through dietary and environmental methods. The message is to make dietary changes as early as possible, ideally in pregnancy, to reduce the risk of obesity in a child.

Bioactive Foods

The science of epigenetics has clarified how dependent we are on the plant world to protect the very essence of life, the genome and epigenome. This interdependence has evolved over the millennium in conjunction with our environment and certainly should give us pause about how we care for the earth, because our health is entwined with the plant kingdom in many ways.

Much of the research presented in this section utilizes isolated phytonutrients from food, which in an experimental setting allows for an easier assessment of effect. However, it is much preferred and more practical to use the whole food source (drinking green tea rather than taking EGCG as a nutraceutical) as a means of preventing epigenetically driven illness. The research often focuses on reversing cell changes that have already occurred, such as in cancer cells, by employing isolated nutrients, such as sulforaphane from soybeans. Everyone should have as a goal to prevent these illnesses through the information we can glean from these studies. A quote from the most important text in Chinese medicine *(The Yellow Emperor's Classic of Internal Medicine)* summarizes brilliantly the difference between preventing a disease and treating it once it has occurred: "To fight a disease after it has occurred is like digging a well when one is thirsty, or forging a weapon once a war has begun."

Let's take a more in-depth look at some of the most potent bioactive foods that can protect the epigenome, improve adaptation, and reduce the risk of chronic disease.

Folate and B Vitamins

Folates are a group of water-soluble vitamins found primarily in green leafy vegetables. Folic acid plays a major role as a methyl (CH_3) source for the universal methyl donor S-adenosylmethionine, ultimately acting through the enzyme DNA methyltransferase (see Figure 1). Folate is involved in DNA synthesis, repair, and methylation, all of which maintain genomic stability. Folate deficiency can lead to global hypomethylation, leading to expression of many genes that should be silenced, increasing risk for colon, breast, ovarian, pancreatic, brain, lung, and cervical cancers. For example, Duthie (2011) reviewed the research on folate and colon cancer and found that the majority of human studies suggest that people who consume the highest levels of folate have significantly lower risk of developing colon polyps or cancer.

In addition, folic acid impacts many other aspects of health. It is needed to metabolize homocysteine to methionine, and for the synthesis of monoamine neurotransmitters, including dopamine and epinephrine, which affect mood and energy. Folic acid is needed for the synthesis of melatonin, which promotes restful sleep, and has antioxidant and anticancer properties; and folate is needed for the synthesis of red blood cells. It is critical that pregnant women supplement their diet with folate to prevent birth defects, including spina bifida. Inadequate intake of folic acid is commonly seen with the standard American diet that is woefully short on folate-rich dark green vegetables.

Excessive use of alcohol or medications, including antacids, aspirin, oral contraceptives, and antibiotics, can further deplete folic acid levels. It is not uncommon in the elderly to find lower folate levels and heightened homocysteine levels, leading to abnormal methylation and accelerated aging phenomena. Homocysteine is a metabolite of the amino acid methionine, the key methyl donor in epigenetic regulation. It gets metabolized to cysteine if there are adequate cofactors, including folic acid, B12, zinc, and selenium. If the metabolic conversion is inadequate from lack of folic acid or other factors, a range of health effects is possible, including increased risk of heart disease, strokes, blood clots, osteoporosis, and possibly dementia.

If supplementation with folic acid is needed because of poor diet, malabsorption, or the use of medications, there is reason to consider a novel form of folic acid: 5-methyltetrahydrofolate or 5-MTHF. Up to 30 percent of the U.S. population carries a mutation in the gene that is needed for the conversion of dietary folic acid to its active form, 5-MTHF. This mutation increases the risk of heart disease by 20 percent. The conversion takes several steps and if inadequate, combined with the typically low dietary intake of folic acid in most Americans, a person would be functionally low in folate activity, leading to higher risk for cancer through epigenetic mechanisms as well as increased risk of heart disease through poor metabolism of homocysteine.

Blood tests (5-MTHFR gene assay) are available to measure folate metabolism mutations. Two mutations can be identified: C677T and A1298C. If a person has two pairs of the C677T allele, then they are especially vulnerable to folate metabolism issues and should use the 5-MTHF form of folate. The A1298C mutation does not appear to be as problematic. In my practice, I routinely test for homocysteine, a risk factor for heart disease, stroke, blood clots, and osteoporosis. If homocysteine levels are elevated, I will also measure the 5-MTHFR gene and prescribe 5-MTHF as a form of folate in doses of 1,000 micrograms daily if there are no contraindications.

If homocysteine levels are elevated, in addition to folate, other B vitamins, including B2, B12, and B6, are needed to lower the homocysteine levels. Normal levels are often reported as up to 13 micromoles per liter (μmol/L). However, ideal levels are lower (closer to 8 μmol/L). Although there is conflicting evidence about whether homocysteine is the cause of increased risk for heart disease, or just a bystander, the risk of heart disease doubles if homocysteine levels are above 13 μmol/L.

As noted, B vitamins, including folate, B2, B6, and B12, act as cofactors in methylation reactions and are crucial for maintenance of DNA integrity and DNA methylation. These one-carbon methylation pathways may modify associations between environmental toxicants and the risk for disease such as Alzheimer's and the health of the brain in general. Folate supplementation is associated with reduced risk of several cancers; however, once disease is present, it is possible that a relative increase in one-carbon nutrients may speed disease progression. A recent study (Christensen and Marsit 2011) showed that methylation patterns found in the cells of larger breast tumors were associated with higher folate intake. (It is possible that a confounding variable in the use of folic acid and not the active metabolite 5-methyltetrahydrofolate is the reason for these findings.)

It has been found that green tea (EGCG) provides an anticancer effect through inhibition of folate metabolism, leading to demethylation of DNA through reduced folic acid levels. These studies confirm the complex nature of folic acid supplementation in which individuals who are deficient will show lower cancer risks if they take folic acid supplements, whereas those who are already high in folate will increase the cancer risk with excess use. There is a U-shaped curve in regards to folic acid use, with the goal being in the middle of the curve. Because of these findings, I suggest that most people obtain their folic acid from their diet unless there is an indication of deficiency (high homocysteine or 5-MTHFR polymorphism) or situations like pregnancy where supplemental folate is recommended. High doses of folate can also mask B12 deficiency and disrupt zinc function. As in all nutritional therapies, a balanced approach is needed, which would include the use of B12 and other B vitamins with high-dose folic acid treatment.

In addition to low intake of folate-rich foods, alcohol is known to reduce folic acid levels and disrupt the liver release of folate as well as interfere with several steps of methionine metabolism needed for methylation. Alcohol use is associated with colon and breast cancer, and every alcoholic drink per day is associated with a 10 percent excess risk for the disease. Epigenetic mechanisms might explain this association.

Food Item	Folate Amount
Cooked chicken liver (75 g)	420 mcg
Fresh spinach (1 cup)	262 mcg
Fresh asparagus (1 cup)	262 mcg
Boiled beets (1 cup)	136 mcg
Fresh papaya (1 cup)	115 mcg
Cooked Brussels sprouts (1 cup)	94 mcg
Enriched pasta (½ cup)	92 mcg
Fresh avocado (1 cup)	90 mcg
Fresh strawberries (1 cup)	90 mcg
Cooked collard greens (½ cup)	88 mcg
Canned garbanzo beans (½ cup)	80 mcg
Hazel nuts (½ cup)	58 mcg
Tofu (¾ cup)	53 mcg
Cooked broccoli (1 cup)	50 mcg
Cooked rice (½ cup)	50 mcg
Shredded romaine lettuce (½ cup)	40 mcg

Table 2: Folate-Rich Foods

Sulforaphane and Cruciferous Vegetables

Eat your broccoli, kids! We all heard this as children, though broccoli and other cruciferous vegetables are often not a favorite of children or even adults. (Think President George H. W. Bush, who famously said he didn't like broccoli.) The very reason for the unique taste of these foods is what makes them so powerful in affecting our health and protecting the epigenome: sulforaphane. Broccoli and other cruciferous vegetables, including Brussels sprouts, cabbage, kale, and cauliflower, are known to have many health-enhancing benefits. Sulforaphane (SFN), one of the most active compounds found in cruciferous vegetables, especially broccoli sprouts, has been shown to improve detoxification pathways and reduce the risk of developing several cancers.

Sulforaphane as an isolated phytonutrient has been used in most of the studies on the epigenetic effect of broccoli. It is derived from freshly germinated broccoli sprouts, which contain 30 to 50 times the concentration of sulforaphane as mature broccoli. Sulforaphane works to prevent cancer by inhibiting Phase I (liver) metabolism that creates carcinogens while increasing Phase II metabolism that promotes the excretion of carcinogens (see Chapter 3 on detoxification). In addition, SFN inhibits the growth of abnormal cells and reduces angiogenesis (the growth of new blood vessels), a crucial factor in preventing the spread of cancer. It supports cell cycle arrest and apoptosis, reduces central nervous system inflammation, and improves cardiovascular function. In addition, in a study by Bhamre and colleagues (2009), SFN improved the expression of tumor suppressor genes through acetylation and inhibition of DNA methyltransferase. This was identified in colon cancer cells, prostate cancer cells, and breast cancer cells.

In a study by Hsu and colleagues (2011), sulforaphane was found to restore normal cell function through normalizing epigenetic markers of methylation and histone configuration in prostate cancer cells. SFN allowed silenced genes to be expressed, a critical aspect of reversing cancer progression. Meeran and colleagues (2010) found similar effects of SFN in breast and colon cancer cells.

An important study in 2010 by Li and colleagues found that broccoli sprout extract was the only substance to inhibit breast cancer stem cells and potentially prevent the disease from starting. Breast cancer is generally initiated from and maintained through a small population of breast cancer stem cells. Any substance that can target these cells could truly prevent the disease.

SFN from broccoli influences both DNA methylation and histone deacetylase (HDAC) inhibition, promoting normal cell function and cell surveillance through tumor suppressor genes. SFN is unusual in the degree that it affects both these factors as well as improves detoxification and reduces angiogenesis. It is almost a complete anti-cancer nutrient as well as contributing to a healthy cardiovascular system and reducing inflammation.

DNA methylation is a normal process of turning off genes, and it helps to control what DNA material gets read as part of genetic communication within cells. In cancer that process gets altered. These same disrupted processes appear to play a role in other diseases, including obesity, cardiovascular disease, immune function disorders, neurodegenerative disease, and even aging. SFN and other bioactive foods restore the balance of these cellular control processes, critical steps in adapting well and staying healthy.

One cup of broccoli, Brussels sprouts, or another cruciferous vegetable per day changes DNA methylation in blood cells two hours after ingestion, producing beneficial epigenetic effects. For therapeutic purposes, supplements that contain sulforaphane might be required. A typical daily dose of 30 to 100 milligrams of sulforaphane from broccoli sprout extract is recommended.

Curcumin

It is known that the incidence of Alzheimer's disease in India is significantly lower than in the United States. Researchers have postulated that the reason for this lower incidence is the presence of turmeric, a spice widely used in Indian cuisine. Curcumin, the yellow pigment present in turmeric *(Curcuma longa)*, is thought to be the critical phytonutrient.

Curcumin has been used in Ayurvedic medicine for centuries and has been found to have many health-enhancing properties, which include reducing inflammation, inhibiting blood vessel growth (especially in cancers), and antioxidant effects. Curcumin produces anti-inflammatory effects by inhibiting the inflammatory pathways COX-2, TNF-alpha, and NF-kB activity. (These pathways are also the target of many common drugs like ibuprofen as well as a range of prescription medications used in asthma, arthritis, and autoimmune disease.) Curcumin has been used for many years in Ayurvedic medicine in the treatment of joint and gastrointestinal problems and shows promise in reducing reoccurrence of ulcerative colitis. In my practice I have seen beneficial results using curcumin as an anti-inflammatory for joint and muscle pain as well as for general immune system effects.

There has been a tremendous amount of research done on curcumin, much of it reported in Indian medical journals. It is one of the safest botanicals and can be used both in food as yellow curry spice and as a supplement. Curcumin has shown antitumor activity against leukemias, lymphomas, multiple myeloma, brain cancer, melanoma, and skin, lung, prostate, breast, ovarian, liver, gastrointestinal, pancreatic, and colorectal epithelial cancers. Curcumin inhibits the growth of cancer cells and induces cell death (apoptosis), including cancer stem cells and their progenies.

Curcumin is particularly protective of the brain and neurological system, where its antioxidant and anti-inflammatory properties are very important. It has an effect on amyloid plaques in Alzheimer's disease, with studies showing protection against the toxicity induced by amyloid plaques. As mentioned above, population studies have shown a significantly lower incidence of Alzheimer's disease in India.

Curcumin is a powerful epigenetic nutrient, inhibiting histone deacetylase (HDAC) in cancer models, leading to increased apoptosis in cancer cells. Fu and Kurzrock (2010) found that curcumin also inhibits DNA methyltransferase. Curcumin is a potent hypomethylating (gene-activating) agent, which reflects its broad-based impact on inflammation, cancer, diabetes, and other diseases. In addition, curcumin has been shown to decrease differentiation of pre-adipocytes into fat cells, justifying its folk name, "killer of fat," providing another tool in the fight against obesity.

There have been thousands of studies investigating the role of curcumin in health, though its use in the United States has been slow to be embraced. The effects of curcumin are many, making it one of the most important bioactive foods in the nutritional arsenal in maintaining high-level wellness and adaptation.

Following is a summary of key curcumin studies:

- Curcumin reduces amyloid plaques in the brain in animal models, improving cognitive function.
- Curcumin can improve mood, as a natural monoamine oxidase inhibitor, increasing dopamine and serotonin.
- Curcumin improves neurogenesis (the growth of new nerves) in the hippocampus and frontal cortex, reversing stress-related behavior in animal studies.
- It is anti-inflammatory, inhibiting multiple inflammation pathways, including TNF-alpha and interleukins, and modulating T-cell and B-cell activity.
- Curcumin reduces arthritis symptoms, acting as an anti-inflammatory.
- It has beneficial effects on the kidneys, liver, and heart.
- Curcumin has anticancer effects through epigenetic mechanisms.

Employing turmeric in the diet as a spice will raise the curcumin level in the body; however, unless turmeric has been used over a long period, such as in traditional Indian diets, it might be wise to use a supplement of curcumin to achieve therapeutic benefits. Absorption of curcumin from supplements can be difficult; therefore, the forms that I have found most useful are complexed with phytosomes or bioperene, an extract from black pepper. Therapeutic doses range from 500 to 1,000 milligrams several times a day. Using curcumin in a therapeutic mode should be under the supervision of a health care provider.

Tea Polyphenols: Epigallocatechin-3-gallate (EGCG)

For many years evidence has mounted that drinking green tea is a good idea. As discussed in Chapter 6, it has antioxidant effects and can even enhance fat burning. However, the potency of green tea as a regulator of the epigenome is just now being appreciated. Tea has been a staple drink in many cultures for centuries. Green tea is essentially unfermented tea, whereas black tea is fermented. After water, tea is the most consumed beverage in the world. The tea plant, *Camellia sinensis,* is cultivated in more than thirty countries, particularly in Asia. Besides the social and ceremonial use of tea, it has broad-based therapeutic properties, with the phytonutrient polyphenolic compounds present in tea possibly reducing the risk of coronary heart disease, cancer, and other degenerative conditions.

Green tea contains between 30 and 40 percent polyphenols, whereas black tea contains between 3 and 10 percent. A recent Japanese study (Tomata et al. 2012) of fourteen thousand people found that three to four cups per day of green tea lowered risks of stroke, dementia, and osteoporosis. In addition, it lowered the incidence of depression and loss of muscle strength.

The most abundant polyphenol compound in green tea is catechins; of these, epigallocatechin-3-gallate (EGCG) accounts for more than 50 percent of the total polyphenol content. EGCG protects cells, including neurons, against stress-induced cell death. Like curcumin, EGCG activates Nrf2, an enzyme system that increases detoxifying effects, especially in the brain. Green tea polyphenols protect red blood cells from oxidative stress; support healthy insulin activity through reduction of inflammatory cytokine hormones, preventing free-radical damage; and promote fat oxidation and possible weight loss.

Green tea has been shown to induce apoptosis and cell cycle arrest in many cancer cells without affecting normal cells. Its epigenetic effects include inhibition of DNA methyltransferase (DNMT), leading to demethylation and reactivation of tumor suppressor genes silenced by methylation in esophageal, prostate, and oral cancers. Landis-Piwowar, Milacic, and Dou (2008) showed that long-term low-dose exposure to EGCG and genistein (from soy) resulted in the epigenetic alteration of gene expression, and reduced growth and caused cellular apoptosis in breast cancer cells; EGCG also regulates gene expression through changes in histone modification.

Yuasa and colleagues (2009) reviewed studies that strongly correlate dietary habits, including green tea intake, as well as physical activity, to epigenetic reactivation of several anticancer genes, including tumor suppressor genes. They demonstrated in patients with stomach cancer that past lifestyle and dietary habits, including consumption of cruciferous vegetables and green tea polyphenols, improved the methylation status of several genes, such as CDX2 and BMP-2, which are important for preventing gastric cancer.

Another crucial effect of green tea is its protective quality against toxic pollutants that have disruptive epigenetic effects. Loest and colleagues (2002) found that green tea catechins decrease absorption of lipids (fats) and lipid-soluble compounds, including toxic chemicals. Green tea consumption lowers plasma levels and increases fecal excretion of fat-soluble chemicals termed persistent organic pollutants (POPs), according to a study by Morita and colleagues in 1997. Green tea inhibits the intestinal absorption and enhances the elimination of lipids and fat-soluble organic compounds, including POPs, a critical property in protecting the epigenome from the effects of toxic chemicals.

Three to four cups of green tea per day is recommended as a preventive amount for epigenetic purposes. For therapeutic purposes an intake of green tea polyphenols equivalent to ten cups of tea, or about 600 milligrams as a capsule containing 18 percent EGCG, is recommended. If using this amount of EGCG, supplement with folic acid (5-MTHF) unless there is a current cancer diagnosis, in which case consult a health practitioner who is an expert in nutritional medicine.

Benefits of Green Tea

• Powerful antioxidant

• Protects against DNA damage and hypermethylation

• Induces detoxifying enzymes

• Affects gene signaling, regulating cell growth and apoptosis

• Selectively improves intestinal bacteria functioning

• Inhibits intestinal absorption of fat-soluble organic pollutants (POPs)

• Is thermogenic and helps to burn excess fat

Genistein

Asians who eat a traditional Asian diet have a lower incidence of heart disease and breast and prostate cancer compared to Asians eating a Western diet. The difference has been attributed to fermented soy products. In 2005 Fang and colleagues reported on Asian immigrants who maintained a traditional diet after immigrating to the United States. Comparing this group with Asian women who had adopted a typical American diet, they found a much lower incidence of breast cancer in the women with the traditional Asian diet, which is rich in fermented soy products such as tofu, miso, and tempeh. Prostate cancer incidence has also been shown to be lower in those eating traditional Asian diets. (See Chapter 6 for more details on genistein.)

Nutrient	Food Source	Epigenetic Role
Methionine	Sesame seeds, Brazil nuts, fish, peppers, spinach	SAM synthesis for methylation
Folic Acid	Leafy vegetables, sunflower seeds, nutritional yeast, liver	Methionine synthesis, DNA methylation
Vitamin B12	Meat, liver, shellfish, milk	Methionine synthesis
Curcumin	Turmeric, yellow curry spice	Removes methylation, turns on protective genes, decreases inflammation
Choline	Egg yolks, liver, soy, cooked beef, chicken, veal, and turkey	Methyl donor to SAM
Betaine	Wheat, spinach, shellfish, and sugar beets	Breaks down homocysteine from SAM synthesis
Resveratrol	Red wine, grapes, berries	Removes acetyl groups from histones, activates oncogenes, extends life span in animal studies
Genistein	Soy, soy products	Cancer prevention, Inhibits DNA Methylation
Sulforaphane	Brussels sprouts, cabbage, broccoli, kale	Histone modification, increased histone acetylation turning on anticancer genes, inhibits DNA methylation, improves detoxification
Butyrate	A compound produced in the intestine when dietary fiber is fermented	Increased histone acetylation turning on "protective" genes

Table 3: Bioactive Foods and Nutrients

Nutrient	Food Source	Epigenetic Role
Diallyl Disulfide (DADS)	Garlic	Increased histone acetylation turning on anticancer genes
EGCG	Green tea	Inhibits DNA methylation, activates tumor suppressor genes, reduces inflammation

Table 3: Bioactive Foods and Nutrients (continued)

Genistein is the most abundant isoflavone in soybeans, fava beans, and kudzu root, and has been the focus of considerable research in epigenetics and cancer prevention. Genistein isoflavones have a strong effect on regulating the epigenome and have been found to affect tumor growth through epigenetic mechanisms. Like other bioactive foods, genistein activates tumor suppressor genes, which affect cancer-cell survival through DNA methylation inhibition and chromatin histone remodeling. Genistein has been shown to reactivate silenced tumor suppressor genes in esophageal, colon, prostate, and breast cancer cells. It selectively induced apoptosis (cell death) in cancer cells but not normal cells. Genistein increased histone acetylation that also activated tumor suppressor genes in prostate cancer cells, leading to cell cycle arrest and cancer-cell death.

Bernal and Jirtle (2010) found that genistein was able to protect mice in utero from epigenetic alterations caused by bisphenol A exposure. One of the damaging effects of toxic chemicals, including bisphenol A (found in plastic bottles, tin cans, and food storage containers), is epigenetic methylation and the silencing of tumor suppressor genes. This is of great concern due to the massive amounts of this chemical and other endocrine disruptors now in the environment, and its effects on pregnant women and their babies.

In pregnant Agouti mice, genistein activated a return to normal methylation in the offspring, as seen in the brown coat color of the pups from mothers who were supplemented with a high soy diet during pregnancy. Even more stunning was the apparent protection of the offspring against obesity in adulthood. These studies indicate that a transgenerational impact from dietary genistein is possible, though the science is still not settled.

Apart from its epigenetic effects, genistein is considered to be a phytoestrogen (a plant-based substance that can stimulate human estrogen receptors), because it concentrates in estrogen receptors, particularly in breast tissue. It is thought that phytoestrogens are protective, because they are extremely weak stimulants of the receptors and do not allow the stronger stimulation from estradiol (the strongest human estrogen) to activate the receptors and increase the risk for breast cancer. This might also add to genistein's possible effects on preventing breast cancer and prostate cancer. (There are estrogen receptors in the prostate that some researchers feel contribute to the development of prostate cancer from elevated estrogen levels.) There has been some concern about excessive soy use overstimulating estrogen receptors, though the majority of the epigenetic studies strongly support the use of genistein to inhibit and prevent cancer-cell growth. All the population studies on the beneficial effects of soy and genistein are with the traditional forms of this food: tempeh, tofu, miso, and roasted soybeans, not soy milk and soy yogurt. To obtain the benefit and reduce the possible risks of excessive use, I suggest consuming only the food sources of genistein that have been used over thousands of years, the aged soy products.

Other Bioactive Food Factors

Dietary fiber (especially soluble fiber) is a critical factor in the health of the epigenome. Butyrate, a fatty acid that forms in the colon from the fermentation of dietary fiber by probiotic bacteria, affects histone modulation. Histone deacetylase (HDAC) inhibition and increased acetylation of histones have been reported in several cell lines that were treated with butyrate. These alterations in histones have been associated with beneficial changes, including normalization of cells, cell cycle arrest of abnormal cell cycles, apoptosis (cell death), and inhibition of invasion and metastasis.

The typical American diet is woefully low in fiber. The recommended amount of dietary fiber is between 20 and 35 grams per day, with the average American consuming only 12–18 grams, while many children and teens consume less than 20 percent of what is recommended. Foods high in soluble fiber include beans and other legumes, whole grains, fruits, and vegetables.

Butyrate levels are also dependent on normal colonic bacteria (flora), which are easily disrupted by antibiotic or anti-inflammatory medications. Organic yogurt (preferably unsweetened) with live lactobacillus cultures is one good source of beneficial bacteria. Other sources are kefir and other cultured dairy and aged foods such as sauerkraut. Supplementing with probiotics as well as increasing dietary soluble fiber to enhance butyrate production is another step to take to protect the epigenome.

Foods high in soluble fiber needed for butyrate production include:

- Legumes (all beans, split peas, lentils)
- Oats, rye, barley, chia seeds
- Prunes, plums, berries, apples, bananas, and pears
- Broccoli, carrots, artichokes
- Root vegetables like sweet potatoes, yams, rutabaga
- Psyllium seed husks and flaxseeds
- Almonds, walnuts, and other nuts, raw and unsalted

Choline (an essential nutrient often grouped with the B vitamins) and its metabolites are a core part of the methylation pathway and have a major impact on epigenetic methylation. The 2012 study by Jiang and colleagues, mentioned earlier in this chapter, discussed the epigenetic effect of choline on cortisol levels in the offspring of mothers given additional choline in pregnancy. The researchers compared the effects of 930 milligrams of choline against a typical dietary intake of 480 milligrams over a twelve-week period. They measured DNA methylation levels of the genes that control cortisol production in umbilical cord blood, placental tissue, and maternal blood and found a significant decrease in gene expression through epigenetic methylation from the higher choline intake. This is an important finding, suggesting that maternal diet can impact the stress responsiveness and adaptation ability in the offspring through epigenetic mechanisms. So if you blame your mother for making you a stress responder, it could have started when you were still in the womb. This data should make every woman who is in her childbearing years consider not only adequate dietary folic acid but choline as well.

Choline is needed for other physiological purposes: structural integrity (supporting the bilipid cell-membrane structure and mitochondrial membranes) and signaling roles for cell membranes; neurotransmission (acetylcholine synthesis); and as a major source for methyl groups. Most adults need between 400 and 500 milligrams per day. Following are the foods with the highest levels of choline:

- Beef liver (pan-fried) 100 grams (about 3.5 ounces): 418 mg
- ½ pound cod fish: 190 mg
- ½ pound chicken: 150 mg
- Whole large egg (in the yolk): 112 mg
- Beef (ground) 80 percent lean/20 percent fat (3.5-ounce patty): 81 mg
- Cauliflower ¾ cup cooked (1-inch pieces): 62 mg
- Navy beans ½ cup cooked: 48 mg
- Tofu 100 grams (about 3.5 ounces): 28 mg
- Almonds ½ cup sliced: 26 mg
- Peanut butter 2 tablespoons: 20 mg

Betaine, a metabolite of choline, functions closely with other nutrients like S-adenosylmethionine (SAM), folic acid, and vitamins B6 and B12 to break down homocysteine and reduce toxic levels

---

An Epigenetic Feast

Next time you ask, "What's for dinner, honey?," help to answer this question with epigenetically minded food choices. Here is an example of one of my favorite meals and its bioactive components.

A cup of green tea (EGCG)

Stir-fry of tofu (genistein and choline) with turmeric (curcumin) and garlic (allyl) as spices, sesame seeds (methionine), and vegetables, including broccoli, kale, and Brussels sprouts (sulforaphane)

A salad with greens like spinach, chard, and asparagus (folic acid), beets (betaine)

A glass of red wine (resveratrol)

Other foods to add to the stir-fry could be fish, whole eggs, or chicken (choline and methionine).

Using organic foods as much as possible will protect a healthy epigenome, because foods like eggs and animal protein can harbor high levels of POPs if not organically raised.

---

of this substance in the bloodstream. Betaine is found in wheat, spinach, shellfish, and beets.

In addition to these foods, other fruits and vegetables have also been reported to have epigenetic targets, either through DNA methyltransferase (DNMT) inhibition or histone modifications. These bioactive foods include: garlic, which contains allyl compounds that improve histone configuration; celery and parsley with apigenin; tomatoes with lycopene; milk thistle with silymarin; and red wine, red grapes, berries, and peanuts containing resveratrol.

Resveratrol deserves special mention because it has received so much attention as one of the few phytonutrients found to increase longevity in animal studies by enhancing mitochondrial regeneration (see Chapter 6). Resveratrol was found to also have strong anticancer properties by modulating pathways that control cell division and growth, apoptosis, inflammation, angiogenesis, and metastasis. Resveratrol has been shown to inhibit proliferation of a wide variety of human tumor cells in skin, breast, prostate, lung, and colon cancers.

The Environment, Toxins, and Epigenetics

As a physician practicing environmental medicine for the past thirty-five years, I have seen the impact that toxic chemicals and heavy metal contamination have had on the health of my patients. The extent of the damage these chemicals create is only now beginning to be appreciated. Researchers have discovered that some of the harmful effects of these toxins occur through epigenetic mechanisms. The amount of pollutants and toxins that are threatening the health of everyone, especially the unborn, is staggering. All the answers are certainly not in, but it is not too hard to imagine that sometime in the future we will see the connection between environmental toxins and every chronic and degenerative disease that is present today.

Environmental epigenetics reflects the constant interplay between nutritional state, detoxification pathways, hormonal status, and environmental toxicants, all impacting the epigenome. Environmental toxins (including persistent organic pollutants like PCBs and bisphenol A) and toxic metals (including arsenic, cadmium, and lead) are widely distributed around the planet and can be found in some amount in almost every person. I routinely measure heavy metals in provoked urine samples (the procedure includes a chelating medication given before a urine collection) and find in my practice, despite being in a relatively pristine setting with almost no industrial exposures, elevated levels of lead, mercury, arsenic, or cadmium in more than half the patients tested.

In 2005 the Centers for Disease Control measured the levels of a variety of toxins and metals in a sample of the U.S. population.

Shockingly, they found 148 different environmental chemicals in blood and urine samples. Included were heavy metals, phytoestrogens, polycyclic aromatic hydrocarbons, dioxin-like compounds, polychlorinated biphenyls (PCBs), phthalates, and pesticides. Many of these toxicants have powerful dysregulating effects on the epigenome, leading to increased risk for cancer, heart disease, obesity, and other serious health consequences. Toxicants affect DNA methylation and histone modifications, the same markers that are vulnerable to poor dietary habits.

One of the main avenues for increased tissue levels and body burden of these toxicants is food. For example, PCBs, which are endocrine disruptors and a POP (persistent organic pollutant), were used as insulation material for electrical transformers and transmission lines. Because of their toxicity, the use of this group of chemicals in open or dissipative sources was banned in the United States in 1973. In 1979 the U.S. Congress banned the domestic production of PCBs, although some use continues in closed systems such as capacitors and transformers. A worldwide ban of PCB production was put into effect by the Stockholm Convention on Persistent Organic Pollutants in 2001.

Despite this ban, PCBs are still found in soils and in food. Dairy cows and cattle eating feed contaminated with PCBs concentrate this toxin in fats, which we consume as dairy products and meat. PCBs are absorbed through the digestive tract and accumulate in fatty tissue. POP exposure found in the fat of obese individuals might actually increase the risk for diabetes more than obesity itself.

The risks from toxicants can't be fully explained by damage directly to genes, because they are modulated by other nongenetic factors, especially the epigenome. Up until recently the determination of environmental risks from these chemicals has been based on the effect they have on the genome and DNA. Government regulations on acceptable levels of exposure were determined by the amount of DNA damage found in animal studies. However, as we now know, the effect of these toxicants goes beyond DNA damage, altering the state of the epigenome. The ultimate cost of an increased body burden of both toxic metals and POPs might not be known for many decades as changes in a person's epigenome increase the risk for cancer, heart disease, and diabetes that might persist through several generations. One example is a study by Dolinoy and colleagues (2007) that showed bisphenol A causing global hypomethylation, leading to increased cancer risk in subsequent generations of animals. In addition, each person has a differing capacity to detoxify these pollutants, based on their own genetics and nutritional state.

As I pointed out in Chapter 3, the U.S. Environmental Protection Agency, the Centers for Disease Control and Prevention, and other government agencies involved with monitoring these substances have assessed the health effects of each toxicant one by one, and allow a certain level of all these chemicals to be in food and water. However, as the 2009 CDC study found, many different chemicals are found in every person, with additive effects on the epigenome and overall health. Research into the effects of these chemicals is further complicated by the fact that there is widely varying individual susceptibility to these toxicants based on genetics and diet. Combining exposure to these toxins with the average American diet, inadequate in folic acid from vegetables, and fiber to generate butyrate, insufficient broccoli or other crucifers, and little or no curcumin, can cause havoc at the level of DNA methylation and histone modification. It is not hard to see how these POPs can contribute to the epidemic of chronic disease and obesity.

The good news is that bioactive foods can reverse the methylation changes induced by chemicals like bisphenol A (BPA). Dolinoy and colleagues (2007) found that genistein and folic acid supplementation reversed the methylation effects in utero of BPA exposure in mice. The complex interaction between bioactive foods, environmental toxicants, and the epigenome ultimately goes a long way in determining a person's future health. Those who eat wisely and reduce their toxic exposures will profit from this knowledge.

One more important area to explore is the impact of epigenetic marks on aging. Shen and colleagues (2005) found an overall trend of increased methylation of normal human prostate and colon tissue in several genes associated with aging. Increased methylation turns off tumor suppressor genes and contributes to the onset of cancer and other diseases of aging. The research seems clear that inadequate dietary intake of bioactive foods and excess exposure to toxicants accelerate the aging process through methylation and histone changes, as well as increase the risk of major disease through epigenetic phenomena.

Toxic Heavy Metals

There are many toxic metals contributing to health problems, including lead, cadmium, arsenic, and mercury, which persist almost indefinitely in the environment. For example, in polar ice in Greenland, lead levels have been identified that are linked to pollution from Greek and Roman civilizations two thousand years ago. Lead levels skyrocketed in the United States after tetraethyl lead was added to gasoline in the 1920s. According to a 1988 congressional report, sixty-eight million children had toxic exposures to lead from 1927 to 1987. In my practice the frequency of elevated lead levels after a chelation challenge is almost 50 percent. Much of this contamination is from lead stored in bones, where it makes a home along with calcium. When bone breaks down as we age, the lead is released into the rest of the body, contributing to health effects on the immune system, heart, and brain. Lead is especially dangerous in children, where it is associated with reduction in IQ and learning deficits.

All the toxic metals contribute to a more rapid aging of tissues, and increased risk for heart disease and cancer. A common mechanism for all these toxins is depletion of antioxidant protection as they create free-radical damage. Glutathione, the key cell-membrane antioxidant, as well as other antioxidants, including vitamin E and lipoic acid, is depleted by oxidative stress from toxic metals, leaving cells more vulnerable to membrane damage and chronic disease.

Diseases such as autoimmune conditions, kidney disease, memory defects, muscle weakness, and thyroid disorders all can have a heavy metal trigger. Much of this damage is going unnoticed by most doctors, mainly because the focus of academic medicine has been on toxic effects of acute large exposures to metals such as industrial accidents and not on the subtle lifelong accumulation that most people experience.

In addition to these deleterious effects, it is now becoming clear that several of these metals can cause epigenetic alterations. The metals most studied regarding epigenetic effects are arsenic, cadmium, and mercury. Let's look a little closer at these toxins.

Arsenic

Organic and inorganic arsenic is found throughout the environment. Inorganic arsenic is combined with elements other than carbon and is emitted into the air and deposited in water and soil from industrial sources, including smelting and mining, as well as from forest fires and volcanic eruptions. Arsenic is used in the semiconductor industry, strengthening alloys of copper and lead, as well as in pesticides. It is linked to cancers of the skin, bladder, prostate, liver, and lungs.

The major source of exposure to arsenic is through drinking water from contaminated wells and from rice products from contaminated water. This is especially true in Asia. In a paper by Bagchi in 2007 it was estimated that more than 137 million people in seventy countries have been exposed to high levels of arsenic. Arsenic in food or water decreases uptake of iron, manganese, copper, and zinc. Arsenic in fish and shellfish is usually the nontoxic organic form, though it could interfere with essential minerals as well.

Aggressive bladder cancers were seen in individuals with excess arsenic exposure in drinking water, which leads to abnormal methylation. It appears that depletion of S-adenosylmethionine and disruption of methylation from arsenic is the mechanism that creates arsenic-related cancers. In addition, Marsit and colleagues (2006) found a link between arsenic and bladder cancer, associated with repression of tumor suppressor genes.

Arsenic has also been linked to increased risk of cardiovascular disease. In Taiwanese villages with high arsenic levels in drinking water, there was an increase in the incidence of heart disease with elevated arsenic levels of more than 200 percent. Like the other toxins, the cellular burden of arsenic depletes the body of the protective antioxidants, including glutathione.

The good news is that folic acid supplementation lowers blood arsenic levels and can repair the depletion of the methyl donor SAM, limiting the damage that arsenic as well as other heavy metals inflict on the epigenome. It is possible to measure arsenic and other toxic metal levels through blood or urine testing to assess their tissue levels and body burden. If these levels are elevated, a course of chelation therapy can reduce an individual's burden and protect their epigenome. In addition, antioxidant therapy with vitamin C, vitamin E, and alpha lipoic acid is needed.

Cadmium

Cadmium exposure occurs from proximity to coal-burning power plants, the manufacturing of nickel-cadmium batteries, and other industrial processes. Air, water, and soil can be contaminated with cadmium, which is known to be carcinogenic in humans and animals. A primary source of cadmium exposure is through one's diet, including fish, shellfish, and other foods. Painters can be exposed from red paint dye. Another major source is exposure to cigarette smoke, even secondhand smoke.

Cadmium mimics the important nutrients zinc and calcium and concentrates in the liver and kidneys. Cadmium is linked to lung, prostate, pancreatic, kidney, liver, stomach, and bladder cancers. Cadmium exposure increases DNA methylation of tumor suppressor genes that were turned off, leading to the increased incidence of cancer. Cadmium has also been linked to an increased incidence of hypertension and heart disease.

Mercury

A lot has been written about mercury toxicity and the dangers it poses, especially to pregnant women. The FDA has issued warnings to limit the intake of large predatory fish during pregnancy because of the elevated exposure to mercury from these fish and its effects on the fetus. Mercury is released into the atmosphere from coal-fired power plants and other industrial sources as elemental, particle-bound oxidized mercury. It is also released from gold mining operations, smelters, cement production, and waste disposal. Mercury vapor is released from dental amalgams and absorbed into the central nervous system. Though mercury-containing dental amalgam fillings are banned in many European countries, they are still in use in the United States.

Mercury is found in the world's oceans, where it is converted by bacteria to methyl mercury, a highly toxic compound. It then enters the food chain through fish and shellfish. Mercury levels concentrate higher up the food chain, moving from plankton to larger predatory fish. Shark, swordfish, king mackerel, albacore tuna, and tilefish have the highest levels of methyl mercury. The lowest levels of mercury are found in salmon, shrimp, catfish, and pollack.

On an epigenetic level, mercury, like other toxins, causes abnormal DNA methylation, leading to altered cell metabolism and increased oxidative stress. As many as 40 percent of my patients have demonstrated elevated urinary mercury levels after a chelation challenge with either DMSA or EDTA. The first step in reducing one's mercury burden is avoiding fish with high mercury content. In addition, it is wise to remove amalgam filings containing mercury. (I refer my patients to a dentist skilled in amalgam removal who uses suction devices and other means to prevent reabsorption of the mercury vapors from drilling.) If needed, chelation therapy with DMSA or EDTA can be employed to enhance removal of this toxin.

Mercury carries other risks as well, including increased oxidized cholesterol, increased platelet aggregation (clotting), hypertension, and endothelial dysfunction, leading to a greater incidence of heart disease. Some researchers even postulate that elevated mercury levels are as great a risk as cigarette smoking in regards to heart disease. In a study by Sørensen and colleagues (1999), elevated umbilical cord blood mercury of newborns was associated with increased blood pressure in children at age seven. Mercury also increases autoimmunity, including thyroiditis, and other conditions.

As is the case with other heavy metals, the human body has limited capacity to remove and excrete this toxin. In fact, the average human (150 pounds) has 13 milligrams of mercury in his or her body that disrupts antioxidant protection significantly. Mercury can reduce immune system function, increase vascular inflammation, increase cell death (apoptosis), disrupt mitochondrial membranes (leading to increased fatigue), and stimulate inflammatory hormone production in the vascular system. It is possible to protect against some of these toxic changes through the use of selenium as a supplement (selenomethionine 200 milligrams) and oral micronized glutathione (under the guidance of your physician).

We are only now scratching the surface in understanding the impact these heavy metals have on the epigenome and human health in general. To protect the precious inheritance that is the genome, it is prudent for everyone to reduce exposure to these metals as much as possible and to seek medical evaluation to assess and reduce the body burden of these toxicants.

Endocrine Disruptors and Persistent Organic Pollutants (POPs)

Endocrine disruptors are a group of chemicals (PCBs, DDT, BPA, phthalates) that interfere with hormonal system function in humans and animals, often attaching to hormonal receptor sites throughout the body. They are among the persistent organic pollutants (POPs) that have enormously long half-lives and continue to pollute the environment for decades, even after banned from use. Because many of these pollutants are fat soluble, foods that are high in fat contain higher levels of POPs than even fruits and vegetables. It is thought that 90 percent of the PCB and DDT (a pesticide banned in the United States in 1972) burden found in humans is from dietary sources. Fortunately, ingestion of antioxidant-rich and anti-inflammatory fruits and vegetables with bioactive compounds can partially protect against the epigenetic effects of POPs.

Other endocrine disruptors include bisphenol A (BPA), commonly found in polycarbonate plastic bottles, food containers, and tin cans; DDT and its metabolite DDE; phthalates found in some toys, flooring, cosmetics, and medical equipment; and polybrominated diphenyl ethers (PBDEs) used as flame retardants in electronics, bedding, clothing, and cars.

Phthalates are used to soften polyvinyl chloride and are found in adhesives and glues, agricultural adjuvants, building materials, personal care products such as nail polish, liquid soap, and perfumes, medical devices, vinyl floors, shower curtains, detergents, packaging, toys, pharmaceuticals, food products, and textiles. More than six million tons of plasticizers are produced worldwide every year. Phthalates are classified as endocrine disruptors because of their estrogenic effects and may adversely affect male reproductive organs in children. Exposure to phthalates, like other POPs, occurs mainly through the diet; however, they can be absorbed through the skin via personal care products and even through the lungs. In 2009, the U.S. Centers for Disease Control (CDC) published the *Fourth National Report on Human Exposure to Environmental Chemicals,* which included a study of 298 adults that found levels of a metabolite of the phthalate DBP in the urine of everyone tested during the years 1999–2004. Though the exposure to phthalates is ubiquitous, the CDC and the FDA have not found a clear connection between these POPs and negative health effects. Unfortunately, the information on the websites of these agencies does not discuss the disruptive epigenetic impacts that have been found in repeated studies.

For example, in breast cancer cells, exposure to phthalates led to the demethylation of estrogen receptor genes, which increased estrogen stimulation of the tissue. Phthalate exposure in utero has been associated with elevated body mass index (BMI) during the first three years of life, a disturbing finding considering the epidemic of childhood obesity. In addition, a variety of developmental abnormalities have been found as a result of phthalate exposure. There is also concern that exposure in utero to phthalates can lead to children with behavioral problems.

Bisphenol A (BPA) is also considered to be an endocrine disruptor and can accumulate in adipose (fat) tissue. It is now thought to be similar in potency to estradiol (the most active human estrogen) in stimulating a cellular response. BPA is used in the production of plastics and resins that are found in food and drink containers, flame retardants, dental sealants, and in the recycling of thermal paper. BPA is one of the highest-volume chemicals produced worldwide. The *Fourth National Report on Human Exposure to Environmental Chemicals* detected BPA in the urine of 93 percent of those tested. The greatest exposure to BPA is through the food chain.

Doherty and colleagues (2010) found that pregnant mice exposed to BPA developed alterations that led to reduced methylation in their offspring. This caused overexpression of a gene (EZH2) associated with breast cancer, and reduced expression of DNA-repair mediator genes in the pups. Exposure to BPA led to higher body weight, increased breast and prostate cancer, and altered reproductive function in the offspring. Prostate tissues in the offspring showed consistent methylation changes as a result of BPA exposures, suggesting that the prostate epigenome is permanently altered by exposure to BPA either in utero or early in life, increasing the risk of prostate cancer with aging. In humans, exposure to BPA and other endocrine disruptors early in life may predispose the mammary and prostate glands to pre-cancerous lesions in adult life, possibly explaining the dramatic increase in breast and prostate cancer in recent decades. Even though BPA and phthalates are rapidly excreted, the sheer volume of exposure has kept essentially all Americans with detectable levels of these endocrine disruptors. As noted earlier, maternal supplementation with folic acid and genistein may counteract the hypomethylating effects of BPA.

In addition, learning disabilities, attention deficit disorder (ADD), cognitive and brain development problems, feminizing effects, and other sexual-development changes have all been linked to endocrine-disrupting chemicals, possibly through epigenetic mechanisms. Though there has been an attempt by the chemical industry to downplay the impact of these toxicants, the research on the epigenetic effects of these chemicals is particularly disturbing. Synergistic mechanisms exist between deficiencies of essential nutrients and exposure to environmental toxins that amplify the damage done by these chemicals. Many children and adults bear the double burden of nutrient deficiencies and exposure to heavy metals, PCBs, BPA, phthalates, lead, and arsenic, leading to disruptive epigenetic impacts. These effects can be modified with better dietary habits and education to reduce toxin exposure. In addition to toxicants, chronic inflammation and poor diet can lead to abnormal methylation in aging tissue, leading to greater risk for obesity as well as cancer and other diseases of aging.

There is ample evidence that pesticides, which are known to be endocrine disruptors, can also have negative impacts on the epigenome. Choosing to use organic foods whenever possible and avoiding the foods with the highest level of pesticide contamination can help protect the expression of genes both in utero and throughout life.

Using fruits and vegetables that have heavy pesticide exposure can lead to unacceptable levels of these chemicals, as demonstrated in a study conducted by the European Parliament. In evaluating just eight foods, they found twenty-eight different pesticide residues, including ten known carcinogens, three neurotoxins, eight endocrine disruptors, and three developmental toxins. Table 4 is a list compiled by the Environmental Working Group of the most and least contaminated fruits and vegetables.

Most Contaminated (use only organically grown)	Lowest in Pesticides
1. Apples	1. Onions
2. Celery	2. Sweet corn
3. Strawberries	3. Pineapples
4. Peaches	4. Avocado
5. Spinach	5. Asparagus
6. Nectarines (imported)	6. Sweet peas
7. Grapes (imported)	7. Mangoes
8. Sweet bell peppers	8. Eggplant
9. Potatoes	9. Cantaloupe (domestic)
10. Blueberries (domestic)	10. Kiwi
11. Lettuce	11. Cabbage
12. Kale/Collard greens	12. Watermelon

Table 4: Pesticide Contaminants in Food (from the Environmental Working Group)

Not only does dietary deficiency of the key bioactive foods compromise the health of the epigenome, ingestion of pro-inflammatory omega-6 fatty acids, such as linoleic and arachidonic acids (found in red meat and processed foods), leads to further inflammation and epigenetic changes. Heavy metals and organic pollutants that contribute to lower levels of antioxidants likely aggravate inflammatory states when an individual's intake of omega-3 essential fatty acids (from fish and vegetable sources) and polyphenols (like flavonoids in fruit, tea, and vegetables) is limited. This combination of dietary factors and environmental toxicants contributes to the heightened state of inflammation found in many people who have poor dietary habits. Inflammation itself is a risk factor for cancer and, as noted earlier in the book, for elevated cortisol and diseases of aging, including heart disease, diabetes, arthritis, and allergies, and is a major contributor to obesity.

Toxin Solutions

The ability to clear toxins varies from individual to individual, depending on several factors: the nutritional sufficiency of the cofactors needed for the detoxification pathways (see Chapter 3); the efficiency of enzyme systems and proteins needed for detoxification; the antioxidant status in the liver and other organs, especially in regards to glutathione; the state of the gastrointestinal tract and the health of the microbiota (beneficial bacteria such as bifidobacter and acidophilus); and the dietary intake of fiber and other nutrients.

Increasing excretion of POPs and heavy metals can be accomplished through some simple behaviors: drink more water; increase exercise, which stimulates liver detoxification enzymes and promotes excretion through the kidneys and skin; and use saunas to remove some of the POPs through sweat. Diet plays a major role in reducing the toxic load. Using whole, organic foods, including nuts, seeds, deeply colored vegetables, and whole grains, provides many of the needed nutrients to support detoxification pathways. Drinking three to four cups of green tea a day reduces absorption and increases elimination of many fat-soluble POPs. Adding the detoxifying nutritional supplements discussed in Chapter 3, especially alpha lipoic acid, N-acetylcysteine (NAC), and vitamin C, will enhance the removal of POPs and heavy metals.

Improving the detoxification function is within the reach of everyone. Knowing the source of the persistent organic pollutants and heavy metals and changing behaviors to reduce exposure to them add additional protection. A great resource for identifying sources of toxic chemicals is an internet guide to 74,000 products, produced by the Environmental Working Group. Below are the key points for reducing the toxic load of POPs and heavy metals and protecting the epigenome.

More than 90 percent of the U.S. population has detectable levels of BPA. Higher levels were found with the use of soda, school lunches, and meals prepared outside the home. Packaging and containers are the biggest sources of BPA, though not all sources are

---

Bisphenol A

- Do not use plastic water bottles and other containers (unless the container states BPA free).
- Avoid microwaving food in plastic containers (polycarbonate containers that contain BPA usually have a #7 on the bottom).
- Limit canned foods and packaged foods. BPA levels went down 50-70 percent when eating only fresh foods (Rudel et al. 2011).
- Store food in glass, porcelain, or steel containers.
- Limit exposure to thermal paper and carbonless copy paper (such as credit card receipts).

---

known. Supplements that specifically help in clearing BPA include N-acetylcysteine (NAC), alpha lipoic acid, and milk thistle.

Phthalate exposure comes from multiple sources, including diet, especially fatty foods such as milk, butter, and red meat. Avoiding these foods unless they are organically produced will reduce phthalate levels. Avoid as well the use of plastic storage containers. Exposure also occurs through absorption through the skin and the inhalation of volatile phthalates. When possible, use phthalate-free personal care products, including liquid soap, perfumes, nail polish, eye shadow, and hair spray. Children are especially at risk from infant care products such as baby shampoos, powder, and lotions. Avoid any products that mention "fragrance" as an ingredient, because that might include phthalates or paraben, another product in cosmetics that could disrupt metabolism. Protective supplements include alpha lipoic acid, NAC, and vitamins E and C.

PCBs, though banned, are still found in the food chain, especially in fatty foods, including dairy, red meat, poultry, and some fish. Using organically raised products (both animal protein and vegetables) can lower exposure to PCBs. A diet rich in detoxifying phytonutrients like broccoli, garlic, onions, kale, and other darkly colored vegetables is especially important to reduce PCB levels. Saunas, exercise, and increased water intake can help as well.

Toxic metals are especially difficult to remove from the body because they can be stored in bone (especially lead), fat, and even the brain (mercury). Chelation therapy, as prescribed by a physician experienced in this procedure, can rapidly remove many of the heavy metals. (See referral list in Appendix G.) In addition, certain foods and nutrients have been recommended to reduce heavy metal loads, including cilantro (either fresh or in capsules), garlic (two to three cloves or equivalent in capsules), and chlorella algae (in capsule form). Supplements should include lipoic acid, zinc, selenium, NAC, and taurine. Increasing dietary fiber intake is very important in clearing heavy metals.

Though POPs, heavy metals, and other pollutants pose a serious risk to the health of not only those alive today but future generations, the evidence that bioactive foods can modify the harmful impact of these toxicants is of some comfort. Including adequate amounts of these protectors of the epigenome, including green tea, folic acid from dark green vegetables, genistein from soy, sulforaphane from broccoli, and curcumin from turmeric, is going to be more critical than ever as we continue to pollute our environment. This new information from epigenetics enables every one of us to make dietary and behavioral changes to increase the likelihood of optimum health for ourselves and our children.

10

Conclusion

My clinical experience has taught me that food can have a great impact on the ability to adapt to stressful circumstances. These ideas have had such a significant effect on my patients that I wanted to share these insights with others. Increasing cortisol production and the stress response through the consumption of bad fats, food allergens, and high-glycemic-index carbohydrates leads to greater vulnerability to the inevitable stress that accompanies our lives. It is my job as a physician to not only help people recover from illness, but to do everything possible to optimize well-being and reduce the likelihood of chronic disease. Modern research has demonstrated conclusively that one of the greatest risks for developing the major diseases of our time—diabetes, heart disease, cancer, infections, and arthritis—is allostatic load and abnormal stress-hormone levels.

With the breakthroughs in epigenetics, as described in Chapter 9, we know even more about the importance of diet on cortisol and health. Empowering every person to learn to enhance adaptation and preserve a healthy genome through the use of good nutrition and bioactive foods is the ultimate goal of this book. I have presented compelling research about the impact that environmental toxins, including heavy metals and chemicals (POPs), have on the genome and the risk for chronic disease. Though there is little public awareness and almost no government oversight of the epigenetic effects of these toxins, it is possible with the information in this book for every person to make appropriate choices to reduce their toxic load, improve adaptation, and increase the chances for a robustly healthy life and healthier children.

To maintain adaptation and high-level wellness, proper food choices and dietary supplements need to be supported by good self-care. After all, it is estimated that up to 75 percent of medical visits have a stress-related component. Relaxation and adequate rest, meditation techniques, exercise and outdoor time, intimacy and laughter, time with friends and family, a rich spiritual life, healthy expression of emotions and needs, and health-promoting attitudes and behaviors are all part of adaptation and longevity. A detailed discussion of all these areas is beyond the scope of this book; however, all of these areas are critical to maintain adaptation.

Exercise is such an important component of adaptation that it warrants a brief word. When I ask my patients what they do to decrease their stress, most reply that they work out at a gym or do other forms of aerobic exercise, the more intense the better. There certainly is benefit from aerobic exercise, including improved insulin sensitivity and blood-sugar levels, higher HDL cholesterol, lower total cholesterol, better weight management, and improved blood pressure. However, from the perspective of regulating cortisol, this is not always a great solution. In fact, the response to aerobic exercise or weight lifting is a temporary increase in cortisol, which is needed to reduce the inflammation triggered by the workout. This is why so many people who already might be marginal in their adrenal reserve do badly with this type of exercise.

If you feel that the result of an aerobic workout does relax you and doesn't trigger excess fatigue, then stick with it. However, for many people, walking at a brisk pace (three separate ten-minute walks a day has been shown to have tremendous benefit if time does not permit longer walks), low-intensity cycling, or swimming are better cortisol regulators. Better yet are yoga, tai chi, or qigong techniques. These exercises directly improve cortisol function through breathing techniques, slow movement, qi generation, and a feeling of slowing down and grounding. Including one of these ancient arts with a meditation technique that can be done at home is a powerful approach to adaptation.

Beyond diet and exercise, changing the way you manage stress and how you think about stressful situations can have a dramatic adaptive impact. One example of the effect of attitudes on life experience is the quality of optimism. Optimists live longer, stay healthier, and are generally happier. Though optimism is considered a trait that one either possesses or doesn't, it is possible for anyone to adopt the qualities of optimists. Optimists take responsibility for their actions but not for what they can't control. Having a positive view of life events, optimists feel in control of their lives and expect success and happiness to be theirs. They feel they have the ability to fix what is wrong, deal more directly with stress, and eventually overcome difficult situations.

Another key attitude is feeling in control of one's life. Even more than other factors, maintaining a sense of control in a stressful situation can reduce allostatic load and help regain adaptation. The attitude that one can affect the course and destiny of one's life has been shown to improve healthy aging. A belief that difficult situations can be effectively managed reduces feelings of helplessness and hopelessness, leading to lower cortisol levels and improving resistance to many chronic diseases. Control means that you are not at the mercy of circumstances that you can't impact. At the very least, you can control your reaction to a situation.

Simple changes in attitudes like these can go a long way toward adaptation and health. For some of my patients, adopting proper dietary practices was not possible because of underlying issues, such as feeling out of control or being pessimistic. However, eating better brings about less depression and anxiety and empowers people to make the needed changes to maintain health. It is a classic chicken-and-egg phenomenon: poor control of cortisol leads to mental states that prevent some people from making the right choices to improve cortisol regulation, leading to continued allostatic load.

I have presented a very simple way of breaking out of this dilemma. If the first step can be taken by doing the initial elimination and detoxification diet, then in the majority of people there will be an immediate reduction in allostatic load and better cortisol management. This often leads to an improved mental state and a greater chance to make the long-term changes of the Adaptation Diet and succeed in controlling cortisol, losing weight, and increasing longevity.

Through measurement of salivary cortisol in many of my patients, I have been able to track improvement in their allostatic load from the Adaptation Diet. However, I don't think the average person needs to do cortisol testing to know when they are better adapted. As soon as the aches and pains reduce, digestive symptoms disappear, energy improves, and the mood stabilizes, you can be assured that biochemical adaptation is occurring. And as an extra bonus, losing weight generally follows improved adaptation. Reducing stress and cortisol through the Adaptation Diet is a step in maintaining health and aging well. Combining this with other effective self-care approaches is the answer to adaptation and health.

Appendixes

The seven separate appendixes will make it easier to apply the suggestions of the Adaptation Diet. Recipes are included for both the maintenance Adaptation Diet and for specific requirements, including anti-yeast, wheat-free, and rotation diets.

Appendix A: Glycemic Index

The glycemic index is a ranking of foods based on their effect on raising blood-glucose levels. The index compares the level of blood sugar after eating a portion of food with the glucose levels after either straight glucose ingestion or eating a slice of white bread. The impact a food will have on blood-sugar levels depends on other factors as well, including the size of a standard portion, fiber content, and dietary fat levels. The glycemic index is meant to be a guide to food selection to be used in conjunction with other good dietary practices.

Appendix B: Recipes for Phases One and Two of the Adaptation Diet

A graph is included to help organize symptoms that might occur as you change your diet. Symptoms can occur due to withdrawal from food allergens. It is also useful to use this graph to track symptoms when foods are reintroduced during the challenge period of Phase Two.

Also included in this appendix are sample recipes of allowed foods during Phases One and Two of the Adaptation Diet. These recipes are adapted from patient guides by Metagenics®. Feel free to expand on these recipes as long as you adhere to the foods in Table 1 in Chapter 4.

Appendix C: Recipes for Maintenance Phase Three of the Adaptation Diet

Recipes included here are from a variety of sources. Nancy Brown, a skillful nutritionist, has worked with me for many years and kindly offered some menus ideas and recipes. Some of these recipes are from patient handouts designed by Metagenics®. In addition, I have added selected recipes from Mediterranean diets that are widely available online and in multiple books. I have included a large variety of vegetarian recipes that should be used frequently in the Adaptation Diet.

Appendix D: Rotation Diet

For those people who have identified multiple food allergies during the challenge phase, a rotation diet is essential to reduce allostatic load. I have included a sample four-day rotation menu, recipes, and a grocery list, kindly provided by Carol Buuck, as well as food families lists. It is beyond the scope of this book to give all the needed information to be successful at rotating, but the American Academy of Environmental Medicine (see Appendix G) has ample resources to help with this aspect of the diet. Rotation diets strongly regulate cortisol if done correctly.

Appendix E: Wheat-Free Diet

If there is a concern about wheat allergy or gluten intolerance, I have included wheat- and gluten-free recipes. All these recipes are from Nancy Brown, nutrition consultant. If there is a concern about celiac disease, consult your physician before making any dietary changes.

Appendix F: Anti-Yeast Diet

Many of my patients with food allergies and digestive problems do better on a yeast- and wheat-free diet. If you tested positive to yeast in the food challenge or are curious whether you have candida overgrowth, a yeast-free diet will often enhance well-being in a few weeks. Included is the anti-yeast diet I use in my practice and suggestions on yeast-free foods.

Appendix G: Resources

Organizations are listed that maintain referral lists of physicians who practice integrative medicine and would generally approach patient issues with ideas similar to those presented in this book.

A

Glycemic Index

Glycemic Index

Slow Acting	Moderately Acting	Fast Acting
Breads: Barley kernel bread Multigrain bread Rye kernel bread Whole-wheat kernel bread	50% oat bran bread Cracked-wheat kernel bread Whole-grain pumpernickel bread Whole-wheat bread	Bagels Pita bread Rye-flour bread White bread
Breakfast Cereals: All-bran Rice bran	Toasted muesli Oat bran Oatmeal (slow-cooked)	Cheerios Chex Corn flakes Cream of Wheat Grape-nuts Life Nutri-Grain Oatmeal, instant Puffed wheat Shredded wheat
Cereal Grains: Barley Rice, long-grain parboiled Rye, whole-kernel Wheat, whole-kernel	Brown rice Bulgur Corn Cracked barley	Buckwheat Cornmeal Millet Rolled barley White rice
Dairy: Unsweetened low- fat yogurt	Low-fat fruit yogurt	Frozen yogurt
Fruit: Apple Cherries Grapefruit Peach Pear Plum	Apple juice (unsweetened) Apricots, dried Grapes Oranges Pears, canned in juice	Banana Kiwi Mango Orange juice Papaya Peaches, canned in syrup Pineapple Raisins Watermelon

Glycemic Index

Slow Acting	Moderately Acting	Fast Acting

Legumes:
  Baby lima beans
  Chickpeas
  Green beans
  Kidney beans
  Lentils
  Red beans
  Soybeans
  Split peas
	Black-eyed beans
	Chickpeas, canned
	Navy beans
	Pinto beans
	Romano beans
		Baked beans, canned
		Broad beans
		Green beans, canned

Pasta:
  Fettuccine, egg
    enriched
  Spaghetti, protein
    enriched
  Spaghetti, whole
    meal
	Capellini,
	  whole-grain
	Macaroni,
	  whole-grain
	Spaghetti,
	  whole-grain
		Macaroni and
		  cheese (boxed)
		Rice pasta, brown
		Spaghetti

Root Vegetables:
  Radishes
  Turnips
	Beets
	Carrots
	Rutabagas
	Sweet potatoes
	Yam
		French fries
		Instant potatoes
		New potatoes
		Parsnips
		Russet potatoes
		Sweet potatoes

Snack Foods:
  Almonds
  Peanuts
  Walnuts
		Cookies
		Corn chips
		Crackers
		Jelly beans
		Life Savers
		Mars bars
		Muesli bars
		Popcorn
		Potato chips

Soups: Tomato	Lentil, canned	Black bean, canned Green pea, canned
Sugars: Fructose	Lactose	Glucose Honey Maltose Sucrose

Glycemic Index

Slow Acting	Moderately Acting	Fast Acting

Vegetables:
  Artichokes
  Asparagus
  Broccolis
  Cauliflowers
  Cucumbers
  Dark leafy greens
  Zucchinis
	Green peas
	Tomatoes
		Pumpkin
		Sweet corn

B

Recipes for Phases One and Two of the Adaptation Diet

T his is a sample graph that can be used to track symptoms due to withdrawal of food allergens from the diet. It can also be used when these foods are reintroduced during the challenge period of Phase Two.

Symptom Chart

Instructions: Please grade the severity of your symptoms each day from 0 (none) to 10 (very severe).

Name:_____ Date:_____

Weight before starting: morning _____ evening_____

Weight Day 10:   morning _____ evening_____

Symptoms	Before	Day 1	Day 2	Day 3	Day 4	Day 5	Day 6	Day 7	Day 8	Day 9	Day 10
Headache											
Nausea											
Vomiting											
Abdominal pain											
Diarrhea											
Lousy											
Depression											
Irritability											
Insomnia											
Lethargy											
Backache											
Aching limbs											
Restless legs											
Morning resting pulse											

Sample Recipes for Phase One and Phase Two

(See page 27 for a list of allowed foods.)

Beans and Greens Soup

(serves 4-5)

> 2 tablespoons olive oil
> 1 large onion, chopped
> 2 medium cloves garlic, crushed
> 1–2 stalks celery, diced
> 1–2 medium carrots, diced
> 1 teaspoon salt
> Black pepper to taste
> 5 cups water or vegetable broth
> 1 bay leaf
> 2 cups cooked white beans
> ½ pound fresh chopped mixed greens: kale, collards, spinach, and escarole
> Freshly grated nutmeg

In a saucepan, add oil and sauté the onions and garlic over low heat. When onions are soft, add celery, carrot, salt, and pepper. Stir and sauté another 5 minutes. Add broth or water and bay leaf. Cover and simmer about 20 minutes. Add cooked beans and greens. Cover and continue to simmer, over very low heat, another 15–20 minutes. Garnish as desired with grated nutmeg.

Kasha

(serves 2)

> 1 teaspoon olive oil
> ¼ cup chopped onion
> 1 celery stick, diced
> ½ cup uncooked kasha (buckwheat groats)
> 1 cup water
> Salt and pepper to taste

Sauté onion and celery in oil. Add buckwheat grouts and water and bring to boil. Reduce heat and simmer 20 minutes. Season with salt and pepper as desired.

Vegetable Dal Curry

(serves 2)

> 1 teaspoon olive oil
> ¼ cup chopped onion
> 1 teaspoon turmeric powder
> ¼ teaspoon coriander powder
> Dash cumin
> 1 sliced carrot
> 1 cup cauliflower pieces
> ⅓ cup red lentils
> 1 cup water
> Salt to taste

Heat olive oil and add onion, turmeric powder, coriander powder, and cumin. Sauté. Add carrot and cauliflower; stir to coat. Add lentils and water. Bring to a boil, reduce heat, and simmer about 40 minutes. Add salt to taste.

Ratatouille

(serves 6)

> ½ cup olive oil
> 2 large onions, sliced
> 3 garlic cloves, minced
> 1 medium eggplant, cut into 1-inch cubes
> 2 green bell peppers, chopped
> 3 zucchini, cut into ½-inch slices
> 1 28-ounce can whole tomatoes, drained
> 1 teaspoon salt
> ¼ teaspoon pepper
> 1 teaspoon oregano
> ½ teaspoon thyme

In a 6-quart pot, sauté onion and garlic in oil for 3 minutes. Add eggplant and stir-fry for 5 minutes. Add peppers and cook 5 minutes. Add zucchini and cook for 5 more minutes. Add tomatoes and seasonings. Cover and simmer for 30 minutes.

Rice/Oat Pancakes

(serves 4-5)

1½ cups rice milk
1½ tablespoons lemon juice
1½ cups rice flour
½ cup oat flour
½ teaspoon salt
2 teaspoons baking powder
½ teaspoon baking soda
1 tablespoon apple butter
1 tablespoon cold-pressed safflower oil
Egg substitute to equal 2 eggs

Mix rice milk and lemon juice together and allow to sit for 5 minutes until curds form. Mix dry ingredients together and set aside. In large mixing bowl, beat apple butter, oil, egg, and milk mixture. Add dry mixture and stir gently. Be careful not to overmix. Makes approximately 14 (4-inch) pancakes.

Cauliflower Salad

(serves 10-12)

1 small head cauliflower
3–4 cloves garlic, minced
½ cup chopped pecans
1 tablespoon olive oil (for sautéing)
2 tablespoons olive oil (for dressing)
2 tablespoons flaxseed oil
2 tablespoons vinegar
2 tablespoons each freshly snipped parsley and chives
Salt and pepper to taste

Cut cauliflower into medium-sized florets, and lightly steam. Meanwhile, sauté garlic and pecans in 1 tablespoon olive oil over very low heat until slightly brown. Mix with remaining oils, vinegar, parsley, and chives. In a large bowl, mix cauliflower together and toss with garlic/pecan mixture. Add salt and pepper to taste. Flavor is enhanced the longer this salad sits.

Lentil Salad

(serves 4)

⅔ cup uncooked lentils, well rinsed
1 bay leaf
2 cups water
1 tablespoon chopped fresh basil or 1 teaspoon dried basil
¼ cup finely diced red or green onions
1 whole carrot, grated
¼ cup finely chopped black olives
¼ cup raisins or currants

Simmer lentils and bay leaf in water for about 25 minutes or until tender. Drain and discard bay leaf. In a large bowl, gently toss lentils with basil, onions, grated carrot, chopped olives, and raisins or currants. Mix in Basic Salad and Veggie Dressing (see recipe below) to taste. Gently toss and serve slightly chilled or at room temperature.

Semi-Greek Salad

(serves 4)

3 cups mixed greens
½ cup carrot, shredded
½ cup cabbage, shredded
½ cup green onions, shredded
1 cup cooked garbanzo beans
Few sliced black olives
Few red onion ringlets

Toss together all ingredients. Mix in Basic Salad and Veggie Dressing (see recipe below), making sure to add dry mustard, and toss with greens and veggies.

Basic Salad and Veggie Dressing

(serves 6)

¼ cup each flaxseed and olive oils

3–4 tablespoons vinegar (apple cider, tarragon, rice, red wine, balsamic, or ume plum)

1 tablespoon water

Garlic, whole cloves or minced

Oregano, basil, or other herbs of choice to taste

1 teaspoon dry mustard (optional) whisked into liquid

Mix all ingredients together well in a shaker jar. (Store any leftovers in refrigerator—dressing will solidify in the fridge.)

Oat Bran Muffins

(serves 8)

¾ cup almond milk

1 tablespoon lemon juice

½ cup oat bran

1¾ cups whole oats

1 teaspoon baking powder

½ teaspoon baking soda

¼ teaspoon salt

¼ cup chopped walnuts or almonds

¾ cup unsweetened applesauce

½ cup dates or dried apples

Preheat oven to 400°. Spray muffin cups with oil and set aside. Combine almond milk and lemon juice in a cup and allow to set about 10 minutes or until curds form. Combine dry ingredients in a large bowl. Add almond milk/lemon juice combination and applesauce, mixing gently with a spoon until completely moistened. Stir in dried fruit but do not overmix. Spoon into prepared muffin tin, filling about ¾ full. Bake 20–25 minutes until lightly browned. Allow to cool for 10 minutes before removing from pan.

Split Pea Soup

(serves 6)

    3 cups dry split peas
    2 quarts water
    1 bay leaf
    2 onions, finely chopped
    4 cloves garlic, minced
    3 stalks celery, diced
    2 medium carrots, sliced
    Salt and black pepper to taste
    3 tablespoons apple cider or rice vinegar

Place all ingredients, except for salt, pepper, and cider or vinegar, in Dutch oven. Bring to boil and lower heat to simmer partially covered for about 60 minutes, stirring occasionally. Add more water as needed. Add salt, pepper, and cider or vinegar to taste.

Quinoa Vegetable Soup

(serves 4-6)

    ¼ cup quinoa (well rinsed)
    ½ cup carrots, diced
    ¼ cup celery, diced
    2 tablespoons onion, chopped
    ¼ cup green bell pepper, diced
    2 cloves garlic, chopped
    1 teaspoon olive oil
    4 cups water
    ½ cup tomatoes, chopped
    ½ cup cabbage, chopped
    1 teaspoon salt
    Parsley

Sauté quinoa, carrots, celery, onions, green bell pepper, and garlic in oil until golden brown. Add water, tomatoes, and cabbage and bring to a boil. Simmer 20–30 minutes or until tender. Season with salt to taste and garnish with parsley.

For variations, try adding some of your other favorite vegetables, chopped and sautéed.

Millet Pâté

(serves 4)

½ cup cooked millet

½ cup silken extra-firm tofu

¼ cup carrot, grated

1 tablespoon tahini

1½ tablespoons light yellow miso

3 tablespoons nutritional yeast

⅛ teaspoon each celery seed and savory

Place all ingredients in a bowl and mix well. Serve as a spread on rice cakes.

Stir-Fry Vegetables and Chicken

(serves 2)

1 teaspoon sesame oil

2 teaspoons fresh ginger, grated

Any combination of the following vegetables:

2 carrots, diced

1 stalk celery, diced

1 cup bok choy, chopped

½ cup diced onion

½ cup chopped broccoli and/or cauliflower

½ cup snow peas

¼ cup mung bean sprouts

3 ounces boneless organic chicken, cut into strips or cubes

Freshly chopped basil to taste (optional)

1 teaspoon flaxseed oil

Heat sesame oil and ginger in a wok and stir-fry your choice of vegetables for about 5 minutes. Add chicken pieces and continue to stir-fry until cooked through. If desired, add freshly chopped basil just before removing from heat. Add flaxseed oil upon completion of cooking. Serve with Pecan Rice (see recipe below).

Pecan Rice

(serves 4)

> 2½ cups water
> 1 cup wild and brown rice mix
> 2 tablespoons chopped pecans
> 1 teaspoon walnut or olive oil

Bring water to a boil and add rice, stirring to mix well. Cover and simmer rice for about 45 minutes or until all liquid has been absorbed. Do not stir while cooking. While rice is cooking, sauté pecans in oil over low heat until lightly browned. Toss pecan mixture with cooked rice and serve immediately.

Sassy Beans

(serves 1)

> 1 teaspoon olive oil
> 1 tablespoon chopped scallions
> 1 clove garlic, minced
> ½ cup chopped onion
> ½ cup vegetarian refried beans
> ¼ cup cilantro, chopped (optional)
> Chopped black olives (optional)
> ¼ avocado (optional)

Sauté scallions, garlic, and onion in olive oil. Add refried beans. Remove from heat. If desired, garnish with cilantro, black olives, and avocado. Serve with Pecan Rice (see recipe above).

C

Recipes for Maintenance

*Phase Three of the
Adaptation Diet*

Vegan Roasted Red Pepper Hummus (*V)

(serves 6-8)

> 1 15-ounce can chickpeas (garbanzo beans), drained
> 1 roasted red pepper (see note below)
> 3 tablespoons lemon juice
> ½ tablespoon sesame tahini
> 1 clove garlic, minced
> ½ teaspoon ground cumin
> ½ teaspoon red chili powder or cayenne pepper
> Kosher salt to taste
> Extra-virgin olive oil (optional)

Purée chickpeas, roasted red pepper, lemon juice, sesame tahini, garlic, cumin, and red chili powder together in a blender or food processor. The mixture should be thick and smooth but grainy. Add kosher salt to taste. If serving as dip, drizzle with olive oil before serving.

Note: For the roasted red pepper, buy them canned (or in a jar) or simply grill or broil them until black on each side. Once they cool, the blackened outside simply rubs off.

Summer Chicken Salad with Garden Herbs

(serves 6-8)

> 1 3½-pound whole chicken
> Water
> ¼ cup chopped fresh chives
> 3 tablespoons white or red wine vinegar

2 tablespoons capers
2 tablespoons thyme
1 teaspoon oregano
4 teaspoons extra-virgin olive oil
½ teaspoon salt, preferably sea salt
½ teaspoon freshly ground pepper
2 cloves garlic, minced

Place chicken in a stockpot; cover with water and bring to a boil. Reduce heat and simmer 50 minutes or until tender. Drain, reserving broth for another use. Cool chicken completely, then remove skin from chicken and discard. Remove chicken from bones and discard bones and fat. Chop chicken into bite-sized pieces.

Combine chives and remaining ingredients in a large bowl. Add chicken; toss well to coat.

Note: To save 50 minutes of cooking time, just stop by the grocery store and pick up a chicken that's already roasted. This is a huge time-saver and delicious too.

Mediterranean Chicken and Rice Bake

(serves 6)

1¾ cups chicken broth
¼ cup chopped fresh parsley
¼ cup sliced pitted ripe olives
1 tablespoon lemon juice
¼ teaspoon ground black pepper
1 can (about 14½ ounces) stewed tomatoes
1¼ cups uncooked regular long-grain brown rice
6 skinless, boneless chicken breasts
½ teaspoon garlic powder
Paprika

Mix broth, parsley, olives, lemon juice, black pepper, tomatoes, and rice in 3-quart shallow baking dish. Cover. Bake at 375° for 20 minutes.

Top with chicken. Sprinkle with garlic powder and paprika. Bake an additional 30 minutes or until chicken and rice are done.

Grilled Salmon with Mustard and Herbs

(serves 3-4)

2 lemons, thinly sliced, plus 1 lemon cut into wedges for garnish
20–30 sprigs mixed fresh herbs
1 clove garlic
¼ teaspoon salt
1 tablespoon Dijon mustard
2 tablespoons chopped mixed herbs
1 pound center-cut salmon, skinned (see Tip)

Preheat grill to medium-high.

Lay two 9-inch pieces of heavy-duty foil on top of each other and place on a rimless baking sheet. Arrange lemon slices in two layers in the center of the foil. Spread herb sprigs over the lemons. With the side of a chef's knife, mash garlic with salt to form a paste. Transfer to a small dish and stir in the mustard and chopped mixed herbs. Spread the mixture over both sides of the salmon. Place the salmon on the herb sprigs.

Slide the foil and salmon off the baking sheet onto the grill without disturbing the salmon/lemon stack. Cover the grill; cook until the salmon is opaque in the center, 18 to 24 minutes. Wearing oven mitts, carefully transfer foil and salmon back onto the baking sheet. Cut the salmon into 4 portions and serve with lemon wedges (discard herb sprigs and lemon slices).

Tip: To skin a salmon fillet, place salmon fillet on a clean cutting board, skin-side down. Starting at the tail end, slip the blade of a long knife between the fish flesh and the skin, holding down firmly with your other hand. Gently push the blade along at a 30° angle, separating the fillet from the skin without cutting through either.

Asian Gazpacho (*V)

(serves 6)

6 tomatoes, seeded and finely chopped, or 1 28-ounce can chopped tomatoes

2 cups vegetable broth

1 teaspoon dry sherry

2 tablespoons fresh cilantro, chopped

1 tablespoon light soy sauce

4 scallions, white part only

4 thin slivers of fresh ginger

¼–½ teaspoon Chinese chili sauce, to taste

2 limes

Place the tomatoes in a 2- or 3-quart saucepan, over low heat. Add the vegetable broth, sherry, cilantro, soy sauce, scallions, and ginger. Bring the mixture to a simmer and cook for 20 minutes. Remove from the heat and allow to cool for a few minutes. Purée in a food processor or blender. Chill. Just before serving, stir in chili sauce. Grate the peel of one lime and add to the soup. Squeeze the juice from both of the limes into the soup.

Creamy Cold Tomato Soup (*V)

(serves 5)

1 cucumber, chopped

1 scallion, chopped

1 clove garlic

4 cups tomato juice

1 green bell pepper, chopped

½ teaspoon dill weed

Salt and pepper to taste

1 cup plain yogurt

Sliced mushrooms or tomato chunks for garnish

Combine the first six ingredients, put small amounts at a time in blender, and blend until smooth. Use salt sparingly, if needed, and add pepper. Whisk in yogurt. Chill several hours before serving and garnish as desired with mushrooms or tomatoes.

Hummus Wrap (*V)

(serves 1)

2 small or 1 large low-carb tortilla(s)
¼ cup hummus
8–10 cherry tomatoes
¼ avocado, slivered

Spread 2 tablespoons hummus on each tortilla. Top with 4–5 cherry tomatoes on each and garnish with slivers of avocado.

Cold Salmon with Raita

(serves 8)

2 pounds salmon fillets (about 1½ inches thick)
1–2 tablespoons olive oil

Preheat oven to 275°. Place salmon skin-side down in ovenproof pan. Brush with olive oil. Roast uncovered until salmon flakes with a fork, about 25–30 minutes. Do not allow it to overcook. Serve at room temperature. Can make a day ahead and refrigerate, but bring to room temperature before serving. Serve topped with Raita (see recipe below).

Raita

(serves 8)

1 cucumber, chopped into small dice
1 medium carrot, grated
¼ cup chopped onion
1 tomato, chopped into small dice
⅛ teaspoon salt
1 cup plain, low-fat yogurt
2–3 tablespoons chopped fresh cilantro or mint or 1 teaspoon
    ground cumin (optional)

In a mixing bowl, mix cucumbers, carrots, onions, and tomatoes with salt and allow to sit for 15–30 minutes. Drain well. Combine with yogurt and optional ingredient, if desired. Chill for 20 minutes. Serve with salmon.

Crustless Vegetable Quiche (*V)

(serves 8)

5 eggs

½ cup nonfat or 1 percent low-fat milk

12 ounces (¾ cup) nonfat or low-fat cottage cheese

½ cup part-skim mozzarella cheese, grated

10 ounces frozen chopped broccoli, thawed

10 ounces frozen chopped spinach, thawed

1 tablespoon olive oil

½ teaspoon salt

¼ teaspoon freshly ground pepper

Beat eggs in a medium-sized bowl. Add milk and beat some more. Add remaining ingredients and stir vigorously to blend. Pour into a deep, lightly oiled casserole, and place it in a 9 × 13-inch pan filled partway with hot water. Bake in a 375° oven for about 35–45 minutes, or until a knife, inserted into center of the quiche, comes out clean.

Fish Creole

(serves 4)

1 tablespoon olive oil

1 onion, chopped

½ cup thin-sliced celery

¼ cup green bell pepper, chopped

1 garlic clove, minced

2 tablespoons fresh parsley or 2 teaspoons dried parsley

1 bay leaf

¼ teaspoon rosemary, chopped

1 28-ounce can tomatoes with liquid

1 pound fish fillets

2 cups cooked brown rice

Heat oil in a large saucepan and lightly sauté the onion, celery, pepper, and garlic until soft. Add parsley, bay leaf, rosemary, and tomatoes. Simmer, uncovered, about 20 minutes. Add fish fillets in small pieces and simmer until cooked through, about 5–10 minutes more. Remove bay leaf. Serve over brown rice.

Grilled Leg of Lamb

(serves 4 per pound)

2 cups red wine

2 teaspoons poultry seasoning

1 teaspoon salt

3 cloves garlic, cut in slivers

1 leg of lamb (boned and butterflied by butcher)

Mix red wine, poultry seasoning, salt, and garlic. Pour mixture over leg of lamb, and place in covered container in the refrigerator to marinate for 12–24 hours.

Grill over hot coals approximately 20 minutes on each side. Baste occasionally while grilling. This is a delicious replacement for steak!

Lentil-Barley Stew (*V)

(serves 8)

2 tablespoons olive oil

4 medium carrots, diced

2 medium leeks (with 3 inches of green left on), diced

2 celery stalks, diced

2 medium zucchini, diced

1 large onion, diced

2 garlic cloves, minced

1 cup dried lentils, rinsed

½ cup barley

1 teaspoon dried thyme

6–8 cups chicken or vegetable broth

2 cups diced tomatoes

1 cup chopped fresh basil leaves

Salt and pepper to taste

½ cup chopped parsley

Heat olive oil in a large, heavy pot and add carrots, leeks, celery, zucchini, onion, and garlic. Cook over low heat, stirring occasionally, for about 10 minutes until vegetables have softened. Add lentils, barley, thyme, and 6 cups broth. Bring to a boil and reduce heat to a simmer. Cook uncovered about 30 minutes, stirring often. Add remaining 2 cups of broth as needed if dry. Add tomatoes and basil, and salt and pepper to taste; cook 10 more minutes. Stir in parsley and serve.

Mango Salmon

(serves 6)

2 teaspoons tamari or regular soy sauce

1 tablespoon fresh ginger, minced

1 cinnamon stick (3 inches)

1 teaspoon rice or cider vinegar

1 10-ounce bottle mango nectar

1 teaspoon olive oil

6 salmon fillets, 5 ounces each and 1 inch thick

In a small saucepan, stir together the first five ingredients. Bring to boil, reduce heat, and simmer uncovered for 20–25 minutes or until reduced to about ¾ cup. Pour mixture through a strainer and discard the solids. Return mixture to saucepan and keep warm.

Brush olive oil on broiler pan, place salmon on pan, and broil 5 inches away from heat for 5 minutes. Brush salmon with mango mixture and broil 3 more minutes or until fish flakes with a fork. Serve immediately and allow individuals to garnish salmon with remaining mango mixture as desired.

Roasted Salmon or Red Snapper with Salsa

(serves 8)

4 salmon or red snapper fillets, 8 ounces each

4 teaspoons olive oil

1 tablespoon fresh lime juice

1 tablespoon fresh cilantro, chopped

Salt and pepper to taste

Preheat oven to 400°. Brush 1 teaspoon olive oil on a baking sheet and place fish skin-side down. Combine remaining olive oil, lime juice, and cilantro; brush on each fillet. Sprinkle with salt and pepper to taste. Allow to sit for 15 minutes, then bake for 20 minutes or until just cooked. Garnish with Salsa (see recipe below) and serve immediately.

Salsa

(serves 1)

2 large tomatoes, diced
2 scallions, chopped
1 tablespoon cilantro, chopped
1 clove garlic, chopped
1 tablespoon olive oil
2 teaspoons fresh lime juice

Combine in a bowl.

Spaghetti Squash Topped with Ratatouille (*V)
(serves 6)

One medium spaghetti squash, halved with seeds removed

Place squash cut-side up in an ovenproof dish with ½-inch water and cover with foil. Bake at 375° for about 40 minutes or until easily pierced with a fork. Do not overbake. When squash is cool enough to handle, scrape with a fork to release spaghetti-like strands. Top with Ratatouille (see recipe below).

Ratatouille (*V)
(serves 6)

¼ cup olive oil
2 large onions, sliced
3 garlic cloves, minced
1 medium eggplant, cut into 1-inch cubes
2 green bell peppers, chopped
3 zucchini, cut into ½-inch slices
1 28-ounce can tomatoes, drained (fresh, ripe tomatoes may be substituted when available)

1 teaspoon salt
¼ teaspoon pepper
1 teaspoon oregano
½ teaspoon thyme

In a 6-quart pot, sauté onion and garlic in 1 tablespoon oil for 3 minutes. Add 1 tablespoon oil and eggplant and stir-fry for 5 minutes. Add another tablespoon oil and the peppers and cook 5 minutes. Add the last tablespoon oil and the zucchini; cook for 5 more minutes. Then add tomatoes and seasonings; cover and simmer for 30 minutes. Use to top spaghetti squash or as a vegetable side dish.

Stir-Fried Tofu with Ginger Broccoli (*V)

(serves 4)

1 pound extra-firm tofu
2 tablespoons tamari (low-sodium soy sauce)
2 tablespoons olive oil
2 teaspoons fresh ginger, peeled and minced
2 garlic cloves, minced
1 tablespoon arrowroot or cornstarch
1 tablespoon dry sherry
½ teaspoon cayenne or ¼ teaspoon hot-pepper flakes
2 cups broccoli florets
2 cups mushrooms, sliced
1 red bell pepper, cut into thin strips
¼ cup water
1 teaspoon sesame oil
Salt and pepper to taste

Slice tofu into cubes. Toss with tamari soy sauce and set aside for 5–10 minutes. In a wok or large nonstick skillet, heat 1 tablespoon oil over high heat. When oil is hot, lower heat to medium-high and add ginger and garlic; stir-fry for 30 seconds. Drain tofu, reserving tamari, and add tofu to the wok, stir-frying for 2 more minutes. Remove tofu mixture from wok and set aside.

Using a fork or small whisk, mix reserved tamari with arrowroot or cornstarch, sherry, and cayenne in a small bowl. Set aside.

Heat another 1 tablespoon oil in wok over high heat. Add broccoli, mushrooms, and bell pepper, and stir-fry for 2 minutes. Add ¼ cup water and bring to boil. Cover wok and reduce heat to medium, steaming vegetables about 5 minutes until slightly tender. Return tofu mixture to wok.

Stir reserved tamari mixture into wok, and cook over medium heat until thickened and thoroughly heated; do not overcook vegetables. Add sesame oil, and salt and pepper to taste, and adjust seasonings if you desire a spicier dish. Serve immediately or make ahead and refrigerate until ready to serve. Reheat carefully; flavors are enhanced when the dish sits overnight.

Tofu/Vegetable Stir-Fry (*V)

(serves 4)

> 1 tablespoon sesame oil
> 1 clove garlic, chopped
> 1 tablespoon fresh ginger, grated or chopped
> 2 cups any combination of chopped vegetables, such as bok choy, celery, bean sprouts, Napa cabbage, or blanched broccoli or cauliflower
> 1 cup fresh mushrooms, sliced
> 1 red bell pepper, cut into strips
> 2–4 tablespoons tamari (soy sauce)
> 1 14-ounce package firm tofu, drained and cubed
> 2 cups cooked brown rice

Heat oil in wok over high heat; add garlic and ginger and stir constantly until lightly browned. Add vegetables and cook for 3 or 4 minutes, depending on crispness desired. Add tamari and cubed tofu; cook an additional minute; remove from heat. Serve over brown rice.

Turkey-Bulgur Skillet

(serves 4)

1 pound ground turkey or ¾ pound cubed tofu
1 medium onion, chopped
1 clove garlic, minced
1 cup uncooked bulgur wheat
1 16-ounce can tomatoes, including juice
1 cup water
¼ teaspoon marjoram
½ teaspoon thyme
2 bay leaves
1½ cups frozen peas, defrosted
Salt and pepper to taste

In a large, heavy skillet over medium heat, sauté turkey, onion, and garlic until onion is softened. Drain off excess fat. Add bulgur and cook for 1 minute more. Stir in tomatoes, water, and spices. Cover and simmer for 20 minutes, stirring occasionally to break up tomatoes. Add peas, and salt and pepper to taste.

Vegetarian option: Omit turkey and sauté the onion and garlic in 2 teaspoons olive oil. Add ¾ pound cubed tofu to the skillet along with the bulgur.

Turkey Chili

(serves 8)

2 pounds ground turkey
2 16-ounce cans tomatoes, cut up (undrained)
2 15-ounce cans red kidney beans, drained
1 8-ounce can tomato sauce
1 medium onion, chopped
¼ cup dry red wine (optional)
1 teaspoon dried parsley flakes
¾ teaspoon dried basil, crushed
¾ teaspoon dried oregano, crushed
½ teaspoon black pepper

½ teaspoon ground cinnamon
1 clove garlic, minced
¼–½ teaspoon ground red pepper
1–2 tablespoons chili powder
1 bay leaf

In a 4-quart Dutch oven, cook the turkey until it is no longer pink. Drain off fat. Stir in undrained tomatoes, drained kidney beans, tomato sauce, onion, wine (if desired), and spices. Simmer uncovered for 45 minutes, stirring occasionally.

Vegetarian option: Omit turkey and add 2 cups cauliflower pieces, 1 large chopped potato, 1 chopped green bell pepper, 2 chopped carrots, ½ pound chopped mushrooms, and 3 cups fresh or frozen corn kernels to the ingredients listed above. Bring mixture to a boil. Simmer uncovered until vegetables are tender, about 30 minutes.

Mediterranean Fish Fillets

(serves 2)

1 teaspoon extra-virgin olive oil
1 small onion, thinly sliced
2 tablespoons dry white wine
1 clove garlic, finely chopped
1 cup canned diced tomatoes
4 Kalamata olives, pitted and chopped
⅛ teaspoon dried oregano
⅛ teaspoon freshly grated orange zest
¼ teaspoon salt, divided
¼ teaspoon freshly ground pepper, divided
8 ounces thick-cut, firm-fleshed fish fillets, such as Pacific halibut or mahi-mahi

Preheat oven to 450°. Heat oil in a medium nonstick skillet over medium-high heat. Add onion and cook, stirring often, until lightly browned, 2–4 minutes. Add wine and garlic and simmer for 30 seconds. Stir in tomatoes, olives, oregano, and orange zest. Season with ⅛ teaspoon salt and ⅛ teaspoon pepper.

Season fish with the remaining ⅛ teaspoon each salt and pepper. Arrange the fish in a single layer in a pie pan or baking dish. Spoon the tomato mixture over the fish. Bake, uncovered, until the fish is just cooked through, 10–20 minutes. Divide the fish into 2 portions and serve with sauce.

Mediterranean Lamb Salad

(serves 6)

> 1 pound boneless leg of lamb steaks, 1–1½ inches thick
> 1½ teaspoons kosher salt, divided
> Freshly ground pepper to taste
> 2 medium cucumbers, peeled, halved, seeded, and diced
> 2 large tomatoes, diced
> 1 15-ounce can chickpeas, rinsed
> ½ cup minced red onion
> ¼ cup crumbled feta cheese
> ¼ cup sliced fresh mint leaves
> ¼ cup lemon juice
> 1 teaspoon extra-virgin olive oil

Preheat grill to high. Sprinkle lamb with ½ teaspoon salt, and pepper to taste. Grill the lamb for 2–4 minutes per side for medium, depending on the thickness of the steaks. Transfer to a cutting board and let rest for at least 5 minutes before thinly slicing across the grain.

Meanwhile, place cucumbers, tomatoes, chickpeas, onion, feta cheese, and mint in a large bowl. Add lemon juice, oil, the remaining 1 teaspoon salt, and more pepper to taste; stir to combine. Serve topped with the sliced lamb.

Middle Eastern Chickpea and Rice Stew

(serves 6)

> 1 tablespoon extra-virgin olive oil
> 3 medium onions, halved and thinly sliced (about 3 cups)
> 2 teaspoons ground cumin
> 2 teaspoons ground coriander

1 cup orange juice

4 cups reduced-sodium chicken broth or vegetable broth

2 15-ounce cans chickpeas, rinsed

3 cups peeled and diced sweet potato (about 1 pound)

⅔ cup brown basmati rice

¼ teaspoon salt

¼ teaspoon freshly ground pepper

½ cup fresh cilantro, chopped

Heat oil in a large saucepan over medium heat; add onions and cook, stirring often, until tender and well browned, 10–12 minutes. Add cumin and coriander and stir for about 15 seconds. Add orange juice and broth. Stir in chickpeas, sweet potato, rice, and salt. Bring to a boil; reduce heat to a gentle simmer and cover. Cook, stirring occasionally, until the rice is tender and the sweet potatoes are breaking down to thicken the liquid, about 45 minutes. Season with pepper. (The stew will be thick and will thicken further upon standing. Add more broth to thin, if desired, or when reheating.) Serve topped with cilantro.

Mustard-Crusted Salmon

(serves 4)

1¼ pounds center-cut salmon fillets, cut into 4 portions

¼ teaspoon salt, or to taste

Freshly ground pepper to taste

¼ cup reduced-fat sour cream

2 tablespoons stone-ground mustard

2 teaspoons lemon juice

Lemon wedges

Preheat broiler. Line a broiler pan or baking sheet with foil, then coat it with cooking spray. Place salmon pieces, skin-side down, on the prepared pan. Season with salt and pepper. Combine sour cream, mustard, and lemon juice in a small bowl. Spread evenly over the salmon.

Broil the salmon 5 inches from the heat source until it is opaque in the center, 10–12 minutes. Serve with lemon wedges.

Roasted Cod with Warm Tomato-Olive-Caper Tapenade

(serves 4)

> 1 pound cod fillet
> 3 teaspoons extra-virgin olive oil, divided
> ¼ teaspoon freshly ground pepper
> 1 tablespoon shallot, minced
> 1 cup cherry tomatoes, halved
> ¼ cup cured olives, chopped
> 1 tablespoon capers, rinsed and chopped
> 1½ teaspoons fresh oregano, chopped
> 1 teaspoon balsamic vinegar

Preheat oven to 450°. Coat a baking sheet with cooking spray. Rub cod with 2 teaspoons oil. Sprinkle with pepper. Place on the prepared baking sheet. Transfer to the oven and roast until the fish flakes easily with a fork, 15–20 minutes, depending on the thickness of the fillet.

Meanwhile, heat the remaining 1 teaspoon oil in a small skillet over medium heat. Add shallot and cook, stirring, until it begins to soften, about 20 seconds. Add tomatoes and cook, stirring, until softened, about 1½ minutes. Add olives and capers; cook, stirring, for 30 seconds more. Stir in oregano and vinegar; remove from heat. Spoon the tapenade over the cod before serving.

Seafood Couscous Paella

(serves 2)

> 2 teaspoons extra-virgin olive oil
> 1 medium onion, chopped
> 1 clove garlic, minced
> ½ teaspoon dried thyme
> ½ teaspoon fennel seed
> ¼ teaspoon salt
> ¼ teaspoon freshly ground pepper
> Pinch of crumbled saffron threads

1 cup no-salt-added diced tomatoes, with juice
¼ cup vegetable broth
4 ounces bay scallops, tough muscle removed
4 ounces small shrimp (41–50 per pound), peeled and de-veined
½ cup whole-wheat couscous

Heat oil in a large saucepan over medium heat. Add onion; cook, stirring constantly, for 3 minutes. Add garlic, thyme, fennel seed, salt, pepper, and saffron; cook for 20 seconds.

Stir in tomatoes and broth. Bring to a simmer. Cover, reduce heat, and simmer for 2 minutes.

Increase heat to medium, stir in scallops, and cook, stirring occasionally, for 2 minutes. Add shrimp and cook, stirring occasionally, for 2 minutes more. Stir in couscous. Cover, remove from heat, and let stand for 5 minutes; fluff.

Spiced Turkey with Avocado-Grapefruit Relish
(serves 2)

Avocado-Grapefruit Relish
1 large seedless grapefruit
½ small avocado, peeled, pitted, and diced
1 small shallot, minced
1 tablespoon fresh cilantro, chopped
1 teaspoon red wine vinegar
1 teaspoon honey

Spiced Turkey
1 tablespoon chili powder
½ teaspoon Chinese five-spice powder
⅛ teaspoon salt
2 turkey cutlets (8 ounces)
1 tablespoon canola oil

To prepare relish: Remove the peel and white pith from grapefruit with a sharp knife and discard. Cut the grapefruit segments from the surrounding membrane, letting them drop into a small bowl. Squeeze out remaining juice into the bowl and discard membrane. Add avocado, shallot, cilantro, vinegar, and honey. Toss well to combine.

To prepare turkey: Combine chili powder, five-spice powder, and salt on a plate. Dredge turkey in the spice mixture.

Heat oil in a medium skillet over medium-high heat. Add the turkey and cook until no longer pink in the middle, about 2–3 minutes per side. Serve the turkey with the avocado-grapefruit relish.

Butternut Squash Pilaf (*V)

(serves 8)

2 pounds butternut squash, peeled, halved, and seeded
3 tablespoons extra-virgin olive oil
1 large red onion, finely chopped
1 clove garlic, minced
2 tablespoons water
1 tablespoon tomato paste
1 cup instant or parboiled brown rice
1¾ cups water or 1 14-ounce can vegetable broth
½ cup white wine
½ cup fennel fronds, chopped
2 tablespoons fresh oregano, chopped
1 teaspoon salt
Pinch of cinnamon
Freshly ground pepper to taste

Grate the squash through the large holes of a box grater.

Heat oil in a large cast-iron or nonstick skillet over medium-low heat. Add onion and garlic and cook, stirring, until soft and lightly colored, 10–12 minutes. Combine 2 tablespoons water and tomato paste in a small bowl and stir it into the pan. Add rice and stir to coat. Add the squash, in batches if necessary, and stir until it has reduced in volume enough so that you can cover the pan.

Increase the heat to medium-high, pour in 1¾ cups water (or broth) and wine, cover, and bring to a boil. Reduce the heat to medium-low and cook, covered, stirring once or twice, until the rice has absorbed most of the liquid and the squash is tender, 25–30 minutes.

Add fennel fronds, oregano, salt, cinnamon, and pepper; gently stir to combine. Remove from heat and let stand, covered, for 5 minutes. Serve hot or at room temperature.

Lima Bean Spread with Cumin and Herbs (*V)

(serves 6-8)

1 10-ounce package frozen lima beans
4 cloves garlic, crushed and peeled
¼ teaspoon red pepper, crushed
2 tablespoons extra-virgin olive oil
4 teaspoons lemon juice
1 teaspoon ground cumin
½ teaspoon salt, or to taste
Freshly ground pepper to taste
1 tablespoon chopped fresh mint
1 tablespoon chopped fresh cilantro
1 tablespoon chopped fresh dill

Bring a large saucepan of lightly salted water to a boil. Add lima beans, garlic, and crushed red pepper; cook until the beans are tender, about 10 minutes. Remove from heat and let cool in the liquid.

Drain the beans and garlic. Transfer to a food processor. Add oil, lemon juice, cumin, salt, and pepper; process until smooth. Scrape into a bowl; stir in mint, cilantro, and dill. Good as a veggie dip or spread on crackers.

Parsley Tabbouleh (*V)

(serves 4)

> 1 cup water
> ½ cup bulgur
> ¼ cup lemon juice
> 2 tablespoons extra-virgin olive oil
> ½ teaspoon garlic, minced
> ¼ teaspoon salt
> Freshly ground pepper to taste
> 2 cups (about 2 bunches) flat-leaf parsley, finely chopped
> ¼ cup fresh mint, chopped
> 2 tomatoes, diced
> 1 small cucumber, peeled, seeded, and diced
> 4 scallions, thinly sliced

Combine water and bulgur in a small saucepan. Bring to a full boil, remove from heat, cover, and let stand until the water is absorbed and the bulgur is tender, 25 minutes or according to package directions. If any water remains, drain bulgur in a fine-mesh sieve. Transfer to a large bowl and let cool for 15 minutes.

Combine lemon juice, oil, garlic, salt, and pepper in a small bowl. Add parsley, mint, tomatoes, cucumber, and scallions to the bulgur and stir. Add the dressing and toss. Serve at room temperature or chill for at least 1 hour to serve cold.

Ratatouille à la Casablancaise (*V)

(serves 8)

> 1 large eggplant (1¼–1½ pounds), peeled and cut into ¼-inch cubes
> 1½ teaspoons salt, divided
> 3 tablespoons plus 1 teaspoon extra-virgin olive oil, divided
> 1 medium yellow summer squash, peeled and cut into ¼-inch cubes
> 1 red bell pepper, diced
> 3 medium tomatoes, peeled, seeded, and diced, or 1 cup drained canned diced tomatoes

2 cloves garlic, minced

1¼ teaspoons ground cinnamon

1 teaspoon sugar

¼ teaspoon freshly ground pepper

Place eggplant on a baking sheet and sprinkle with 1 teaspoon salt; let stand for 30 minutes. Rinse and pat dry.

Heat 3 tablespoons oil in a nonstick skillet over medium-high heat. Add the eggplant, squash, and bell pepper. Cook, stirring, until the vegetables are soft, 8–10 minutes. Transfer to a large bowl.

Add the remaining 1 teaspoon oil to the pan. Add tomatoes, garlic, cinnamon, sugar, the remaining ½ teaspoon salt, and pepper. Cook, stirring, until the tomatoes begin to break down, 3–5 minutes. Add to the bowl with the eggplant mixture, and stir to combine. Cool to room temperature before serving for the best flavor.

Red Wine Risotto

(serves 8)

4½ cups reduced-sodium beef broth

2 tablespoons extra-virgin olive oil

1 medium onion, finely chopped

2 cloves garlic, minced

1½ cups arborio, carnaroli, or other Italian "risotto" rice

¼ teaspoon salt

1¾ cups dry red wine, such as Barbera, Barbaresco, or Pinot noir

2 teaspoons tomato paste

1 cup Parmigiano-Reggiano cheese, finely grated, divided

Freshly ground pepper to taste

Place broth in a medium saucepan; bring to a simmer over medium-high heat. Reduce the heat so the broth remains steaming but is not simmering.

Heat oil in a Dutch oven over medium-low heat. Add onion and cook, stirring occasionally, for 5 minutes. Add garlic and cook, stirring, until the onion is very soft and translucent, about 2 minutes. Add rice and salt, and stir to coat.

Stir ½ cup of the hot broth and a generous splash of wine into the rice; reduce heat to a gentle simmer and cook, stirring constantly, until the liquid has been absorbed. Add more broth, ½ cup at a time, along with some wine, stirring after each addition until most of the liquid has been absorbed. After about 10 minutes, stir in tomato paste. Continue to cook, adding broth and wine and stirring after each addition until most of the liquid is absorbed; the risotto is done when you've used all the broth and wine and the rice is creamy and just tender, 20–30 minutes more.

Remove the risotto from the heat; stir in ¾ cup cheese and pepper. Serve sprinkled with the remaining ¼ cup cheese.

Roasted Root Vegetables with Chermoula (*V)

(serves 6)

¼ cup extra-virgin olive oil

3 cloves garlic, minced

2 teaspoons paprika, preferably sweet Hungarian

2 teaspoons ground cumin

1 teaspoon salt

1 medium baking potato, peeled and cut into 1-inch chunks

1 medium sweet potato, peeled and cut into 1-inch chunks

1 medium turnip, peeled and cut into 1-inch chunks

1 medium rutabaga, peeled and cut into 1-inch chunks

2 medium carrots, cut into ½-inch slices

8 ounces butternut squash, peeled, seeded, and cut into 1-inch chunks

Preheat oven to 425°. Place oil, garlic, paprika, cumin, and salt in a food processor or blender and pulse or blend until smooth.

Place potato, sweet potato, turnip, rutabaga, carrots, and squash in a large bowl and toss with the spiced oil mixture until well combined. Place the tossed vegetables in a roasting pan large enough to accommodate the pieces in a single layer.

Roast the vegetables, stirring once or twice, until tender, 45–50 minutes.

Roasted Eggplant and Feta Dip (*V)

(serves 12)

1 medium eggplant (about 1 pound)
2 tablespoons lemon juice
¼ cup extra-virgin olive oil
½ cup crumbled feta cheese, preferably Greek
½ cup red onion, finely chopped
1 small red bell pepper, finely chopped
1 small chili pepper, such as jalapeño, seeded and minced (optional)
2 tablespoons fresh basil, chopped
1 tablespoon flat-leaf parsley, finely chopped
¼ teaspoon cayenne pepper, or to taste
¼ teaspoon salt
Pinch of sugar (optional)

Position oven rack about 6 inches from the heat source; preheat broiler.

Line a baking pan with foil. Place eggplant in the pan and poke a few holes all over it to vent steam. Broil the eggplant, turning with tongs every 5 minutes, until the skin is charred and a knife inserted into the dense flesh near the stem goes in easily, 14–18 minutes. Transfer to a cutting board until cool enough to handle.

Put lemon juice in a medium bowl. Cut the eggplant in half lengthwise and scrape the flesh into the bowl, tossing with the lemon juice to help prevent discoloring. Add oil and stir with a fork until the oil is absorbed. (It should be a little chunky.) Stir in feta, onion, bell pepper, chili pepper (if using), basil, parsley, cayenne, and salt. Taste and add sugar if needed.

Sautéed Spinach with Pine Nuts and Golden Raisins (*V)

(serves 2)

2 teaspoons extra-virgin olive oil

2 tablespoons golden raisins

1 tablespoon pine nuts

2 cloves garlic, minced

1 10-ounce bag fresh spinach, tough stems removed

2 teaspoons balsamic vinegar

⅛ teaspoon salt

1 tablespoon shaved Parmesan cheese

Freshly ground pepper to taste

Heat oil in a large nonstick skillet or Dutch oven over medium-high heat. Add raisins, pine nuts, and garlic; cook, stirring, until fragrant, about 30 seconds. Add spinach and cook, stirring, until just wilted, about 2 minutes. Remove from heat; stir in vinegar and salt. Sprinkle with Parmesan and pepper, and serve immediately.

Adzuki Bean Soup (*V)

(serves 4-6)

3 cups adzuki beans

2 teaspoons extra-virgin olive oil

1 small onion, diced

3 small stalks celery, diced

1 ear corn (optional)

2 tablespoons garlic, chopped

1 tablespoon Spike

1 tablespoon Chinese five-spice powder

1½ tablespoons molasses

¼ cup tomato paste

Arrowroot as needed

Sea salt (unrefined) to taste

⅓ cup cilantro, chopped

Soak beans overnight and discard water. Add fresh water and cook beans until tender. In a separate pan cook onions and celery in olive oil over medium heat until tender. Then add corn, garlic, Spike, Chinese five-spice powder, molasses, and tomato paste, stir together, and simmer for 10 minutes. Add this mixture to the cooked beans. (Hint: First remove and reserve some of the beans' water to adjust consistency later.) Bring soup to a simmer and thicken with an arrowroot slurry. Adjust flavor with salt to taste. Add cilantro at the very end.

Crusty Herbed Cauliflower (*V)

(serves 4-6)

Cold-pressed olive oil

1 medium cauliflower head (about 2 pounds)

2 eggs

½ teaspoon sea salt

1 tablespoon Spike

1 cup dry whole-grain bread crumbs

½ cup fresh basil, chopped

¼ cup parsley leaves, chopped

3 tablespoons wheat flour

1 tablespoon butter, melted

Preheat oven to 300°. Coat baking sheet with cold-pressed olive oil.

Cut cauliflower into medium-sized florets. Cook in steamer basket over simmering water in covered saucepan for 5–10 minutes or until tender. Remove.

Meanwhile, beat together eggs and sea salt in a mixing bowl. Toss Spike, bread crumbs, basil, and parsley in another mixing bowl. Place flour in bag. Add cauliflower florets to the bag in batches, shaking to coat. Dip florets in egg mixture, then in crumb mixture, turning to coat. Place on prepared baking sheet. Drizzle with butter.

Bake for 30 minutes or until golden and crispy. Serve hot.

Hearty Lentil Loaf (*V)

(serves 4-6)

8 cups water, divided

2 cups lentils, rinsed

1 bay leaf

1 cup uncooked fine bulgur wheat

1 cup soft whole-wheat bread crumbs

1 egg, beaten

1 tablespoon tomato paste

1 medium onion, chopped

1 clove garlic, crushed

1 teaspoon thyme, dried and crumbled

1 teaspoon tarragon, dried and crumbled

1 teaspoon sea salt

2 teaspoons oregano, dried and crumbled

3 tablespoons tomato paste or tomato sauce

Preheat oven to 350°. Combine lentils and bay leaf in a saucepan with 6 cups water. Bring to a boil, reduce heat, cover, and simmer until lentils are soft and most of the water has been absorbed, about 45 minutes.

Combine bulgur and 2 cups water in a medium saucepan. Bring to a boil, reduce heat, cover, and simmer for 15 minutes. Transfer lentils to a large mixing bowl. Add bulgur and remaining ingredients except tomato paste or sauce. Mix well with your hands until thoroughly combined. Pat mixture into a 9-inch loaf pan. Bake for 40 minutes until firm, but not dry. During the last 5 minutes of baking, brush top with tomato paste or sauce. Let cool for 15 minutes. Cut into slices and serve warm.

Stuffed Cabbage (*V)

(serves 6-8)

½ cup uncooked kasha

½ cup uncooked brown rice mixed with wild rice, or just brown rice

1 tablespoon curry powder

1 teaspoon ground ginger

1 teaspoon savory

1 teaspoon sea salt

1 tablespoon cold-pressed olive oil

1 cup mushrooms, finely chopped

1 small onion, chopped

3 large heads of cabbage

¼ cup currants

½ cup cubed pineapple (canned or fresh)

Preheat oven to 300°. Cook kasha and rice separately, then cool. In mixing bowl, blend together all ingredients, including kasha and rice, except cabbage. Prepare cabbage by steaming heads, then place in cool water. Peel back leaves. Roll ¼–½ cup of mixture in each cabbage leaf with the large part of the stem rolling forward. Bake for 45 minutes.

Sweet and Sour Tempeh (*V)

(serves 6)

½ cup almonds

2 12-ounce blocks tempeh

4 tablespoons tamari

1 large onion

1 large green bell pepper

1 large red bell pepper

1 stalk celery

1 large carrot

Olive oil

1 cup fresh pineapple chunks

1½ tablespoons honey

2 tablespoons apple cider vinegar

1¼ cups vegetable stock or water

1½ tablespoons arrowroot

Toast almond pieces in a dry skillet over medium heat and set aside.

Cut tempeh into 2-inch cubes and marinate 1 hour in 2 tablespoons tamari. Cut onion across center and down into wedge-shaped slices. Cut green and red bell pepper in pointy wedges, and celery and carrot in thin diagonal slices. Stir-fry vegetables in olive oil until crisp tender. Add pineapple after 2–3 minutes.

Combine honey, vinegar, and 1 cup of the vegetable stock, and add to vegetables along with tempeh. Dissolve arrowroot in remaining ¼ cup stock and the remaining 2 tablespoons tamari. Add arrowroot mixture to vegetables to thicken sauce. Cook for 3–4 minutes more. Garnish with toasted almonds. Serve with brown rice.

Tofu Enchiladas (*V)

(serves 4-6)

Preheat oven to 350°.

Enchilada Sauce

1 cup tomato sauce
¼ cup onion, chopped
1 tablespoon chili powder
1 tablespoon garlic
1 tablespoon cumin
1 tablespoon apple cider vinegar
1 teaspoon Vege-Sal
1 tablespoon Spike

Blend in a blender until smooth. Heat and reserve.

Enchilada Mix

14 ounces tofu, crumbled
½ large carrot, chopped
1 stalk celery, chopped
½ squash (any kind), chopped
½ onion, chopped

¼ cauliflower, chopped

1 tablespoon oregano

1 tablespoon cumin

1 teaspoon Vege-Sal

6 whole-wheat tortillas

Combine enchilada mix and roll mixture into whole-wheat tortillas. Place enchiladas in a baking dish, top with enchilada sauce, and bake for 30 minutes.

Eggplant Tabbouleh (*V)

(serves 4-6)

Olive oil

1 eggplant, sliced thinly, lengthwise

Sea salt

1 cup hot vegetable broth

1 cup couscous

2 Roma tomatoes, diced

¼ leek, julienne-cut

2 tablespoons basil, chopped

Preheat oven to 400°. Lightly brush a cookie sheet with olive oil. Place eggplant on greased cookie sheet. Lightly brush eggplant with olive oil. Sprinkle eggplant with sea salt. Roast eggplant in oven for 5–8 minutes or until supple. Remove from oven, then reduce heat in oven to 350°.

Lightly brush an ovenproof bowl with olive oil, and drape eggplant over sides and in bottom of bowl, reserving some of the eggplant.

Heat vegetable broth to the boiling point. Put couscous in a bowl and pour hot broth over it. Stir in tomatoes, leek, and basil. Pour couscous mixture into eggplant "bowl" and cover top with more eggplant.

Bake for 15 minutes. Turn out onto a plate, cut like a pie, and serve.

Black Bean Soup (*V)

(serves 4-6)

½ cup black beans
4 cups water
1 leek, chopped
1 carrot, chopped
2 stalks celery, chopped
1 tablespoon garlic, chopped
Sea salt to taste
1 quart soup stock
1 15-ounce can diced tomatoes
2 tablespoons tomato paste
Cilantro, chopped (garnish)

Soak beans in 4 cups water overnight. Discard water.

In a soup pot, sauté all veggies (except tomato products), as well as the garlic and sea salt, in a little bit of water. When veggies are slightly tender, add soup stock and beans and simmer, stirring occasionally. When beans are tender, add tomato products and continue to simmer for 20 minutes. Serve with cilantro garnish.

Spinach Soufflé (*V)

(serves 8)

2 cups mushrooms, chopped
1 teaspoon ground thyme
1 tablespoon ground basil
1 tablespoon lemon juice
1 tablespoon garlic, chopped fine
½ cup olive oil
⅔ cup tamari
3 whole eggs, beaten
1 whole red onion, chopped
1–2 bunches uncooked spinach, chopped medium in food
    processor

7 slices whole-grain bread, chopped into medium-sized bread crumbs

1 cup cashews or Brazil nuts, chopped fine in food processor

6 egg whites, beaten

Combine mushrooms, thyme, basil, lemon juice, and garlic; sauté in oil.

In large mixing bowl, combine sautéed mixture, tamari, whole eggs, onion, spinach, bread crumbs, and cashews.

Mix, by hand, and fold in egg whites. Place mixture in 2-inch-deep buttered baking dish. Bake at 350° for 45 minutes.

Mixed Grain and Nut Pilaf (*V)

(serves 4-6)

2 cups mushrooms, finely chopped

1 cup red onion, finely chopped

½ cup celery, finely chopped

½ cup wild rice

1 teaspoon olive oil

2 cups brown rice

½ cup chopped nuts

3 tablespoons Braggs Liquid Aminos

Water as needed

Preheat oven to 350°. Sauté mushrooms, onion, celery, and wild rice in olive oil until the veggies are tender. Add these to the remaining ingredients except the water, and stir together. Place in casserole dish and spread the mixture out evenly. Add water to the dish so you cover the rice by ½ inch, and place uncovered in the oven. Check after 30 minutes to see if you need to add more water. The wild rice takes longer to cook, so sample it to test for doneness.

Lima Bean Casserole (*V)

(serves 4-6)

6 cups lima beans (soaked, drained, and cooked) and reserve liquid
3 cups Roma tomatoes, seeded and chopped
3 cups baby spinach
1 cup soy Parmesan cheese
2 tablespoons garlic, chopped
Unrefined sea salt to taste

Bread Crumb Mixture

3 cups whole-grain bread crumbs
¼ cup thyme, chopped
¼ cup Italian parsley, chopped
1 stick butter, melted
½ cup soy cheese, grated (optional)

Mix the first group of ingredients together, and taste. If you like it, place the mixture in an uncovered casserole dish. Bake slowly at 275–300°, letting the beans absorb the juices. Adjust liquid as needed to avoid the mixture drying or becoming too much like soup. Top with bread crumb mixture 20 minutes before the casserole is finished. Let rest for 15 minutes before serving so that the beans will soak up the extra juice.

Eggplant Casserole (*V)

(serves 4-6)

2 cups eggplant, pared and cubed
1 cup tomato sauce
½ cup green bell pepper, chopped
1 cup onion, chopped
2 cups whole-grain bread crumbs
1 teaspoon sea salt
1 tablespoon oregano
1 tablespoon basil
1 teaspoon thyme

1 tablespoon nutmeg

1 teaspoon fresh garlic, chopped

1 cup soy cheese, grated

Combine all ingredients (except soy cheese) and pour into casserole dish. Bake in oven at 350° for 45 minutes. Sprinkle soy cheese on top of casserole and bake another 15 minutes.

D

Rotation Diet

Menu Suggestions for Four-Day Rotation Diet

Day One

Breakfast

Cereal: Pearl barley, kamut, or milo; walnuts, pecans, or macadamias; pineapple, banana, or papaya; and goat yogurt

Green blender drink: Pineapple or banana with romaine lettuce

Lunch

Sautéed mahi-mahi or ahi with walnuts and shiitake mushrooms

Asparagus or okra with walnut oil

Baked sweet potato

Salad of romaine or other lettuce; jicama; diced pineapple, apple, or pear; pecans or walnuts

Dinner

Tuna salad with pineapple, diced apple, pear, or kiwi; diced jicama; and walnuts

Day Two

Breakfast

Cereal: Teff or buckwheat; mango, grapes, or blueberries; yogurt; pistachios, cashews, or Brazil nuts

Green blender drink: Kale with mango or grapes

Lunch

Baked turkey dogs with sauerkraut, mustard, and cashew cheese or mozzarella on rye bread

Steamed broccoli and cauliflower garnished with cashews or pistachios

Steamed spicy cabbage with sea salt, cinnamon, and vinegar

Dinner

Arugula, mango, and cashew salad

Turkey and cheese wraps with arugula, mango or grapes, and cashews; or buffalo patty melts with provolone and mustard on rye bread

Day Three

Breakfast

Cereal: Quinoa; berries, diced apple, or diced pear; pine nuts, sesame seeds, or peanuts; and sheep yogurt

Green blender drink: Chard with apple, strawberries, or raspberries

Lunch

Sautéed filet of sole with parsley and sesame seeds; or lamb patties with dill sauce made with sheep yogurt

Snow pea pods or boiled beets

Salad of beet greens with sesame seeds; or strawberry and spinach salad with pine nuts

Dinner

Guacamole

Apple wedges with tahini

Cinnamon applesauce

Bean soup with leftover or frozen vegetables

Day Four

Breakfast

Cereal: Whole-grain or steel-cut oatmeal with peaches, apricots, nectarines, cherries, or plums; and almonds, sunflower seeds, or pumpkin seeds

Green blender drink: Cantaloupe or watermelon smoothie with fennel, celery, and carrots

Lunch

Sautéed salmon with capers and stone-ground mustard

Slaw made from grated zucchini, crookneck squash, carrots, coconut, and almonds

Steamed parsnips, zucchini, crookneck squash, and baby carrots

Dinner

Salmon quesadillas

Celery sticks with almond butter

Recipes for Four-Day Rotation Diet

(All recipes serve 2 people.)

Day One

Breakfast

Dressed-Up Barley Hot (or Cold) Cereal

½ cup pearl barley

1 cup water

Walnuts, pecans, or macadamias

Pineapple, banana, or papaya

Goat yogurt

Combine barley and water the night before. In the morning, bring to a boil. Simmer 15 minutes. (May also be cooked the same day by combining 1½ cups water and ½ cup barley. Bring to a boil and simmer 35–40 minutes. If you have an early-morning rush, grains may be cooked the night before or up to a week ahead and refrigerated. All cooked cereals are good cold too.) Serve with walnuts, pecans, macadamias, diced pineapple, sliced banana, papaya, or goat yogurt, as desired. Other grains for this day are kamut and milo, which can be prepared according to producer's instructions and served as above.

Pineapple/Banana Breakfast Smoothie

1 cup pineapple (or 1 banana or both)

4–5 large romaine lettuce leaves

2 cups water (can include vegetable cooking water from day before)

Blend all ingredients in a blender and serve. (Best if blended until very smooth with a good blender, such as Vita-Mix.)

Lunch

Sautéed Mahi-Mahi or Ahi with Walnuts and Shiitake Mushrooms
2 tablespoons walnut or macadamia oil
8–12 ounces cod (or mahi-mahi)
⅓ cup walnuts (or macadamias or pecans)
2–3 large shiitake mushrooms, sliced
1 teaspoon garlic powder or 1–2 cloves garlic, crushed
Sea salt

Put oil in small frying pan and heat on medium-low. Add fish and sauté for a few minutes. Add nuts, shiitakes, and seasonings and cook, covered, until fish is flaky (approximately 10–15 minutes). If you are trying to eliminate calories from oil, you can easily poach the fish by substituting 1 cup water for oil and cook on medium-low until flaky. You can also bake the fish at 350° for 20–30 minutes or until flaky.

Herbed Asparagus
½ bunch asparagus (or okra)
½ cup water
1 tablespoon walnut oil
1 tablespoon vinegar
Oregano or Italian seasoning (optional)
Sea salt

Steam asparagus in water until fork tender. Pour off water and reserve for breakfast smoothies. Rinse asparagus in cold water to halt cooking. Sprinkle other ingredients over asparagus and roll in pan to coat.

Baked Sweet Potato
1 large sweet potato

Thoroughly wash a sweet potato. Cut off both ends and split down the middle. Place in covered baking dish. Bake at 350° until fork tender, approximately 1 hour. (You may coat outside of skin with coconut oil prior to cooking for a nice flavor.)

Romaine Salad with Pineapple, Jicama, and Pecans

4–5 leaves romaine (or other lettuce)

¼ jicama, diced

½ pineapple (or apple or pear), diced

1 tablespoon walnut oil

1 tablespoon vinegar

¼ cup pecans (or walnuts)

Chill all ingredients in covered salad bowl. (You can store oil and vinegar in bottom of bowl, under salad, until ready to toss. If tossed too long before serving, greens will wilt.) Toss just before serving.

Dinner

Tuna Salad with Pineapple, Walnuts, and Jicama

1 can tuna

2 tablespoons mayonnaise

1 tablespoon vinegar

1 clove fresh garlic, crushed, or garlic powder

Sea salt

4 cups (or more) chopped lettuce

½ pineapple (and/or apple, pear, kiwi), diced

¼ jicama, diced

⅓ cup walnuts

Mix tuna with mayo (can substitute oil if necessary) and seasonings. Place lettuce in individual bowls and garnish with pineapple, jicama, and walnuts. Place a scoop of tuna mixture on each salad.

Day Two

Breakfast

Fancy Teff Breakfast Cereal

½ cup teff (or buckwheat)

1 cup water

Mango, grapes, blueberries

Nonfat plain cow yogurt (optional)

Pistachios, cashews, Brazil nuts

Combine teff and water in saucepan. Bring to boil. Simmer 15–20 minutes. (Teff will then need to be stirred, since it tends to separate at first.) Serve with diced mango, grapes, cow yogurt, pistachios, cashews, and/or Brazil nuts. (Blueberries may be used for any fruits today and provide great nutrition!) Buckwheat also makes a nice cereal.

Mango-Grape Kale Breakfast Smoothie

4–5 medium kale leaves

1 peeled, coarsely chopped mango and/or 1 cup grapes

Blend until smooth and serve.

Lunch

Turkey Sauerkraut Melt

2 slices rye bread

Coarsely ground mustard

1 cup sauerkraut

3–4 turkey dogs (or 1½ cups sliced turkey)

4 slices cashew cheese or mozzarella (optional)

Preheat oven to 350°. In a greased baking dish, place the 2 slices of rye bread. Spread coarsely ground mustard over each slice. Place half of sauerkraut on each slice. Place turkey dogs (split down middle, lengthwise) on sauerkraut. Top with slices of cheese. Bake for 20 minutes until hot or cheese is melted.

Steamed Broccoli and Cauliflower

1 small broccoli crown

¼ small head cauliflower

1 cup water

Sea salt to taste

Cashews or pistachios (optional)

Clean broccoli and cauliflower and cut into florets. Place in saucepan with water. Bring to boil on medium. Reduce heat, cover, and steam 10 minutes or until fork tender. Do not overcook, or vegetables lose color and nutrients. Season with sea salt to taste. Garnish with cashews or pistachios.

Steamed Spicy Cabbage

¼ head red cabbage

1 cup water

Sea salt to taste

¼ teaspoon cinnamon

1 tablespoon vinegar

Clean cabbage and thinly slice. Place in pan with water and bring to a boil. Simmer 10 minutes or until fork tender. Reserve water for breakfast smoothies. Season with sea salt, cinnamon, and vinegar.

Dinner

Arugula, Mango, and Cashew Salad

4 cups arugula (or watercress)

½ mango, peeled and diced

¼ cup cashews

1 tablespoon canola oil

1 tablespoon vinegar

Clean arugula and place in salad bowl. Garnish with mango and cashews. Chill. Just before serving, toss with oil and vinegar.

Turkey and Cheese Wraps

2 whole-wheat tortillas

Stone-ground mustard

4 slices roasted turkey

4 slices cashew cheese or mozzarella

1 cup arugula

½ cup mango, diced, or ½ cup grapes

½ cup cashews

Sea salt to taste

Heat dry griddle or frying pan on medium heat. Warm tortillas to soften. Spread each with stone-ground mustard. On each tortilla place 2 slices turkey, 2 slices cheese, ½ cup arugula, ¼ cup mango or grapes, and ¼ cup cashews. Season with sea salt. Roll up burrito-style. Can be eaten with knife and fork or wrapped in napkin.

or

Buffalo Patty Melts

2 buffalo patties

Olive oil

4 slices provolone (or other cheese)

2 slices rye bread

Stone-ground mustard

Sauté patties with olive oil in frying pan until brown. Melt cheese on top. Serve on rye bread, spread with mustard. Great with sauerkraut or leftover steamed vegetables.

Day Three

Breakfast

Quinoa Hot Cereal with Berries and Sheep Yogurt

½ cup quinoa

1 cup water

Berries, diced apple, or diced pear

Pine nuts, sesame seeds, or peanuts

Sheep yogurt

Place quinoa and water in saucepan. Bring to a boil. Reduce heat and simmer 15–20 minutes. Serve with any combination of berries, diced apple, diced pear, pine nuts, sesame seeds, peanuts, and sheep yogurt.

Green Magic Smoothie

4 large chard leaves

2 cups water

1 apple, cored (or 1 cup strawberries or raspberries)

Blend until smooth and serve. Delicious!

Lunch

Sautéed Filet of Sole with Parsley and Sesame Seeds

2 tablespoons olive oil

8–12 ounces filet of sole

Parsley

Sesame seeds

Heat olive oil in sauté pan on medium heat. Add filet of sole, lower heat, and cook, covered, until flaky. (This fish cooks very quickly.) Garnish with parsley and sesame seeds. (This recipe is great with mushrooms added to the sauté, if you haven't had them in four days.)

or

Lamb Patties with Dill Sauce for Main Dish or Wrap

½ pound ground lamb

1 clove garlic, crushed

⅛ teaspoon cayenne pepper

⅛ teaspoon fennel seed

⅛ teaspoon cinnamon

⅛ teaspoon cumin seed

⅛ teaspoon coriander seed

⅛ teaspoon oregano

Sea salt to taste

½ cup sheep yogurt

½ teaspoon dill weed

Preheat oven to 350°. Thoroughly mix lamb, garlic, cayenne pepper, fennel seed, cinnamon, cumin seed, coriander seed, and oregano in a bowl with clean hands. (I usually mix the spices in a larger quantity, such as 2 teaspoons of each, and keep in a jar. Then all I have to do is add ¾ teaspoon of the mixture to the lamb.) Shape into two patties. Place uncovered in baking dish.

Bake 20 minutes or until desired doneness is reached. (Juices will run over down the edges when thoroughly cooked.) Season cooked patties with sea salt. Mix yogurt and dill weed and serve as sauce over the top.

These patties can be served with vegetables or in a wrap. For the wrap, place on a warmed tortilla 1 sliced lamb patty, 2–3 tablespoons yogurt sauce, a handful of pine nuts, and some spinach leaves. Season with salt and wrap up. Delicious!

Snow Pea Pods and Garden Peas

20 snow pea pods
½ cup frozen peas
½ cup water
Sea salt to taste

Place pea pods, peas, and water in saucepan. Bring to boil over medium heat. Simmer approximately 5 minutes or until fork tender. Season with sea salt.

Beautiful Beets

2 small beets
1 cup water
Sea salt to taste

Wash, peel, and quarter beets. Put in saucepan with water. Boil 15 minutes or until fork tender. Season with sea salt.

Tasty Beet Greens

1 bunch beet greens
1 cup water
1 tablespoon vinegar
1 tablespoon sesame oil
Sea salt to taste
Sesame seeds

Thoroughly wash greens and stems. Slice across greens and stems in ½-inch strips. Place in pan with water. Bring to a boil over medium heat. Simmer 5 minutes or until wilted. Pour off water and reserve for breakfast drink. Season with vinegar, oil, and sea salt. Garnish with sesame seeds.

Strawberry and Spinach Salad with Pine Nuts

2 cups spinach

½ cup strawberries (or raspberries), sliced

⅓ cup pine nuts

1 tablespoon olive oil

2 tablespoons vinegar (balsamic, rice wine, red wine, etc.)

Place spinach in salad bowl. Garnish with berries and pine nuts. Chill. Before serving, toss with oil and vinegar.

Dinner

Easy Guacamole

1 mashed avocado

2 tablespoons salsa

Sea salt to taste

Juice of ½ orange (optional)

Juice of ½ lemon (optional)

2 tablespoons onion (optional)

Mix all ingredients and serve with eggs.

Apple Wedges with Tahini

2 apples, cut in wedges

4 tablespoons tahini (sesame butter) or peanut butter

Serve apple wedges with tahini as a side dish or snack.

Easy Old-Fashioned Cinnamon Applesauce

2 apples

1 cup water

½ teaspoon cinnamon

Peel and thinly slice apples and place in saucepan with water. Simmer until mushy. Break up with spoon or potato masher. Season with cinnamon.

Day Four

Breakfast

Whole-Grain Oatmeal with Sliced Peaches and Sunflower Seeds

½ cup whole-grain or steel-cut oats

1½ cups water

Peaches, apricots, nectarines, cherries, or plums

Almonds, sunflower seeds, or pumpkin seeds

Place oats and water in saucepan. Bring to boil. Simmer 50–60 minutes. Serve with sliced peaches, apricots, nectarines, cherries, or plums and almonds, sunflower or pumpkin seeds, or any combination of these that you like.

Melon Slush Smoothie

½ cantaloupe with rind and seeds removed

1 stalk fennel, with leaves

1 large stalk celery, or equivalent amount of celery leaves

2 cups water

⅓ cup baby carrots

Blend all ingredients until smooth and serve. This recipe is also delicious with watermelon as a substitute for the cantaloupe. We also like to use beet juice from previous day for part of the water. This really makes a beautiful color!

Lunch

Sautéed Salmon with Capers and Stone-Ground Mustard

2 tablespoons coconut oil

8–12 ounces wild salmon

2 tablespoons stone-ground mustard

Sea salt to taste

1 tablespoon capers

Heat oil in sauté pan. Add salmon and cook, covered, on medium-low until flaky, about 10 minutes. In a small bowl, combine mustard, salt, and capers. Top salmon with mustard/caper mixture.

Coconut, Carrot, Squash Slaw

1 small zucchini, grated
1 small crookneck squash, grated
1 large carrot, grated
¼ cup unsweetened coconut, grated
½ cup almonds, soaked
2 tablespoons vinegar
¼ teaspoon stevia
2 tablespoons almond oil

Combine all ingredients and chill until ready to serve.

Steamed Parsnips, Carrots, and Squash

1 parsnip, peeled and sliced
1 small zucchini, sliced
1 small crookneck squash, sliced
1 cup baby carrots
1 cup water
Sea salt to taste

Place all ingredients except sea salt in saucepan. Bring to a boil. Reduce to simmer and cook approximately 10 minutes or until fork tender. Season with sea salt before serving.

Dinner

Salmon Quesadillas

Olive or coconut oil
1 can good-quality salmon
2 rice tortillas
4 slices soy cheese (optional)

Lightly grease an iron grill or heavy frying pan with coconut or olive oil. Mash salmon in bowl until thoroughly mixed. On medium heat, grill warm tortilla to soften. Fill tortilla with half of salmon and half of soy cheese. Fold tortilla in half and place on grill, lightly covered with flat lid. Cook on medium until lightly browned. Flip over and brown the other side. You can cook 2 quesadillas at once.

Celery Sticks with Almond Butter

3 large stalks celery, sliced lengthwise and cut into 2-inch lengths
4 tablespoons almond butter

After cutting, chill celery in covered container until ready to serve. Serve with almond butter.

Helpful Hints for Rotation Diet

- Modify the grocery list to fit your plan. Store staples such as seeds, nuts, nut butters, oils, grains, flours, breads (freeze), and frozen fruits/vegetables to have on hand. When shopping, stick to whole, unprocessed foods to avoid allergenic ingredients.
- Organize refrigerator and freezer and label shelves 1, 2, 3, and 4 for each day. This makes it easier to find what you and family members can eat on that day.
- Each day, check for ingredients needed for the following day and defrost as needed.
- Do all cooking for each day at one time by preparing fruits, vegetables, salad, and other ingredients and refrigerating on shelf for that day.
- Use masking tape and marking pen to label refrigerator and freezer dishes with 1, 2, 3, or 4 and name of food.

The following grocery list and food families lists are provided to help you design a four-day rotation diet. It can be helpful to rotate food by family if food allergies are a significant problem. For example, amaranth and quinoa are both in the amaranth family and can be eaten on the same day, but four days should separate their use. Generally it is not necessary to be that strict with the rotation;

amaranth and quinoa can be eaten on separate days. However, some of my patients who are extremely food sensitive need to rotate foods based on food family.

FOOD	DAY ONE	DAY TWO	DAY THREE	DAY FOUR
Meat/Fish/ Poultry	Turkey, pheasant, chicken, Cornish hen, quail, duck, goose, ostrich, grouse, partridge, eggs of birds, herring, sardine, snapper (red and other types), anchovy, scallops	Beef, buffalo, moose, venison, oysters, clams, crab, lobster, crayfish, shrimp, mussels	Rabbit, cod, haddock, ocean perch, albacore tuna, mackerel, flounder, sole, turbot, marlin, bass, catfish, eel	Pork, goat, lamb, salmon, trout, smelt, whitefish, perch, walleye, pike, pickerel, snails, squid, octopus
Nuts/Seeds	Hazelnuts, pine nuts, sunflower seeds, macadamia nuts, chestnuts	Pumpkin seeds, poppy seeds, acorn, almond	Walnut, pecan, hickory, peanut, cashew, pistachio, caraway seed, sesame seed	Brazil nut, litchi nut, psyllium seeds, coconut, flax seeds
Grains/ Starchy Vegetables	Buckwheat, artichoke, lotus, chestnut (starch, flour, breads, and pastas), arrowroot, malanga (Oriental potato or eddoes), tapioca, cassava	Rice, wild rice, corn, millet, teff, Job's tears (flour, breads, and pastas)	Soy, lentil, chickpea, carob, kudzu, guar gum, water chestnut, quinoa, amaranth, yam (flour, breads, and pastas)	Wheat, oats, rye, barley, spelt, kamut, sago, flax (flour, breads, and pastas)
Vegetables	Potato, tomato, eggplant, green/ yellow/red bell peppers, artichoke, lettuce (Boston or romaine, etc.), endive, radicchio	Cucumber, squash, pumpkin, zucchini, asparagus, onion, garlic, leek, chives, shallots, bamboo shoots	Peas, beans, carob, soy, tofu, alfalfa, carrot, celery, parsley, fennel, parsnip, green/black olives, plantain, water chestnuts, yam, sweet potato, spinach, beets, Swiss chard	Cabbage, cauliflower, broccoli, Brussels sprouts, radish, turnip, rutabaga, rapini, collards, kale, kohlrabi, bok choy, cress, arugula, okra, yucca, mushroom

FOOD	DAY ONE	DAY TWO	DAY THREE	DAY FOUR
Fruit	Strawberry, raspberry, blackberry, boysenberry, rhubarb, blueberry, cranberry, huckleberry	Cantaloupe, casaba, honeydew, watermelon apricot, cherry, chokecherry, peach, prune, nectarine, plum, avocado	Mango, gooseberry, currants, banana, orange, lemon, lime, grapefruit, tangerine, uglifruit, kumquat, guava, persimmon, fig, mulberry, breadfruit	Grape, raisin, pineapple, pomegranate, kiwi, papaya, apple, pear, quince, dates
Herbs/Spices/	Paprika, juniper, wintergreen, tarragon, salsify, mint, oregano, sage, thyme, allspice, basil, savory, rosemary, chocolate, black pepper	Lemongrass, poppy seed, capers, clove, allspice, bay leaf, cinnamon, almond extract	Anise, caraway, chervil, coriander, cumin, dill, fennel, ginger, cardamom, turmeric, nutmeg, mace, carob, tamarind	Paprika, cream of tartar, mustard, horseradish, vanilla
Beverages	Potato milk, teas (chamomile, chicory, mint, spearmint, peppermint), cranberry juice	Teas (cinnamon, sassafras, or aloe vera), almond milk, rice milk, cow's milk, coffee	Teas (ginger or alfalfa), soy milk, cashew milk, orange juice, lemonade, apricot juice, peach juice, prune juice	Teas (rose hip, vanilla, black, or green), papaya juice, grape juice, apple juice, pineapple juice, coconut milk, goat milk
Oils/Fats	Sunflower oil, safflower oil	Almond oil, hemp oil	Sesame oil, olive oil	Canola oil, flaxseed oil, coconut oil
Snacks	Potato chips, sunflower seeds	Corn chips, popcorn, rice crackers	Carob bars, soy "nuts," sesame seeds	Dates, raisins, granola
Sweetener	Stevia, frozen concentrated raspberry or cranberry juice	Rice syrup, molasses	Maple sugar or syrup, frozen concentrated citrus juices	Kiwi sweetener, frozen pineapple, apple, or grape juice, honey, date sugar

Grocery List
for Four-Day Rotation Diet
(numbers, 1,2,3,4 refer to the day)

VEGETABLES
❑ __Artichoke-1
❑ __Arugula-2
❑ __Asparagus-1
❑ __Avocado-3
❑ __Beans-3
❑ __Beets-3
❑ __Broccoli-2
❑ __Brussels sprouts-2
❑ __Cabbage-2
❑ __Carrots-4
❑ __Cauliflower-2
❑ __Celery-4
❑ __Chard-3
❑ __Cucumbers-4
❑ __Endive-1
❑ __Fennel-4
❑ __Jicama-1
❑ __Kale-2
❑ __Lettuce-1
❑ __Mushrooms-2
❑ __Okra-1
❑ __Parsley-4
❑ __Parsnips-4
❑ __Peppers-1
❑ __Potatoes-1
❑ __Pumpkin-4
❑ __Radicchio-1
❑ __Romaine-1
❑ __Spinach-3
❑ __Squash-4
❑ __Watercress-2
❑ __Zucchini-4

FRUIT
❑ __Apples-3
❑ __Apricots-4
❑ __Bananas-1
❑ __Berries-3
❑ __Cherries-4
❑ __Figs-2
❑ __Grapefruit-3
❑ __Grapes-2
❑ __Kiwi-1
❑ __Lemons-3
❑ __Limes-3

MISCELLANEOUS

❑ __ Mango-2
❑ __ Melon-4
❑ __ Nectarines-4
❑ __ Oranges-3
❑ __ Papaya-1
❑ __ Peaches-4
❑ __ Pears-3
❑ __ Persimmons-1
❑ __ Pineapple-1
❑ __ Plums-4
❑ __ Tangerines-3

GRAINS/NUTS
❑ __ Almonds-4
❑ __ Amaranth-1
❑ __ Barley-1
❑ __ Beans-3
❑ __ Brazil nuts-2
❑ __ Buckwheat-2
❑ __ Cashews-2
❑ __ Filberts-3
❑ __ Hazelnuts-3
❑ __ Kamut-1
❑ __ Lentils-3
❑ __ Macadamia nuts-1
❑ __ Millet-3
❑ __ Oats-4
❑ __ Peanuts-3
❑ __ Pecans-1
❑ __ Pine nuts-3
❑ __ Pistachios-2
❑ __ Pumpkin seeds-4
❑ __ Quinoa-3
❑ __ Rice-4
❑ __ Rye-2
❑ __ Sesame seeds-3
❑ __ Spelt-3
❑ __ Split peas-3
❑ __ Sunflower seeds-4
❑ __ Teff-2
❑ __ Walnuts-1
❑ __ Wheat-3

DAIRY
❑ __ Butter-2

❑ _____
❑ _____

❑ __Cow yogurt-2
❑ __Eggs-3
❑ __Goat yogurt-1
❑ __Sheep yogurt-3

CHEESES
❑ __Cow-2
❑ __Cream-2
❑ __Goat-1
❑ __Sheep-3
❑ __Soy-4

MEAT, FISH, AND POULTRY
❑ __Ahi/Tuna-1
❑ __Beef-4
❑ __Buffalo-2
❑ __Halibut-3
❑ __Lamb-3
❑ __Mahi-mahi-1
❑ __Orange roughy-4
❑ __Pork-1
❑ __Red snapper-2
❑ __Salmon-4
❑ __Sea bass-2
❑ __Sole-3
❑ __Turkey-2

CONDIMENTS
❑ __Almond butter-4
❑ __Almond oil-4
❑ __Canola oil-2
❑ __Cashew butter-2
❑ __Coconut oil-4
❑ __Grapeseed oil-2
❑ __Macadamia nut butter-1
❑ __Mayonnaise-3
❑ __Mustard-2
❑ __Olive oil-3
❑ __Palm oil-1
❑ __Peanut butter-3
❑ __Safflower oil-1
❑ __Sesame oil-3
❑ __Sunflower oil-4
❑ __Tamari-4
❑ __Walnut oil-1

❑ _____
❑ _____

Food Families Index

The Food Families Index identifies the botanical family of each food.

FOODS	FAMILY	FOODS	FAMILY
Alfalfa	Legume	Cherry	Rose
Almond	Rose	Chicken	Pheasant
Amaranth	Amaranth	Chili Pepper	Potato
Apple	Rose	Cinnamon	Laurel
Asparagus	Lily	Clam	Mollusk
Avocado	Laurel	Clove	Myrtle
Baker's Yeast	Fungi	Cocoa/Chocolate	Sterculia
Banana	Banana	Coconut	Palm
Barley	Grass	Cod	Codfish
Basil	Mint	Coffee	Madder
Beef	Bovine	Corn	Grass
Beet	Goosefoot	Cow's Milk	Bovine
Bell Pepper	Potato	Crab	Crustacean
Black Pepper	Pepper	Cranberry	Heath
Brazil Nut	Sapucaia	Egg	Pheasant
Brewer's Yeast	Fungi	Eggplant	Potato
Broccoli	Mustard	Flounder	Flounder
Brussels Sprouts	Mustard	Garlic	Lily
Buckwheat	Buckwheat	Ginger	Ginger
Cabbage	Mustard	Goat's Milk	Bovine
Cane Sugar	Grass	Grape	Grape
Cantaloupe	Gourd	Grapefruit	Rue (Citrus)
Carrot	Carrot	Green Bean	Legume
Cashew	Cashew	Haddock	Codfish
Cauliflower	Mustard	Halibut	Flounder
Celery	Carrot	Herring	Herring
Cheese	Bovine/Fungi	Kidney Bean	Legume
Lamb	Bovine	Quinoa	Amaranth
Lemon	Rue (Citrus)	Radish	Mustard
Lentil	Legume	Rapeseed (Canola)	Mustard

Food Families Index (continued)

Lettuce	Composite	Rice	Grass
Lima Bean	Legume	Rye	Grass
Lime	Rue (Citrus)	Safflower	Composite
Lobster	Crustacean	Sage	Mint
Mackerel	Mackerel	Salmon	Salmon
Millet	Grass	Scallop	Mollusk
Mung Bean Sprouts	Legume	Sesame	Pedalium
Mushroom	Fungi	Shrimp	Crustacean
Mustard	Mustard	Snapper	Snapper
Nutmeg	Nutmeg	Sole	Flounder
Oat	Grass	Soybean	Legume
Olive	Olive	Spinach	Goosefoot
Onion	Lily	Strawberry	Rose
Orange	Rue (Citrus)	Sunflower	Composite
Oregano	Mint	Sweet Potato	Morning Glory
Oyster	Mollusk	Tangerine	Rue (Citrus)
Papaya	Papaya	Tea	Tea
Parsley	Carrot	Tomato	Potato
Pea	Legume	Trout	Salmon
Peach	Rose	Tuna	Mackerel
Peanut	Legume	Turkey	Turkey
Pecan	Walnut	Walnut	Walnut
Perch	Perch	Wheat	Grass
Pineapple	Pineapple	Whitefish	Whitefish
Pinto Bean	Legume	White Pepper	Pepper
Plum	Rose	White Potato	Potato
Pork	Swine	Yam	Yam
Pumpkin	Gourd	Yellow Wax Bean	Legume
Zucchini	Gourd		

Food Families

PLANT

Algae Family
Agar-agar
Carrageen (Irish moss)
Dulse
Kelp

Amaranth Family
Amaranth
Quinoa

Amaryllis Family
Agave
Mescal, pulque
Tequila

Arum Family
Ceriman
   arrowroot
   dasheen (white
     yam)
   malanga arrowroot
   poi
   taro

Banana Family
Arrowroot (Musa)
Banana
Plantain

Beech Family
Chestnut
Chinquapin

Birch Family
Filbert (hazelnut)
Oil of birch
(wintergreen)
(Some wintergreen
flavor is methyl
salicylate.)

Bixa Family
Annatto (natural yellow
   dye)

Borage Family
Borage
Comfrey (leaf and root)

Buckwheat Family
Buckwheat
Garden sorrel
Rhubarb
Sea grape

Buttercup Family
Goldenseal

Cactus Family
Prickly pear

Canna Family
Queensland arrowroot

Caper Family
Caper

Carpetweed Family
New Zealand spinach

Carrot Family
Angelica
Anise
Caraway
Carrot
Celeriac (celery root)
Celery (seed and leaf)
Chervil
Coriander
Cumin
Dill
Dill seed
Fennel
Finocchio

Florence fennel
Gotu kola
Lovage
Parsley
Parsnip
Sweet cicely

Cashew Family
Cashew
Mango
Pistachio
Poison ivy
Poison oak
Poison sumac

Composite Family
Boneset
Burdock root
Cardoon
Celtuce
Chamomile
Chicory
Coltsfoot
Costmary
Dandelion
Endive
Escarole
Globe artichoke
Jerusalem artichoke
Lettuce
Pyrethrum
Romaine
Safflower oil
Salsify (oyster plant)
Santolina (herb)
Scolymus (Spanish
oyster
   plant)
Scorzonera (black
salsify)
Southernwood
Sunflower (seed, meal,
oil, butter

Tansy (herb)
Tarragon (herb)
Witlof chicory (French endive)
Wormwood (absinthe)
Yarrow

Conifer Family
Juniper (gin)
Pine nut

Custard-Apple Family
Cherimoya
Custard-apple
Pawpaw

Cycad Family
Florida arrowroot (zamia)

Dillenia Family
Chinese gooseberry (kiwi berry)

Ebony Family
American persimmon
Kaki (Japanese persimmon)

Flax Family
Flaxseed

Fungi Family
Baker's yeast ("Red Star")
Brewer's yeast
Citric acid (aspergillus)
Mold (certain cheeses)
Morel
Mushroom
Puffball
Truffle

Ginger Family
Cardamom
East Indian arrowroot
Ginger
Turmeric

Ginseng Family
American ginseng
Chinese ginseng

Goosefoot Family
Beet
Chard
Lamb's quarters
Spinach
Sugar beet
Tampala

Gourd Family
Chayote
Chinese preserving melon
Cucumber
Gherkin
Loofah (vegetable sponge)
Muskmelons
  cantaloupe
  casaba
  crenshaw
  honeydew
  Persian melon
Pumpkin (seeds and meat)
Squashes
  acorn
  Boston marrow
  buttercup
  caserta
  cocozelle
  crookneck
  cushaw
  golden nugget
  hubbard varieties
  pattypan
  spaghetti
  straightneck

  turban
  zucchini
Watermelon

Grape Family
Grape
  brandy
  champagne
  cream of tartar
  dried currant
  raisin
  wine
  wine vinegar
Muscadine

Grass Family
Bamboo shoots
Barley
  malt
  maltose
Bran
Bulgur
Corn
  cornmeal
  corn oil
  cornstarch
  corn sugar
  corn syrup
  hominy grits
  popcorn
Couscous
Kamut
Lemongrass
  citronella
Millet
Oat
  oatmeal
Rice, rice flour
Rye
Sorghum
Spelt
Sugarcane
  cane sugar
  molasses
  raw sugar
Sweet corn
Teff

Triticale
Wheat
Wheat germ
Wild rice

Heath Family
Bearberry
Blueberry
Cranberry
Huckleberry

Holly Family
Mate (yerba mate)

Honeysuckle Family
Elderberry
   elderberry flowers

Horsetail Family
Shavegrass (horsetail)

Iris Family
Orris root (fragrance)
Saffron (crocus)

Laurel Family
Avocado
Bay leaf
Cassia bark
Cinnamon
Filé (powdered leaves)
Sassafras

Legume Family
Alfalfa (sprouts)
Beans
   fava
   green
   lima
   mung (sprouts)
   navy
   pinto
   string (kidney)
   yellow wax
Black-eyed peas
(cowpea)

Carob
   carob syrup
Chickpea (garbanzo)
Fenugreek
Gum acacia
Gum tragacanth
Jicama
Kudzu
Lentil
Licorice
Pea
Peanut
Peanut oil
Red clover
Senna
Soybean
   lecithin
   soy flour
   soy grits
   soy milk
   soy oil
Tamarind
Tonka bean
   coumarin

Lily Family
Asparagus
Chives
Garlic
Garlic chives
Leek
Onion
Ramp
Sarsaparilla
Shallot
Yucca (soap plant)

Linden Family
Basswood (linden)

Madder Family
Coffee
Woodruff

Mallow Family
Althaea root
Cottonseed oil

Hibiscus (roselle)
Okra

Malpighia Family
Acerola (Barbados
cherry)

Mint Family
Apple mint
Basil
Bergamot
Catnip
Chia seed
Clary
Dittany
Horehound
Hyssop
Lavender
Lemon balm
Marjoram
Oregano
Pennyroyal
Peppermint
Rosemary
Sage
Spearmint
Summer savory
Thyme
Winter savory

Maple Family
Maple sugar
Maple syrup

**Morning Glory
Family**
Camote
Sweet potato

Mulberry Family
Breadfruit
Fig
Hemp
Hop
Mulberry

Mustard Family
Bok choy
Broccoli
Brussels sprouts
Cabbage
Cardoon
Cauliflower
Chinese cabbage
Collards
Colza shoots
Couve tronchuda
Curly cress
Horseradish
Kale
Kohlrabi
Mustard greens
Mustard seed
Napa
Radish
Rapeseed (canola)
Rutabaga (swede)
Turnip
Upland cress
Watercress

Myrtle Family
Allspice (pimenta)
Clove
Eucalyptus
Guava

Nasturtium Family
Nasturtium (seed, leaf, and flower)

Nutmeg Family
Mace
Nutmeg

Olive Family
Olive
  olive oil

Orchid Family
Vanilla

Oxalis Family
Carambola
Oxalis

Palm Family
Coconut (meal, oil, milk, seed, and leaf)
Date
  date sugar
Palm cabbage
Sago starch

Papaya Family
Papaya

Passion Flower Family
Granadilla (passion fruit)

Pedalium Family
Sesame seed
Sesame oil
  tahini

Pepper Family
Peppercorn
  Black pepper
  White pepper

Pineapple Family
Pineapple

Pomegranate Family
Grenadine
Pomegranate

Poppy Family
Poppy seed

Potato Family
Eggplant
Ground-cherry
Pepino (melon pear)
Pepper (capsicum)
  bell, sweet

cayenne
chili
paprika
pimiento
Potato
Tobacco
Tomatillo
Tomato
Tree tomato

Protea Family
Macadamia (Queensland nut)

Purslane Family
Pigweed

Rose Family
Berries
  blackberry
  boysenberry
  dewberry
  loganberry
  longberry
  tayberry
  youngberry
  raspberry (leaf)
  black raspberry
  red raspberry
  purple raspberry
  strawberry (leaf)
  wineberry
Herb
  burnet (cucumber flavor)
Pomes
  apple
  cider
  crabapple
  loquat
  pear
  pectin
  quince
  rose hips
  vinegar

Stone fruits
  almond
  apricot
  cherry
  peach (nectarine)
  plum (prune)
  sloe

Rue (Citrus) Family
Citron
Grapefruit
Kumquat
Lemon
Lime
Murcott
Orange
Pummelo
Tangelo
Tangerine

Sapodilla Family
Chicle (chewing gum)

Sapucaia Family
Brazil nut
Sapucaia nut (paradise
  nut)

Saxifrage Family
Currant
Gooseberry

Sedge Family
Chinese water chestnut
Chufa (groundnut)

Soapberry Family
Litchi (lychee)

Spurge Family
Cassava or yucca
  cassava meal
Tapioca (Brazilian
    arrowroot)
  castor bean

Sterculia Family
Chocolate (cacao)
Cocoa
    cocoa butter
Kola nut

Tacca Family
Fiji arrowroot

Tea Family
Tea

Valerian Family
Corn salad (fetticus)

Verbena Family
Lemon verbena

Walnut Family
Black walnut
Butternut
English walnut
Heartnut
Hican
Hickory nut
Pecan

Yam Family
Chinese potato (yam)
Ñame (yampí)

ANIMAL

Anchovy Family
Anchovy

Bass Family
Yellow bass

Bear Family
Bear

Bluefish Family
Bluefish

Bovine Family
Beef
Beef by-products
  Gelatin
  Oleomargarine
  Rennin (rennet)
  Sausage casings
  Suet
Buffalo (bison)
Goat
  Milk products
Milk
Milk products
  Butter
  Cheese
  Ice cream
  Lactose
  Spray-dried milk
  Yogurt
Rocky Mountain sheep
Sheep
  Lamb
  Mutton
Veal

Catfish Family
Catfish

Codfish Family
Cod (scrod)
Cusk
Haddock
Pollack

Croaker Family
Croaker
Drum
Sea trout
Silver perch
Spot
Spotted sea trout

Crustacean Family
Crab
Crayfish
Lobster
Prawn
Shrimp

Deer Family
Caribou
Deer (venison)
Elk
Moose
Reindeer

Dolphin Family
Dolphin

Dove Family
Dove
Pigeon (squab)

Duck Family
Duck
Duck eggs
Goose
Goose eggs

Eel Family
American eel

Flounder Family
Dab
Flounder
Halibut
Plaice
Sole
Turbot

Frog Family
Frog

Grouse Family
Ruffed grouse
  (partridge)

Guinea Fowl Family
Guinea fowl
Guinea fowl eggs

Hare Family
Rabbit

Harvestfish Family
Butterfish
Harvestfish

Herring Family
Menhaden
Pilchard (sardine)
Sea herring
Shad
Sprat

Jack Family
Amberjack
Pompano
Yellow jack

Mackerel Family
Albacore
Bonito
Mackerel
Skipjack
Tuna

Marlin Family
Marlin
Sailfish

Minnow Family
Carp
Chub

Mollusk Family
Cephalopods
  Squid
Gastropods
  Abalone
  Snail
Pelecypods
  Clam
  Cockle
  Mussel
  Oyster
  Scallop

Mullet Family
Mullet

Opossum Family
Opossum

Perch and Pike Family
Muskellunge
Pickerel
Pike
Sauger (perch)
Walleye
Yellow perch

Pheasant Family
Chicken
Chicken eggs
Peafowl
Pheasant
Quail

Porgy Family
Northern scup (porgy)

Pronghorn Family
Antelope

Ratite Family
Emu
Ostrich
Rhea

Salmon Family
Salmon
Trout

Scorpionfish Family
Rosefish (ocean perch)

Sea Bass Family
Grouper
Sea bass

Sea Catfish Family
Ocean catfish

Silverside Family
Silverside (whitebait)

Smelt Family
Smelt

Snake Family
Rattlesnake

Snapper Family
Red snapper

Squirrel Family
Squirrel

Sturgeon Family
Sturgeon (caviar)

Sucker Family
Buffalo fish
Sucker

Sunfish Family
Black bass species
Crappie
Sunfish species
  Pumpkinseed

Swine Family
Hog (pork)
  Bacon
  Ham
  Lard
  Pork gelatin
  Sausage
  Scrapple

Swordfish Family
Swordfish

Tilefish Family
Tilefish

Turkey Family
Turkey
Turkey eggs

Turtle Family
Terrapin
Turtle species

Whale Family
Whale

Whitefish Family
Whitefish

E

Wheat-Free Diet

Nancy's High-Fiber Bean and Veggie Burritos (*V)

(serves 2)

¾ cup refried beans (vegetarian-style)
1 cup fresh steamed veggies (carrots, squash, mushrooms, etc.)
2 large corn tortillas
¼ cup fresh salsa
¼ cup low-fat sour cream (optional)

Place beans and veggies in tortillas. Combine salsa and sour cream in a blender and blend until smooth. Divide salsa mixture between two tortillas and roll up burrito-style.

Nancy's Cheesy Corn-Pasta Primavera (*V)

(serves 2-3)

1 cup cooked corn pasta (available in natural-food stores)
2 cups steamed vegetables (broccoli, cauliflower, etc.)
1 tablespoon olive oil or butter
½ cup cottage cheese (or fat-free soy cheese, grated)
1 teaspoon garlic powder or no-salt garlic blend
4 tablespoons Parmesan cheese (or soy Parmesan)

Combine hot cooked pasta with steamed veggies in large bowl. Add oil, cottage cheese, garlic, and only 2 tablespoons of Parmesan cheese into pasta/veggie mix. Top with remaining 2 tablespoons Parmesan. Enjoy!

Soft Rolled Tacos (*V)

(serves 2)

> 1 cup fresh tossed mixed greens or sprouts
> 1 medium carrot, grated
> 1 small tomato, diced
> 2 ounces cooked chicken breast, cut into cubes
>
> or
>
> 4 ounces baked tofu (available at natural-food stores)
> 2 medium unbaked corn tortillas
> 1 recipe Nancy's Fat-Free Spicy Dijon Dressing (blend 4
>   tablespoons vinegar, ½ tablespoon mustard, and ½ tablespoon
>   honey until creamy or mix in a jar and shake to blend)

Mix the first four ingredients together in a small bowl. Stuff tortillas with filling and dressing taco-style.

Nancy's Asian Veggie Stir-Fry (*V)

(serves 2)

> 1 tablespoon oil or water
> 1 teaspoon garlic powder
> 3 ounces chicken, beef, tofu, or shrimp, cut in small pieces
> 2 cups fresh veggies of choice, chopped in small pieces
> 2 tablespoons wheat-free tamari
> 2 teaspoons sesame seeds

In large pan, combine the oil, garlic powder, and meat or tofu and cook until done over medium heat. Add veggies and tamari and cook until veggies are desired texture. Top with sesame seeds.

Mashed Cauliflower (a great substitute for mashed potatoes) (*V)

(serves 6)

> 1 bag frozen cauliflower florets
> 3 tablespoons whole milk or half-and-half
> 4–6 ounces cream cheese to taste

Butter to taste

Salt to taste

Garlic salt, ranch dressing powder, pepper, Parmesan, etc., for flavor (optional)

Microwave the cauliflower in large glass bowl covered with a plate to keep the steam in. Cook until cauliflower is very well done (soft!), approximately 8–10 minutes. Drain.

When cauliflower is cool enough for you to handle, squeeze as much water out of it as possible. Put the cauliflower into a food processor and whir on high just until it gets very smooth. Add the milk, cream cheese, and butter. Mix well. The whole point of this process is to make the cauliflower creamy and smooth. Check the consistency. If it is too thick for you, add a tiny bit of milk, mix, and check again. Too much liquid and you will end up with soup (hence the draining!).

Serve hot/warm; you may need to heat it quickly in the microwave before serving.

For a colorful dish, try adding a small amount of carrots or broccoli to the cauliflower.

Confetti Veggie Salsa and Multi-Bean Chili Pie in a Polenta Chili Relleno Pastry Bowl

(serves 4-6)

Polenta Chili Relleno Pastry Bowl

1 cup nonfat milk

2 tablespoons canola or olive oil or melted butter

1 tablespoon honey or fruit juice concentrate

2 cups plus 2 tablespoons cornmeal (reserve 2 tablespoons for dusting baking dish)

1½ teaspoons baking powder

1 large egg or 2 egg whites (beaten slightly)

¼ cup green chilis (canned, mild)

½ cup low-fat cheddar cheese, grated

Confetti Salsa/Chili Filling

2 tablespoons liquid from drained salsa below

4 cloves fresh garlic, minced

1 cup red onion, diced

1 cup zucchini, diced

1 cup green bell pepper, diced

1 cup corn, frozen or fresh off the cob

½ cup chunky-style salsa (liquid drained)

2 teaspoons cumin

2 teaspoons oregano

3 tablespoons chili powder

1 15-ounce can whole tomatoes, drained

1 15-ounce can black beans, drained and rinsed

1 15-ounce can kidney beans, drained and rinsed

½ pound cooked veggie burger or ground turkey breast, crumbled (optional)

Topping

¼ cup fresh cilantro, chopped

1 cup Mexican Cotija cheese or low-fat cheddar, grated

½ cup Parmesan cheese, grated

Polenta Chili Relleno Pastry Bowl: Combine milk, oil, and honey in saucepan and warm over medium heat until honey melts, or microwave for 20 seconds. Add cornmeal, baking powder, and egg, and mix to form a sticky dough. Fold in chilis and cheese until well mixed. Spray baking dish with nonstick spray, then dust with 2 tablespoons cornmeal. Press dough out evenly to cover baking dish and make outside edge. Bake at 350° for 15 minutes to seal crust.

Confetti Salsa: In large saucepan, add first ten ingredients for filling and cook over medium-high heat for 10 minutes until veggies are slightly tender and flavors are released (this can be done a day before and refrigerated for later).

Add the next four ingredients to the cooked Confetti Salsa and heat over medium-high until hot throughout (about 15 minutes).

Meanwhile, mix the three topping ingredients together in a bowl. Pour salsa/chili filling into partially cooked Polenta Chili Relleno Pastry Bowl, add topping evenly, and bake for 20–30 minutes more.

Wheat-Free Sunflower, Millet, and White Corn Enchiladas with Black Bean and Tomato Garlic Sauce
(serves 6-8)

1 cup cooked millet (cook in 2 cups water until tender)
½ large onion, minced
1 cup white corn, frozen or cut off the cob
¼ cup sunflower seeds (toasted, if desired)
1 teaspoon garlic powder
1 recipe Black Bean and Tomato Garlic Sauce (see below)
½ cup water
1 cup low-fat ricotta cheese
1 cup low-fat jack cheese, grated, divided
½ cup Parmesan cheese, grated, divided
1 can diced green chilies (optional)
1 cup zucchini, shredded (optional)
8 medium corn tortillas

Preheat oven to 350°. Mix cooked millet, onion, white corn, sunflower seeds, garlic powder, 1 cup Black Bean and Tomato Garlic Sauce, and ½ cup water in large skillet. Cook over medium heat just until mix is hot. Remove from heat, mix in the ricotta cheese, all but 2 tablespoons of the jack cheese, and only ¼ cup Parmesan, and add any optional ingredients at this time.

In hot oven, warm tortillas wrapped in foil for 2–3 minutes or microwave for 30 seconds to soften.

To make enchiladas: Spread 1 tablespoon Black Bean and Tomato Garlic Sauce over each warmed tortilla, add ½ cup millet filling, and sprinkle with 2 tablespoons jack cheese. Roll up each tortilla carefully and fit all the tortillas into 8 × 8-inch pan. Cover with remaining sauce and sprinkle with remaining ¼ cup Parmesan. Bake until hot throughout, approximately 20 minutes.

Black Bean and Tomato Garlic Sauce

(serves 3-4)

4 cloves garlic, minced

½ medium red onion, diced

2 tablespoons honey or apple juice concentrate

½ cup carrot or zucchini, shredded

½ cup fresh tomatoes, chopped

1½ cups Italian-style tomato sauce (natural, low-sodium variety)

1 teaspoon dried basil

1 teaspoon dried oregano

1 15-ounce can black beans, rinsed and mashed or left whole
(according to your preference)

Place garlic, onion, juice concentrate, carrot, and tomatoes in large skillet and cook over medium-high heat for 3 minutes. Add Italian-style tomato sauce, basil, oregano, and black beans and bring to a boil. Reduce heat to medium and continue to cook for about 10–15 minutes until it thickens.

Optional: For a heartier sauce, add ½ pound crumbled cooked ground turkey breast or veggie burger.

African Coconut Peanut Tofu

(serves 3-4)

2 cloves fresh garlic, minced

½ cup fat-free chicken or veggie broth

½ large onion, chopped

½ large carrot, chopped

1 stalk celery, chopped

½ large red bell pepper, chopped

1 pound firm-style tofu, cut into large cubes

Sauce

½ cup water or broth

2 tablespoons wheat-free tamari or low-sodium soy sauce

3 cloves garlic, chopped

1 teaspoon turmeric

½ teaspoon ground ginger (or 2 teaspoons fresh ginger, chopped)

⅛ teaspoon cayenne pepper (use more to taste)

4 tablespoons natural peanut butter

2 tablespoons unsweetened coconut, flakes or shredded

1 medium fresh orange (juice only)

Toppings: chopped peanuts, raisins/currants, yogurt (optional)

Stir-fry first six ingredients in large saucepan for 5 minutes or until veggies are slightly tender (add more broth if pan is too dry). Add tofu cubes and cook for 2 more minutes (stir gently so as not to break up tofu). In a small saucepan, add all sauce ingredients and cook over medium-low heat until sauce is smooth and starts to thicken. Note: This sauce can be made ahead and stored in refrigerator. Reheat before serving, adding water if necessary. Add sauce to the cooked veggies/tofu, and toss until well coated. Serve over Ginger Sesame Rice Noodles (see recipe below). Serve optional toppings on the side for an extra touch.

Ginger Sesame Rice Noodles

(serves 4)

2 tablespoons fresh orange juice

2 tablespoons rice or white wine vinegar

2 cloves fresh garlic, minced or crushed

2 tablespoons wheat-free tamari or low-sodium soy sauce

2 teaspoons sesame oil (optional)

1 tablespoon toasted sesame seeds

2 cups rice noodles or any style wheat-free noodles you like, cooked according to package directions

½ cup scallions/green onions, chopped

¼ cup cilantro, chopped

1 tablespoon toasted sesame seeds (topping)

Mix sauce (first six ingredients) together in bowl; set aside. Stir together sauce, cooked noodles, and green onion in large saucepan, and cook over medium heat until hot throughout (about 2–3 minutes). Toss hot noodle mixture with cilantro and remaining sesame seeds and serve.

Serving ideas: Add tofu or veggie burger for a main dish, or serve as side dish.

Nancy's Un-Meatballs and Un-Meatloaf
(serves 12)

2 cups mixed (unsalted) raw nuts (almonds, pecans, etc.)

2 cups oat bran

1 cup oatmeal

2 teaspoons sage

1 teaspoon onion powder

2 teaspoons thyme

1 teaspoon ginger

¼ teaspoon cayenne pepper or to taste

4 tablespoons parsley, chopped

1 cup red onion, chopped

4 cloves garlic, minced

½ cup apple juice

4 tablespoons wheat-free tamari or low-sodium soy sauce

1 cup low-fat ricotta cheese

½ cup low-fat mozzarella cheese, grated

Preheat oven to 350°. Blend nuts in food processor until finely ground. In large bowl, mix oat bran, oatmeal, and ground nuts; add all the spices and chopped parsley and set aside. In iron skillet over medium heat, cook onion and garlic in apple juice and tamari until onions are clear. Add onion mixture to dry mixture and return to food processor; blend until smooth. Add ricotta cheese and mozzarella cheese and continue to blend until well mixed (add some water if too dry to blend). Return to bowl and add enough additional water until the mixture is at a consistency that can be made into meatballs and will hold together well (like meatloaf dough). Dip hands into a clean bowl of water and place 1 tablespoon of mixture at a time into wet hand and roll into balls. Place meatballs onto cookie sheet sprayed with nonstick spray. Bake for 20–30 minutes until crispy brown on outside. Serve over wheat-free pasta and a natural spaghetti sauce, or as appetizers with the natural spaghetti sauce for dipping.

For meatloaf: Place mixture into small bread pans. Baking time will increase by 15–20 minutes.

Sesame Tamari Tangerine Woking Chicken with Crunchy Veggies and 7-Grain Pilaf
(serves 6-8)

2 cups cooked 7-grain mix (Kashi) or brown rice
4 cloves fresh garlic, sliced thin or minced
¼ cup Ginger Tamari Sauce (see recipe below)
2 teaspoons toasted sesame oil (optional)
½ cup scallions, chopped
4 medium boneless, skinless chicken breasts, cut into cubes
1 cup red cabbage, chopped
1 large yellow or red bell pepper, chopped
½ cup Ginger Tamari Sauce (see recipe below)
or
½ cup chicken broth or water
2 small tangerines, peeled, separated, and cut into pieces
or
2 small cans (no sugar added) mandarin oranges, drained
¼ cup toasted sesame seeds
¼ cup cilantro, chopped

Cook 7-grain mix or brown rice according to package directions. This can be done ahead of time.

In wok, iron skillet, or a nonstick pan, place garlic, ¼ cup Ginger Tamari Sauce, sesame oil, scallions, and chicken; cook over medium-high heat until the meat is white throughout. Add cabbage, bell pepper, ½ cup Ginger Tamari Sauce or broth, and cooked 7-grain mix; continue to cook until veggies are desired texture. Add more broth or water if too dry. Stir in remaining ingredients and cook for 3–5 minutes or until heated throughout.

Ginger Tamari Sauce

1 cup wheat-free tamari or low-sodium tamari sauce

½ cup honey or apple juice concentrate

2 tablespoons fresh ginger, finely minced, or 2 teaspoons ground ginger

Add any seasonings that you desire (pepper, herbs, etc.)

In iron skillet, bring all ingredients to a boil. Cook over medium heat for 2 minutes or until mixture starts to thicken. Remove from heat and let cool.

The sauce may be used to marinate food for shish kebabs or for stir-fry (such as tofu, chicken, veggies). Pour sauce over food and place in covered container in the refrigerator overnight to marinate, or add to hot skillet for stir-fry.

This sauce can be made ahead of time and stored in covered container in refrigerator.

Lentil, Brown Rice, and Adzuki Bean Chili

(serves 4-6)

3 15-ounce cans fat-free chicken or veggie broth

2 cups water or carrot juice (for a richer flavor)

1 cup brown rice (uncooked)

1½ cups lentils (if available, red lentils are more colorful)

1 large onion, chopped

3 cloves fresh garlic, minced

3 large carrots, chopped

1 large stalk celery, chopped

1½ tablespoons chili powder

1 teaspoon dried basil

1 teaspoon dried oregano

1 teaspoon dried thyme

1 15-ounce can whole tomatoes with juice

1 15-ounce can adzuki beans or black beans, drained and rinsed
1 cup Italian-style spaghetti sauce (fat-free variety)
½ cup chopped scallions (optional)
½ cup fresh basil or cilantro (optional)
½ cup low-fat cheddar or Parmesan cheese, grated (optional)

In large, heavy saucepan, add first twelve ingredients and bring to a boil. Reduce heat to simmer, cover pan, and cook approximately 40 minutes or until rice and lentils are tender (may need to stir occasionally and add more water if too thick). Remove from heat and add tomatoes, adzuki beans, and Italian-style spaghetti sauce. Return to heat and cook for about 10 more minutes. Top with optional toppings. Serve with crusty wheat-free bread or with warmed corn tortillas. Stores great for 2 weeks in the refrigerator!

Chunky Harvest Vegetable, Bean, and Barley Stew

(serves 8-12)

2 tablespoons white wine or chicken or veggie broth
4 tablespoons wheat-free tamari or low-sodium soy sauce
1 large onion, finely chopped
3 cloves garlic, sliced
1 pound fresh mushrooms, sliced
2 15-ounce cans fat-free chicken or veggie broth
2 cups water (or more broth for a richer flavor)
1 cup pearl barley, uncooked
1 teaspoon thyme leaves, crushed
1 teaspoon tarragon leaves, crushed
2 medium carrots, chopped
1 15-ounce can white beans, drained and rinsed
1 cup fresh-off-the-cob or frozen corn
1 cup frozen green peas
1 cup red pepper, chopped
2 cups cooked chicken breast, shredded (optional topping)
1½ cups firm-style tofu, cubed (optional topping)

In large pan, sauté the first five ingredients until the veggies are tender. Add the remaining ingredients and bring to a boil. Reduce the heat and simmer for about 45 minutes or until barley is tender. Serve with optional toppings (shredded chicken or tofu).

South-of-the-Border Corn, Bean, and Squash Stew

(serves 8-12)

> 1 cup mild salsa (low-sodium variety)
>
> 2 cloves garlic, sliced
>
> 1 medium onion, finely chopped
>
> 2 medium zucchini or yellow summer squash, diced
>
> 2 15-ounce cans fat-free chicken or veggie broth
>
> 1½ cups frozen or fresh-off-the-cob corn
>
> 2 15-ounce cans pinto or black beans (or one can of each)
>
> 3 tablespoons canned green chilis (mild)
>
> 2 teaspoons ground cumin
>
> 1 can evaporated skim milk or soy milk
>
> ½ cup low-fat jack or pepper jack cheese, grated

Optional toppings and additions:

> ½ cup fresh cilantro, chopped
>
> ½ cup fresh tomatoes, diced
>
> ½ cup natural-brand light sour cream
>
> ½ cup natural-brand guacamole

In large pan sauté the first four ingredients for 5 minutes. Stir in the next five ingredients and bring stew to a boil. Reduce heat and allow to simmer for 5 more minutes. Remove from heat and stir in the evaporated milk. Return to medium-low heat until hot throughout (be careful not to burn or curdle). Stir in grated cheese and serve with optional toppings.

Creamy Broccoli and Almond Butter Soup

(serves 6-8)

> 2 15-ounce cans fat-free chicken or veggie broth
>
> 1 cup water

1 cup white potato, diced into small pieces

½ cup green onion, chopped

2 cloves fresh garlic, minced

1 large carrot, chopped

2 cups broccoli, chopped (reserve ½ cup florets)

½ cup almond butter (or peanut butter)

2 teaspoons no-salt seasoning blend (all-purpose blend)

Optional toppings:

¼ cup toasted chopped or sliced almonds

½ cup cilantro, chopped

½ cup carrot, grated

In large saucepan, add first seven ingredients (do not use ½ cup broccoli florets) and bring to a boil. Reduce heat to simmer, cover, and cook for 15 minutes or until veggies are tender. Optional: Blend in food processor for creamy-style.

Remove from the heat and stir in almond butter, seasoning, and reserved ½ cup broccoli florets until completely blended throughout. Return to low heat and allow to simmer for about 3–5 minutes (do not allow to boil).

Serve with optional toppings. Great with crusty bread or with warmed corn tortillas. Stores great for up to 2 weeks in the refrigerator.

Nancy's Crunchy and Colorful Chinese Coleslaw

(serves 8-12)

4 cups red cabbage, chopped or grated

1 large carrot, grated

½ cup green or red bell pepper, chopped

½ cup green onions, chopped

4 tablespoons sliced almonds, toasted*

4 tablespoons sunflower seeds, toasted*

2 tablespoons sesame seeds, toasted*

1 package rice noodles, cooked

½ cup nonfat vanilla or plain yogurt

4 tablespoons rice or balsamic vinegar

2 tablespoons honey or fruit juice concentrate

2 cloves fresh garlic, minced

1 package flavor packet from rice noodles

*To toast nuts/seeds, place in nonstick pan on medium heat and cook for 1–2 minutes until lightly browned. Remove from pan immediately. Be careful not to burn.

Break noodles up into small pieces and cook noodles per instructions on the package; do not add flavor packet. When noodles are done, drain and set aside. Place first seven ingredients in a large bowl and add noodles. In a small jar with a lid or a small mixing bowl, mix yogurt, vinegar, honey, garlic, and flavor packet. Whisk to create dressing. (This is a great dressing for any salad.) Add dressing to noodle/vegetable mixture and chill before serving.

Serving ideas: Add chicken, seafood, or tofu for an excellent main-dish salad for lunch or a light dinner, or stuff in a corn tortilla. Excellent source of beta-carotene and vitamin C.

Nancy's High-Energy Multi-Bean and Rice Bake

(serves 8-12)

2 cups brown rice (regular or quick cooking)

3 15-ounce cans beans (black, kidney, garbanzo, etc.)

½ cup fresh or natural-brand salsa (chunky style)

1 clove garlic, minced

½ large red onion, chopped

2 teaspoons cumin

2 cups natural-brand spaghetti sauce (low-fat and low-sodium style)

10 dashes Tabasco sauce

1 cup fat-free cheddar cheese, grated

½ cup Parmesan cheese, grated

Preheat oven to 350°. Cook rice according to package directions and set aside. Rinse canned beans thoroughly in a colander.

In a large glass baking dish, combine salsa, garlic, onions, and cumin. Cook in microwave on high for 2 minutes until onions are soft (or cook on stove in a nonstick skillet). Add beans, spaghetti sauce, and Tabasco; stir together until mixed.

Place cooked rice in the bottom of a 13 × 9-inch baking pan, cover with bean mixture, and top with grated cheeses. Place in oven and bake 15–20 minutes until hot throughout.

For a quicker method, microwave the casserole for approximately 5 minutes on high.

Spicy Black Bean and Corn Chili

(serves 10-12)

1 medium red onion, chopped
¼ cup chicken broth or apple juice
3 cloves garlic, chopped
1 cup zucchini, chopped
1 cup green bell pepper, chopped
2 cups frozen or fresh-off-the-cob corn
2 15-ounce cans whole tomatoes
½ cup natural-brand chunky-style salsa
2 15-ounce cans black beans
2 tablespoons chili powder
1 teaspoon cumin
1 teaspoon oregano

Rinse beans in colander to remove excess salt.

In a large saucepan or skillet, sauté the first five ingredients over medium-high heat for 2 minutes or until vegetables are softened. Add the remaining ingredients to the pan and bring to a boil. Reduce heat to simmer and continue to cook for 20 minutes, covered, stirring occasionally.

Optional ingredients: Include one of the following ingredients and allow to cook until meat is completely cooked: tofu, chicken breast, or ground turkey breast.

To-Die-For Creamy Carrot Spiced Shakes

(serves 2)

½ medium frozen banana*

1 cup carrot juice (fresh or bottled)

1 cup vanilla nonfat frozen yogurt (or ice milk)

1 tablespoon raisins

1 tablespoon chopped dates

1 teaspoon cinnamon (or less to taste)

1 tablespoon sliced raw almonds

*Peel very ripe banana, wrap in wax paper, and freeze.

Slice the frozen banana into small pieces. Place all the ingredients into blender, and blend until smooth.

Variations: Use any combination of fresh or frozen fruits, juices, and dried fruits. This is a very energizing and flavorful drink!

F

Anti-Yeast Diet

Candida albicans is dependent on simple carbohydrates for growth. You must strictly avoid yeast-containing foods in order to be successful on this diet. The following are guidelines for you to follow.

Sugars

Do not eat sugars or sweets. This includes all products made with honey, molasses, sucrose, or syrup.

Grains

You may eat the following whole grains:

Millet, buckwheat, amaranth, rice, corn, quinoa, and oats. Attempt to use a wide variety of these grains in order to avoid using high-gluten-containing grains. Grains with a high gluten content (wheat, rye, and barley) should be restricted.

Avoid all enriched grains. This means avoid all grains that have been fortified with synthetic nutrients or additives during processing.

Dairy Products

You may eat the following dairy products:

Butter, cream, sour cream, cream cheese, Neufchâtel cheese, cottage cheese, kefir cheese, plain kefir, plain yogurt, and buttermilk.

Avoid all forms of brick cheese, blue cheese, Camembert, etc.

Avoid milk.

Fruit

You may eat up to two pieces of fruit per day. However, fruit juices must be temporarily omitted from the diet. Berries, apples, pears, avocados, and tomatoes are acceptable. Freshness reduces mold buildup.

Avoid citrus fruits and fruits that have high mold content. Melons, especially cantaloupe and the skins of fleshy fruits such as peaches and apricots, fall into this category. Avoid dried fruits such as prunes, raisins, dates, figs, candied cherries, and currants. Avoid canned or frozen fruits, including those containing citric acid.

Nuts

You may eat fresh whole nuts and seeds, including their butters and milks. Avoid peanuts, pistachios, and dry-roasted nuts.

Vegetables

Vegetables are highly encouraged on this diet. You may eat them raw or cooked. Fresh tofu is also acceptable. Avoid mushrooms.

Legumes

You may eat legumes and their sprouts if very fresh. Legumes are beans, peas, pea pods, soybeans, lentils, etc. They can be cooked for soups and stews or cold for salads.

Yeast

Yeast is used in food preparation and handling, so be sure to avoid all commercial breads, rolls, coffee cakes, pastries, etc. Beer, wine, and all other alcoholic beverages should be avoided. Vinegar and vinegar-containing foods such as pickled vegetables, sauerkraut, relish, green olives, and salad dressing should also be avoided. Lemon or lime juice with oil may be used as a salad dressing. Soy sauce, cider, and natural root beer; most commercial soups and barbecue chips; pickled, smoked, or dried meats; fish and poultry, including sausages, salami, tongue, corned beef, pastrami, bacon, and any type of country-style cured pork should all be avoided. Avoid any vitamins or mineral supplements that contain yeast.

Miscellaneous

Dried herb teas and spices are acceptable. Coffee beans are fermented and dried and should be avoided. Coffee and black teas should be avoided due to their caffeine content.

What Is Left to Eat?

- Proteins: Fish, chicken, beef, pork, turkey, duck, seafood of all kinds, eggs, goat, venison, rabbit, frog legs, pheasant, quail, lamb, and veal.
- Vegetables, legumes, grains, and fruit as noted above.

Is It Possible to Eat Out?

Yes! Just order carefully and skip the cocktail. Have oil and lemon juice on your salad. Order chicken, fish, or other animal protein that is prepared without sauces. Broiled or plain items are the safest. Steamed vegetables are perfect. Skip bread, crackers, and dessert.

If you are aware of specific allergies to any of the allowed foods, you must avoid those foods also.

Alternative Foods for a Yeast-Free Diet

FLOURS
Amaranth
Arrowroot
Artichoke (Jerusalem)
Buckwheat
Cassava
Chickpea
Lima bean
Lotus root
Malanga
Nut and seed flours
Oat
Potato
Quinoa
Rice
Sesame
Soybean
Tapioca
Water chestnut
White sweet potato
Yam

LEAVENINGS
Baking powder
Baking soda
Featherweight baking powder

THICKENERS
Agar-agar
Arrowroot starch
Buckwheat flakes
Malanga starch
Potato starch
Rice starch
Tapioca starch

MILK SUBSTITUTES
Almond milk
Goat milk
Milk (cassava, lotus root, malanga, water chestnut, white sweet potato)
Nut or seed milk
Potato milk
Soy milk
Vegetable juices
Zucchini milk

CEREALS AND MEALS
Amaranth (puffed and cereal)
Buckwheat (cereal and flakes)
Creamed cereals (lotus root, amaranth, etc.)
Crispy cereal shreds (malanga, cassava, yam, etc.)
Millet flakes
Quinoa (puffed and cereal)
Rice (cereal and puffed)

PASTAS AND NOODLES
Bifun (rice and potato)
Buckwheat
Green bean noodles
Kuzi Kuri
Mung bean noodles
Pasta (amaranth, cassava, yam, etc.)
Saifun (sweet-potato starch)

VEGETABLE CHIPS
Artichoke chips
Carrot chips
Cassava chips
Malanga chips
Parsnip chips
Potato chips
Rice petals
Sweet-potato chips

OILS
Almond
Apricot kernel
Avocado
Beef drippings
Canola
Chicken fat
Coconut
Cottonseed
Olive
Palm kernel
Pumpkin
Safflower
Sesame
Soy
Sunflower

EGG ALTERNATIVES
Arrowroot mixture
Baking powder mixture
Egg replacer
Flaxseed mixture
Soybean curd

CRACKERS
Amaranth
Brown rice
Cassava
Lotus root
Malanga
White sweet potato
Yam

G

Resources

American Academy of Environmental Medicine

6505 E. Central Avenue, #296
Wichita, KS 67206
Phone: 316-684-5500
Fax: 316-684-5709
Email: administrator@aaemonline.org
Web: www.aaemonline.org

American College for Advancement in Medicine

8001 Irvine Center Drive, #825
Irvine, CA 92618
Phone: 800-532-3668
    949-309-3520
Fax: 949-309-3538
Email: info@acam.org
Web: www.acam.org

American Academy of Anti-Aging Medicine

1801 N. Military Trail, #200
Boca Raton, FL 33431
Phone: 888-997-0112
    561-997-0112
Fax: 561-997-0287
Email: info@worldhealth.net
Web: www.a4m.com

American Holistic Medical Association

27629 Chagrin Boulevard, #213
Woodmere, OH 44122
Phone: 216-292-6644
Fax: 216-292-6688
Email: info@holisticmedicine.org
Web: www.holisticmedicine.org

The Institute for Functional Medicine

505 S. 336th Street, #500
Federal Way, WA 98003
Phone: 800-228-0622
    253-661-3010

Fax: 253-661-8310
Email: client_services@fxmed.com
Web: www.functionalmedicine.org

Environmental Working Group

1436 U Street NW, #100
Washington, DC 20009
Phone: 202-667-6982
Web: www.ewg.org

REFERENCES

Aagaard-Tillery, K.M., Grove, K., Bishop, J., et al. Developmental origins of disease and determinants of chromatin structure: maternal diet modifies the primate fetal epigenome. *J Mol Endocrinol.* 2008;41:91–102.

Abbey, M., Noakes, M., Belling, G.B., Nestel, P.J. Partial replacement of saturated fatty acids with almonds or walnuts lowers total plasma cholesterol and low-density-lipoprotein cholesterol. *Am J Clin Nutr.* 1997;59:995–99.

Abidov, M., Grachev, S., Seifulla, R.D., Ziegenfuss, T.N. Extract of Rhodiola rosea radix reduces the level of C-reactive protein and creatinine kinase in the blood. *Bull Exp Biol Med.* Jul 2004;138(1):63–64.

Adlercreutz, C.H., Golden, B.R., Gorbach, S.L. Soybean phytoestrogen intake and cancer risk. *J Nutr.* Mar 1995;125(suppl 3):S757–70.

Agerholm-Larsen, L., Raben, A., Haulrik, N. Effect of 8-week intake of probiotic milk products on risk factors for cardiovascular diseases. *Eur J Clin Nutr.* Apr 2000;54(4):288–97.

Aggarwal, B.B., Kumar, A., Bharti, A.C. Anticancer potential of curcumin: preclinical and clinical studies. *Anticancer Res.* Jan 2003;23(1A):363–98.

Ahmad, N., Feyes, D., Nieminen, A., Agarwal, R., Mukhtar, H. Green tea constituent epigallocatechin-3-gallate and induction of apoptosis and cell cycle arrest in human carcinoma cells. *J Natl Cancer Inst.* 1997;89:1881–86.

Ahonen, M.H., Tenkanen, L., Teppo, L., Hakama, M., Tuohimaa, P. Prostate cancer risk and prediagnostic serum 25-hydroxyvitamin D levels (Finland). *Cancer Causes Control.* 2000;11:847–52.

al'Absi, M., Lovallo, W.R., McKey, B., Sung, B.H., Whitsett, T.L., Wilson, M.F. Hypothalamic-pituitary-adrenocortical responses to psychological stress and caffeine in men at high and low risk for hypertension. *Psychosom Med.* Jul–Aug 1998;60(4):521–27.

Alele, J.D., Kamen, D.L. The importance of inflammation and vitamin D status in SLE-associated osteoporosis. *Autoimmun Rev.* Jan 2010;9(3):137–39.

Allgood, V.E., Powell-Oliver, F.E., Cidlowski, J.A. The influence of vitamin B6 on the structure and function of the glucocorticoid receptor. *Ann NY Acad Sci.* 1990;585:452–65.

Allgood, V.E., Powell-Oliver, F.E., Cidlowski, J.A. Vitamin B6 influences glucocorticoid receptor-dependent gene expression. *J Biol Chem.* 1990;265:12324–433.

Anagnostis, P., Athyros, V.G. The pathogenetic role of cortisol in the metabolic syndrome: a hypothesis. *J Clin Endocrinol Metab.* May 26 2009;94(8):2692–701.

Anderson, D.A., Shapiro, J.R., Lundgren, J.D., Spataro, L.E., Frye, C.A. Self-reported dietary restraint is associated with elevated levels of salivary cortisol. *Appetite.* Feb 2002;38(1):13–17.

Anderson, J.W., Deakins, D.A., Floore, T.L., Smith, B.M., Whitis, S.E. Dietary fiber and coronary heart disease. *Crit Rev Food Sci Nutr.* 1990;29(2):95–147.

Anderson, J.W., Gustafson, N.J. Hypocholesterolemic effects of oat and bean products. *Am J Clin Nutr.* Sep 1988;48(suppl 3):S749–53.

Anderson, J.W., Gustafson, N.J., Spencer, D.B., Tietyen, J., Bryant, C.A. Serum lipid response of hypercholesterolemic men to single and divided doses of canned beans. *Am J Clin Nutr.* Jun 1990;51(6):1013–19.

Anderson, J.W., Johnstone, B.M., Cook-Newell, M.E. Meta-analysis of the effects of soy protein intake on serum lipids. *N Engl J Med.* Aug 3 1995;333(5):276–82.

Andrew, R., Gale, C., Walker, B., Seckl, J., Martyn, C.N. Glucocorticoid metabolism and the metabolic syndrome: associations in an elderly cohort. *Exp Clin Endocrinol Diabetes.* Sep 2002;110(6):284–90.

Andrews, R.C., Herlihy, O., Livingston, D.E., Andrew, R., Walker, B.R. Abnormal cortisol metabolism and tissue sensitivity to cortisol in patients with glucose intolerance. *J Clin Endocrinol Metab.* Dec 2002;87(12):5587–93.

Anway, M.D., Cupp, A.S., Uzumcu, M., Skinner, M.K. Epigenetic transgenerational actions of endocrine disruptors and male fertility. *Science.* Jun 2005;308(5727):1466–69.

Apostolova, G., Schweizer, R.A., Balazs, Z., Kostadinova, R.M., Odermatt, A. Dehydroepiandrosterone inhibits the amplification of glucocorticoid action in adipose tissue. *Am J Physiol Endocrinol Metab.* May 2005;288(5):E957–64.

Arai, Y., Ohgane, J., Yagi, S., Ito, R., Iwasaki, Y., Saito, K., Akutsu, K., et al. Epigenetic assessment of environmental chemicals detected in maternal peripheral and cord blood samples. *J Reprod Dev.* 57:507–17.

Askari, H., Liu, J., Dagogo, J.S. Energy adaptation to glucocorticoid-induced hyperleptinemia in human beings. *Metabolism.* Jul 2005;54(7):876–80.

Atanasov, A.G., Dzyakanchuk, A.A., Schweizer, R.A., Nashev, L.G., Maurer, E.M., Odermatt, A. Coffee inhibits the reactivation of glucocorticoids by 11beta-hydroxysteroid dehydrogenase type 1: a glucocorticoid connection in the anti-diabetic action of coffee? *FEBS Lett.* Jul 2006;580(17):4081–85.

Aybak, M., Sermet, A., Ayyildiz, M.O., Karakilcik, A.Z. Effect of oral pyridoxine hydrocholoride supplementation on arterial blood pressure in patients with essential hypertension. *Arzneimittelforschung.* 1995;45:1271–73.

Babio, N., Bullo, M., Salas-Salvado, J. Mediterranean diet and metabolic syndrome: the evidence. *Public Health Nutr.* Sep 2009;12(9A):1607–17.

Bagchi, S. Arsenic threat reaching global dimensions. *CMAJ.* 2007;177:1344–45.

Bagot, R.C., Meaney, M.J. Epigenetics and the biological basis of gene x environment interactions. *J Am Acad Child Adolesc Psychiatry.* 2010;49:752–71.

Bahr, V., Pfeiffer, A.F., Diederich, S. The metabolic syndrome X and peripheral cortisol synthesis. *Exp Clin Endocrinol Diabetes.* Oct 2002;110(7):313–18.

Balbio, N., Bullo, M., et al. Adherence to the Mediterranean diet and risk of metabolic syndrome. *Nutr Metab Cardiovasc Dis.* Oct 2009;19(8):563–70.

Baldewicz, T., Goodkin, K., Feaster, D.J., Blaney, N.T., Kumar, M., Kuman, A., et al. Plasma pyridoxine deficiency is related to increased psychological distress in recently bereaved homosexual men. *Psychosom Med.* 1998;60:297–308.

Basu, R., Breda, E., Aberg, A.L. Mechanisms of the age-associated deterioration in glucose tolerance: contribution of alterations in insulin secretion, action, and clearance. *Diabetes.* 2003;52:1738–48.

Bauer, M.E. Stress, glucocorticoids and ageing of the immune system. *Stress.* Mar 2005;8(1):69–83.

Beckman, K.B., Ames, B.N. The free radical theory of aging matures. *Physiol Rev.* 1998;78:547–81.

Behrens, S., Ehlers, C., Bruggemann, T., Ziss, W., Dissman, R., Galecka, M., et al. Modification of the circadian pattern of ventricular tachyarrhythmias by beta-blocker therapy. *Clin Cardiol.* 1997;20:247–53.

Belch, J.J., Ansell, D., Madhok, R. Effects of altering dietary essential fatty acids on requirements for non-steroidal anti-inflammatory drugs in patients with rheumatoid arthritis: a double blind placebo controlled study. *Ann Rheum Dis.* 1988;47(2):96–104.

Belch, J.J., Hill, A. Evening primrose oil and borage oil in rheumatologic conditions. *Am J Clin Nutri.* 2000;71(suppl):S352–56.

Bell, J.T., Tsai, P.C., Yang, T.P., et al. Epigenome-wide scans identify differentially methylated regions for age and age-related phenotypes in a healthy ageing population. *PLoS Genet.* Apr 2012; 8(4):e1002629.

Bernal, A.J., Jirtle, R.L. Epigenomic disruption: the effects of early developmental exposures. *Birth Defects Res A Clin Mol Teratol.* Oct 2010;88(10):938–44.

Bethin, K.E., Vogt, S.K., Muglia, L.J. Interleukin-6 is an essential, corticotropin-releasing hormone-independent stimulator of the adrenal axis during immune system activation. *Proc Natl Acad Sci USA.* Aug 2000;97(16):9317–22.

Bhamre, S., Sahoo, D., Tibshirani, R., Dill, D.L., Brooks, J.D. Temporal changes in gene expression induced by sulforaphane in human prostate cancer cells. *Prostate.* Feb 2009;69(2):181–90.

Bhathena, S.J., Velasquez, M.T. Beneficial role of dietary phytoestrogens in obesity and diabetes. *Am J Clin Nutr.* Dec 2002;76(6):1191–201.

Bhattacharya, S. Anti-stress activity of sitoindosides VII and VIII, new acylsterylglucosides from Withania somnifera. *Phytother Res.* 1987;1:32–37.

Biddle, S.C., Conway-Campbell, B.L., Lightman, S.L. Dynamic regulation of glucocorticoid signaling in health and disease. *Rheumatology (Oxf)*. Mar 2012;51(3):403–12.

Bishayee, A. Cancer prevention and treatment with resveratrol: from rodent studies to clinical trials. *Cancer Prev Res (Phila)*. May 2009;2(5):409–18.

Björntorp, P. Do stress reactions cause abdominal obesity and comorbidities? *Obes Rev*. May 2001;2(2):73–86.

Björntorp, P. Stress and cardiovascular disease. *Acta Physiol Scand*. 1997;640(suppl):144–48.

Björntorp, P. Visceral fat accumulation: the missing link between psychosocial factors and cardiovascular disease? *J Intern Med*. 1991;230:195–201.

Björntorp, P., Holm, G., Rosmond, R. Hypothalamic arousal, insulin resistance and type 2 diabetes mellitus. *Diabetes Med*. 1999;16:373–83.

Björntorp, P., Rosmond, R. The metabolic syndrome: a neuroendocrine disorder? *Br J Nutr*. 2000;83(suppl 1):S49–57.

Black, P.H. The inflammatory consequences of psychologic stress: relationship to insulin resistance, obesity, atherosclerosis and diabetes mellitus, type II. *Med Hypotheses*. 2006;67(4):879–91.

Bland, J.S., Bralley, J.A. Nutritional upregulation of hepatic detoxification enzymes. *J Appl Nutr*. 1992;44:2–15.

Bloedon, L.T., Szapary, P.O. Flaxseed and cardiovascular risk. *Nutr Rev*. Jan 2004;62(1):18–27.

Bollati, V., Baccarelli, A. Environmental epigenetics. *Heredity*. Jul 2010;105(1):105–12.

Bomba, A., Nemcová, R., Gancarcíková, S., et al. The influence of omega-3 polyunsaturated fatty acids (omega-3 pufa) on lactobacilli adhesion to the intestinal mucosa and on immunity in gnotobiotic piglets. *Berl Munch Tierarztl Wochenschr*. Jul 2003;116(7–8):312–16.

Borchers, A.T., Kean, C.L., Gershwin, M.E. The influence of yogurt/ Lactobacillus on the innate and acquired immune response. *Clin Rev Allergy Immunol*. Jun 2002:22(3):207–30.

Boris, M., Mandel, F. Foods and additives are common causes of the attention deficit hyperactive disorder in children. *Ann Allergy.* 1994;72:462–68.

Borkman, M., Campbell, L.V., Chisholm, D.J., Storlien, L.H. Comparison of the effects on insulin sensitivity of high carbohydrate and high fat diets in normal subjects. *J Clin Endocrinol Metab.* 1991;72:432–37.

Braly, J., Holford, P. *Hidden Food Allergies.* Laguna Beach, CA: Basic Health Publications; 2006.

Bramswig, N.C., Kaestner, K.H. Epigenetics and diabetes treatment: an unrealized promise? *Trends Endocrinol Metab.* Mar 2012;23(6):286–91.

Brand-Miller, J.C., et al. Glycemic index and obesity. *Am J Clin Nutr.* 2002;76(1):281S–285S.

Brenneman, J.C. Allergy elimination diet as the most effective gallbladder diet. *Ann Allergy.* 1968;26:83–87.

Brody, S., Preut, R., Schommer, K., Schürmeyer, T.H. A randomized controlled trial of high dose ascorbic acid for reduction of blood pressure, cortisol, and subjective responses to psychological stress. *Psychopharmacology (Berl).* Jan 2002;159(3):319–24.

Brouet, I., Ohshima, H. Curcumin, an anti-tumour promoter and anti-inflammatory agent, inhibits induction of nitric oxide synthase in activated macrophages. *Biochem Biophys Res Commun.* Jan 17 1995;206(2):533–40.

Brown, D., Gaby, A., Reichert, R. Phytotherapeutic and nutritional approaches to diabetes mellitus. *Quarterly Rev Nat Med.* 1998;Winter:329–51.

Bruder, E.D., Raff, H., Goodfriend, T.L. An oxidized derivative of linoleic acid stimulates dehydroepiandrosterone production by human adrenal cells. *Horm Metab Res.* Dec 2006;38(12):803–6.

Brunner, E., Hemingway, H., Walker, B., Page, M., Clarke, P., Juneja, M. Adrenocortical, autonomic, and inflammatory causes of the nested case-control study. *Circulation.* Nov 19 2002;106(21):2659–65.

Bryant, C.S., Kumar, S., Chamala, S., Shah, J., Pal, J., Haider, M., Seward, S., Qazi, A.M., et al. Sulforaphane induces cell cycle arrest by protecting RB-E2F-1 complex in epithelial ovarian cancer cells. *Mol Cancer.* 2010;9:47.

Bujalska, I.J., Kumar, S., Stewart, P.M. Does central obesity reflect "Cushing's disease of the omentum"? *Lancet.* 1997;349:1210–13.

Burgess, J.R., Stevens, L., Zhang, W., Peck, L. Long-chain polyunsaturated fatty acids in children with attention-deficit hyperactive disorder. *Am J Clin Nutri.* 2000;71(suppl):S327–30.

Bustamante, J., Lodge, J.K., Marcocci, L. Alpha-lipoic acid in liver metabolism and disease. *Free Rad Biol Med.* 1998;24(6):1023–39.

Buttner, P., Mosig, S., Lechtermann, A., et al. Exercise affects the gene expression profiles of human white blood cells. *J Appl Physiol.* 2007;102:26–36.

Buydens-Branchey, L., Branchey, M., Hudson, J., Fergeson, P. Low HDL cholesterol, aggression and altered central serotonergic activity. *Psychiatry Res.* Mar 6 2000;93(2):93–102.

Calder, P.C. Mechanisms of action of (n-3) fatty acids. *J Nutr.* Mar 2012;142(3):592S–599S.

Calder, P.C. Omega-3 polyunsaturated fatty acids and inflammatory processes: Nutrition or pharmacology? *Br J Clin Pharmacol.* Jul 6 2012. DOI:10.1111/j. 1365–2125.2012.04374.x.

Calorie Restriction Society website: www.crsociety.org.

Cani, P.D., Delzenne, N.M. The gut microbiome as therapeutic target. *Pharmacol Ther.* May 2011;130(2):202–12.

Cani, P.D., Osto, M., Geurts, L., Everard, A. Involvement of gut microbiota in the development of low-grade inflammation and type 2 diabetes associated with obesity. *Gut Microbes.* Jul 2012;3(4):279–88.

Carr, D.J., Guarcello, V., Blalock, J.E. Phosphatidylserine suppresses antigen-specific IgM production by mice orally administered sheep red blood cells. *Proc Soc Exp Biol Med.* Sep 1992;200(4):548–54.

Carroll, D.N., Roth, M.T. Evidence for the cardioprotective effects of omega-3 fatty acids. *Ann Pharmacother.* 2002;36(12):1950–56.

CDC. Fourth national report on human exposure to environmental chemicals. 2009. www.cdc.gov/exposurereport.

CDC. Fourth national report on human exposure to environmental chemicals, updated tables. Sep 2012. www.cdc.gov/exposurereport /pdf/FourthReport_UpdatedTables_Sep2012.pdf.

Chainani-Wu, N. Safety and anti-inflammatory activity of curcumin: a component of turmeric (Curcuma longa). *J Altern Complement Med.* Feb 2003;9(1):161–68.

Chang, X.X., Yan, H.M., Xu, Q., et al. The effects of berberine on hyperhomocysteinemia and hyperlipidemia in rats fed with a long-term high-fat diet. *Lipids Health Dis.* Jul 4 2012;11(1):86.

Charmandari, E., Weise, M., Bornstein, S., Eisenhofer, G., Keil, M. Children with classic congenital adrenal hyperplasia have elevated serum leptin concentrations and insulin resistance: potential clinical implications. *J Clin Endocrinol Metab.* May 2002;87(5):2114–20.

Chee, K.M., Gong, J.X., Rees, D.M.G., Meydani, M., Ausman, L., Johnson, J., et al. Fatty acid content of marine oil capsules. *Lipids.* 1990;25:523–27.

Chen, J., Stavro, P.M., Thompson, L.U. Dietary flaxseed inhibits human breast cancer growth and metastasis and downregulates expression of insulin-like growth factor and epidermal growth factor receptor. *Nutr Cancer.* 2002;43(2):187–92.

Chen, J., Xu, X. Diet, epigenetic, and cancer prevention. *Adv Genet.* 2010;71:237–55.

Cheung, K.L., Kong, A.N. Molecular targets of dietary phenethyl iso-thiocyanate and sulforaphane for cancer chemoprevention. *AAPS J.* 2010;12:89–97.

Choi, S.W., Friso, S. Epigenetics: a new bridge between nutrition and health. *Adv Nutr (Bethesda).* Nov 2010;1(1):8–16.

Choi, S.W., Friso, S. *Nutrients and Epigenetics.* Boca Raton, FL: CRC Press; 2009.

Christensen, B., Marsit, C. Epigenomics in environmental health. *Front Genet.* Nov 2011;2:84.

Christiansen, E., Schnider, S., Palmvig, B., Tauber-Lassen, E., Pedersen, O. Intake of a diet high in trans monounsaturated fatty acids or satu-rated fatty acids: effects on postprandial insulinemia and glycemia in obese patients with NIDDM. *Diabetes Care.* 1997;20:881–87.

Clarke, J.D., Hsu, A., Yu, Z., et al. Differential effects of sulforaphane on histone deacetylases, cell cycle arrest and apoptosis in normal prostate cells versus hyperplastic and cancerous prostate cells. *Mol Nutr Food Res.* 2011;55:999–1009.

Coiro, V., Casti, A., Rubino, P., Manfredi, G., Maffei, M.L., Melani, A., et al. Free fatty acids inhibit adrenocorticotropin and cortisol secre-tion stimulated by physical exercise in normal men. *Clin Endocrinol (Oxf).* May 2007;66(5):740–43.

Coles, L.S. Table of world-wide living supercentenarians. *J Anti Aging Med.* 2002;5:231–33.

Compton, M.M., Cidlowski, J.A. Vitamin B6 and glucocorticoid action. *Endocr Rev.* 1986;7:140–48.

Connor, W.E. Importance of n-3 fatty acids in health and disease. *Am J Clin Nutr.* 2000;71(suppl):S171–75.

Cornblat, B.S., Ye, L., Dinkova-Kostova, A.T., et al. Preclinical and clinical evaluation of sulforaphane for chemoprevention in the breast. *Carcinogenesis.* Jul 2007;28(7):1485–90.

Corral, A.R., Sierra-Johnson, J., Orban, M., Gami, A.S., Kuniyoshi, R.H.S., Pusalavidyasager, S., et al. Modest fat gain causes endothelial dysfunction in lean healthy humans: a randomized blinded controlled trial. *Circulation.* 2007;116:16(suppl):797.

Costa, R.J., Jones, G.E. The effects of a high carbohydrate diet on cortisol and salivary immunoglobulin A (s-IgA) during a period of increase exercise workload amongst Olympic and Ironman triathletes. *Int J Sports Med.* Dec 2005;26(10):880–85.

Craggs, L., Kalaria, R.N. Revisiting dietary antioxidants, neurodegeneration and dementia. *Neuroreport.* Jan 2011;22(1):1–3.

Creswell, J., Irwin, M.R., et al. Mindfulness-based stress reduction training reduces loneliness and pro-inflammatory gene expression in older adults: a small randomized controlled trial. *Brain Behav Immun.* Oct 2012;26(7):1095–101.

Cynober, L.A. Plasma amino acid levels with a note on membrane transport: characteristics, regulation, and metabolic significance. *Nutrition.* Sep 2002;18(9):761–66.

D'Souza, A.L., Raijkumar, C., Cooke, J., Bulpitt, C.J. Probiotics in prevention of antibiotic associated diarrhoea: meta-analysis. *BMJ.* Jun 8 2002;324(7350):1361.

Dakshinamurti, K., Paulose, C.S., Viswanathan, M., Siow, Y.L. Neuroendocrinology of pyridoxine deficiency. *Neurosci Biobehav Rev.* 1988;12:189–93.

Dakshinamurti, K., Sharma, S.K., Bonke, D. Influence of B vitamins on binding properties of serotonin receptors in the CNS of rats. *Klin Wochenschr.* 1990;688:142–45.

Danescu, L.G., Levy, S., Levy, J. Vitamin D and diabetes mellitus. *Endocrine*. Feb 2009;35(1):11–17.

Darbinyan, V., Kteyan, A., Panossian, A., et al. Rhodiola rosea in stress induced fatigue—a double blind cross-over study of a standardized extract SHR-5 with a repeated low-dose regimen on the mental performance of healthy physicians during night duty. *Phytomedicine*. 2000;7(5):365–71.

Dashwood, R.H., Myzak, M.C., Ho, E. Dietary HDAC inhibitors: time to rethink weak ligands in cancer chemoprevention? *Carcinogenesis*. 2006;27:344–49.

Davis, C.D., Uthus, E.O. DNA methylation, cancer susceptibility and nutrient interactions. *Exp Biol Med (Maywood)*. 2004;229:988–95.

de Kort, S., Keszthelyi, D., Masclee, A.A. Leaky gut and diabetes mellitus: what is the link? *Obes Rev*. Jun 2011;12(6):449–58.

de Prada, T.P., Pozzi, A.O., et al. Atherogenesis takes place in cholesterol-fed rabbits when circulating concentrations of endogenous cortisol are increased and inflammation suppressed. *Atherosclerosis*. Apr 2007;191(2):333–39.

Delarue, J., Matzinger, O., Binnert, C., Schneiter, P., Chiolero, M.R., Tappy, L. Fish oil prevents the adrenal activation elicited by mental stress in healthy men. *Diabetes Metab*. Jun 2003;29(3):289–95.

Delzenne, N.M., Neyrinck, A.M., Backhed, F., Cani, P.D. Targeting gut microbiota in obesity: effects of prebiotics and probiotics. *Nat Rev Endocrinol*. Aug 2011;7(11):639–46.

Delzenne, N.M., Neyrinck, A.M., Cani, D. Modulation of the gut microbiota by nutrients with prebiotic properties: consequences for host health in the context of obesity and metabolic syndrome. *Microb Cell Fact*. Aug 2011;10(S1):S10.

Dhabhar, F.S., Miller, A.H., McEwen, B.S., Spencer, R.L. Effects of stress on immune cell distribution: dynamics and hormonal mechanisms. *J Immunol*. 1995;154:5511–27.

Dhingra, R., Sullivan, L., Jacques, P.F., Wang, T.J., Fox, C.S., Meigs, J.B., et al. Soft drink consumption and risk of developing cardiometabolic risk factors and the metabolic syndrome in middle-aged adults in the community. *Circulation*. Jul 31 2007;116(5):480–88.

Diamanti-Kandarakis, E., Bourguignon, J.P., et al. Endocrine-disrupting chemicals: an Endocrine Society scientific statement. *Endocr Rev*. Jun 2009;30(4):293.

Dixon, R.A. Phytoestrogens. *Annu Rev Plant Biol.* 2004;55:225–61.

Doherty, L., Bromer, J., Zhou, Y., Aldad, T., Taylor, H. In utero exposure to diethylstilbestrol (DES) or bisphenol-A (BPA) increases EZH2 expression in the mammary gland: an epigenetic mechanism linking endocrine disruptors to breast cancer. *Horm Cancer.* 2010;1:146–55.

Dolinoy, D.C. The agouti mouse model: an epigenetic biosensor for nutritional and environmental alterations on the fetal epigenome. *Nutr Rev.* 2008;66(suppl 1):S7–11.

Dolinoy, D.C., Huang, D., Jirtle, R.L. Maternal nutrient supplementation counteracts bisphenol A-induced DNA hypomethylation in early development. *Proc Natl Acad Sci USA.* 2007;104:13056–61.

Dolinoy, D.C., Weidman, J.R., Waterland, R.A., Jirtle, R.L. Maternal genistein alters coat color and protects Avy mouse offspring from obesity by modifying the fetal epigenome. *Environ Health Perspect.* 2006;114:567–72.

Drapeau, V., Therrien, F., Richard, D., Tremblay, A. Is visceral obesity a physiological adaptation to stress? *Panminerva Med.* 2003;45(3):189–95.

Ducasse, M., Brown, M. Epigenetic aberrations and cancer. *Mol Cancer.* 2006;5:60.

Duong, M., Cohen, J.I., Convit, A. High cortisol levels are associated with low quality food choice in type 2 diabetes. *Endocrine.* Feb 2012;41(1):76–81.

Dusek, J.A., Out, H.H., Wohlhueter, A.L., et al. Genomic counter-stress changes induced by the relaxation response. *PLoS One.* Jul 2008;3(7):e2576.

Duthie, S.J. Epigenetic modifications and human pathologies: cancer and CVD. *Proc Nutr Soc.* Feb 2011;70(1):47–56.

Dyerbergt, J., Bang, H.O. Haemostatic function and platelet polyunsaturated fatty acids in Eskimos. *Lancet.* 1979;2(8140):433–35.

Ebbeling, C.B., Leidig, M.M., Sinclair, K.B., et al. Effects of an ad libitum low-glycemic load diet on cardiovascular disease risk factors in obese young adults. *Am J Clin Nutr.* May 2005;81(5):976–82.

Egger, J. Will, J., Carter, C.M. Is migraine food allergy? A double-blind control trial of oligoantigenic diet treatment. *Lancet.* Oct 1983:2(8355):865–69.

Environmental Working Group. www.ewg.org.

Esler, M., Elkelis, N., Schlaich, M., et al. Human sympathetic nerve biology: parallel influences of stress and epigenetics in essential hypertension and panic disorder. *Ann NY Acad Sci.* Dec 2008;1148:338–48.

Esteller, M. Cancer epigenomics: DNA methylomes and histone-modification maps. *Nat Rev Genet.* 2007;8:286–98.

Faggiano, A., Pivonello, R., Melis, D., Alfieri, R., Filippela, M. Evaluation of circulating levels and renal clearance of natural amino acids in patients with Cushing's disease. *J Endocrinol Invest.* Feb 2002;25(2):142–51.

Fairfield, K.M., Fletcher, R.H. Vitamins for chronic disease prevention in adults: scientific review. *JAMA.* 2002;287:3116–26.

Fang, M.Z., Chen, D., Sun, Y., et al. Reversal of hypermethylation and reactivation of p16INK4a, RARbeta, and MGMT genes by genistein and other isoflavones from soy. *Clin Cancer Res.* 2005;11:7033–41.

Fang, M., Chen, D., Yang, C. Dietary polyphenols may affect DNA methylation. *J Nutr.* 2007;137:223S–228S.

Farag, N.H., Moore, W.E., Lovallo, W.R., et al. Hypothalamic-pituitary-adrenal axis function: relative contributions of perceived stress and obesity in women. *J Womens Health (Larchmt).* Dec 2008;17(10):1647–55.

Feinberg, AP. Epigenetics at the epicenter of modern medicine. *JAMA.* 2008;299:1345–50.

Fernandez, M.F., Arrebola, J.P., Taoufiki, J., Navalon, A., Ballesteros, O., Pulgar, R., et al. Bisphenol-A and chlorinated derivatives in adipose tissue of women. *Reprod Toxicol.* 2007;24:259–64.

Fernandez-Real, J.M., Pugeat, M., Grasa, M., Broch, M., Vendrell, J., Brun, J., et al. Serum corticosteroid-binding globulin concentration and insulin resistance syndrome: a population study. *J Clin Endocrinol Metab.* Oct 2002;87(10):4686–90.

Feskens, E.J., Kromhout, D. Cardiovascular risk factors and the 25-year incidence of diabetes mellitus in middle-aged men: the Zutphen Study. *Am J Epidemiol.* 1989;130:1101–8.

Foley, D.L., Craig, J.M., Morley, R., Olsson, C.A., Dwyer, T., Smith, K., et al. Prospects for epigenetic epidemiology. *Am J Epidemiol.* 2009;169:389–400.

Folsom, A.R., Nieto, F.J., McGovern, P.G., et al. Prospective study of coronary heart disease incidence in relation to fasting total homocysteine, related genetic polymorphisms, and B vitamins: the Atherosclerosis Risk in Communities (ARIC) study. *Circulation.* 1998;98:204–10.

Fontana, L., Klein, S., Holloszy, J.O., Premachandra, B.N. Effect of long-term calorie restriction with adequate protein and micronutrients on thyroid hormones. *J Clin Endocrinol Metab.* 2006;91:3232–35.

Fontana, L., Meyer, T.E., Klein, S., Holloszy, J.O. Long-term calorie restriction is highly effective in reducing the risk for atherosclerosis in humans. *Proc Natl Acad Sci USA.* 2004;101:6659–63.

Fortin, P.R., Lew, R.A., Liang, M.H., et al. Validation of a meta-analysis: the effects of fish oil in rheumatoid arthritis. *J Clin Epidemiol.* 1995;48(11):1379–90.

Fries, E., Hesse, J., Hellhammer, J., Hellhammer, D.H. A new view on hypocortisolism. *Psychoneuroendocrinology.* Nov 2005:30(10)1010–16.

Friso, S. Low circulating vitamin B(6) is associated with elevation of the inflammation marker C-reactive protein independently of plasma homocysteine levels. *Circulation.* 2001;103:2788–91.

Friso, S., Choi, S.W. Gene-nutrient interactions and DNA methylation. *J Nutr.* 2002;132;8(suppl):2382S–2387S.

Fruehwald-Schultes, B., Kern, W., Born, J., Fehm, H.L., Peters, A. Hyperinsulinemia causes activation of the hypothalamus in humans. *Int J Obes Relat Metab Disord.* May 2001;25(suppl 1):S38–40.

Fu, S., Kurzrock, R. Development of curcumin as an epigenetic agent. *Cancer.* Oct 2010;116(20):4670–76.

Gaffney, B.T., Hugel, H.M. The effects of Eleutherococcus senticosus and Panax ginseng on steroidal hormone indices of stress and lymphocyte subset numbers in endurance athletes. *Life Sci.* Dec 14 2001;70(4):431–42.

García-Prieto, M.D., Tébar, F.J., et al. Cortisol secretary pattern and glucocorticoid feedback sensitivity in women from a Mediterranean area: relationship with anthropometric characteristics, dietary intake and plasma fatty acid profile. *Clin Endocrinol (Oxf).* Feb 2007;66(2):185–91.

Garland, C., Comstock, G., Garland, F. Serum 25-hydroxyvitamin D and colon cancer: eight year prospective study. *Lancet.* 1989;2:1176–78.

Geurts, L., Everard, A., le Ruyet, P., Delzenne, N.M., Cani, P.D. Ripened dairy products differentially affect hepatic lipid content and adipose tissue oxidative stress markers in obese and type 2 diabetic mice. *J Agric Food Chem.* Feb 2012;60(8):2063–68.

Geurts, L., Lazarevic, V., Derrien, M., et al. Altered gut microbiota and endocannabinoid system tone in obese and diabetic leptin-resistant mice: impact on apelin regulation in adipose tissue. *Front Microbiol.* 2011;2:149.

Gilbert, D.G., Dibb, W.D. Effects of nicotine and caffeine, separately and in combination, on EEG topography, mood, heart rate, cortisol, and vigilance. *Psychophysiology.* Sep 2000;37(5):583–95.

Gilchrest, B.A., Bohr, V.A. Aging processes, DNA damage, and repair. *FASEB J.* 1997;11:322–30.

Gluck, M.E., Geliebter, A., Lorence, M. Cortisol stress response is positively correlated with central obesity in obese women with binge eating disorder (BED) before and after cognitive-behavioral treatment. *Ann NY Acad Sci.* Dec 2004;1032:202–7.

Goldstein, D., McEwen, B.S. Allostasis, homeostasis, and the nature of stress. *Stress.* 2002;5:55–58.

Goleman, D., Gurin, J., eds. *Mind/Body Medicine: How to Use Your Mind for Better Health.* New York: Consumer Reports Books; 1993:80.

Golub, M.D. The adrenal and the metabolic syndrome. *Curr Hypertens Rep.* 2001;3:117–20.

Gonzalez-Bono, E., Rohleder, N. Glucose but not protein or fat load amplifies the cortisol response to psychosocial stress. *Horm Behav.* May 2002;41(3):328–33.

Goralczyk, R. Beta-carotene and lung cancer in smokers: review of hypotheses and status of research. *Nutr Cancer.* 2009;61(6):767–74.

Gowers, I.R., Walters, K., Kiss-Toth, E., et al. Age-related loss of CpG methylation in the tumour necrosis factor promoter. *Cytokine.* Dec 2011;56(3):792–97.

Grant, E.C. Food allergies and migraine. *Lancet.* May 5 1979;1(8123):966–69.

Green, H.R., Jones, R. *Celiac Disease: A Hidden Epidemic.* New York: HarperCollins; 2006.

Hamazaki, K., Itomura, M. Effect of omega-3 fatty acid-containing phospholipids on blood catecholamine concentrations in healthy volunteers: a randomized, placebo-controlled, double-blind trial. *Nutrition.* Jun 2005;21(6):705–10.

Hamazaki, T., Itomura, M. Anti-stress effects of DHA. *Biofactors.* 2000;13(1–4):41–45.

Han, E.S., Evans, T.R., Shu, J.H., Lee, S., Nelson, J.F. Food restriction enhances endogenous and corticotropin-induced plasma elevations of free but not total corticosterone throughout life in rats. *J Gerontol A Biol Sci Med Sci.* 2001;56:391–97.

Han, J., Lin, H., Huang, W. Modulating gut microbiota as an anti-diabetic mechanism of berberine. *Med Sci Monit.* Jul 2011;17(7):RA164–67.

Hanai, H., Ilda, T., Takeuchi, K., et al. Curcumin maintenance therapy for ulcerative colitis: randomized, multicenter, double-blind, placebo-controlled trial. *Clin Gastroenterol Hepatol.* Dec 2006;4(12):1502–6.

Harris, W.S., Park, Y., Isley, W.L. Cardiovascular disease and long-chain omega-3 fatty acids. *Curr Opin Lipidol.* 2003;14(1):9–14.

Hartvig, P., Lindner, K.J., Bjurling, P., Laengstrom, B., Tedroff, J. Pyridoxine effect on synthesis rate of serotonin in the monkey brain measured with positron emission tomography. *J Neural Transm Gen Sect.* 1995;102:91–97.

Hartz, A.J., Bentler, S., Noyes, R., Hoehns, J., Logemann, C., Sinift, S. Randomized controlled trial of Siberian ginseng for chronic fatigue. *Psychol Med.* Jan 2004;34(1):51–61.

He, K., Rimm, E.B., Merchant, A. Fish consumption and risk of stroke in men. *JAMA.* 2002;288(24):3130–36.

Heerwagen, M.J.R., Miller, M.R., Barbour, L.A., et al. Maternal obesity and fetal metabolic programming: a fertile epigenetic soil. *Am J Physiol Regul Integr Comp Physiol.* 2010;299:R711–R722.

Heijmans, B.T., Tobi, E.W., Stein, A.D., Putter, H., Blauw, G.J., Susser, E.S., et al. Persistent epigenetic differences associated with prenatal exposure to famine in humans. *Proc Natl Acad Sci USA.* 2008;105:17046–49.

Heilbronn, L.K., de Jonge, L., Frisard, M.I., et al. Effect of 6-month calorie restriction on biomarkers of longevity, metabolic adaptation, and oxidative stress in overweight individuals: a randomized controlled trial. *JAMA*. 2006;295:1539–48.

Hennig, B., Ettinger, A.S., Jandacek, R., et al. Using nutrition for intervention and prevention against environmental chemical toxicity and associated diseases. *Environ Health Perspect*. 2007;115:493–95.

Hennig, B., Reiterer, G., et al. Modification of environmental toxicity by nutrients: implications in atherosclerosis. *Cardiovasc Toxicol*. 2005;5(2):153–60.

Herceg, A. Epigenetics and cancer: towards an evaluation of the impact of environmental and dietary factors. *Mutagenesis*. 2007;22:91–103.

Herrera, B.M., Keildson, S., Lindgren, C.M. Genetics and epigenetics of obesity. *Maturitas*. May 2011;69(1):41–49.

Herrick, K., Phillips, D.I., Haselden, S., Shiell, A.W., Campbell-Brown, M., Godfrey, K.M. Maternal consumption of a high-meat, low-carbohydrate diet in late pregnancy: relation to adult cortisol concentrations in the offspring. *J Clin Endocrinol Metab*. Aug 2003;88(8):3554–60.

Herrschaft, H., Nacu, A., Likhachev, S., Sholomov, I., Hoerr, R., Schlaefke, S. Ginkgo biloba extract EGb 761Ò in dementia with neuropsychiatric features: a randomized, placebo-controlled trial to confirm the efficacy and safety of a daily dose of 240 mg. *J Psychiatr Res*. Jun 2012;46(6):716–23.

Hertog, M.G., Feskens, E.J., et al. Dietary antioxidant flavonoids and risk of coronary heart disease: the Zutphen Elderly Study. *Lancet*. Oct 23 1993;342(8878):1007–11.

Heudorf, U., Mersch-Sundermann, V., Angerer, J. Phthalates: toxicology and exposure. *Int J Hyg Environ Health*. 2007;210:623–34.

Higdon, J.V., Delage, B., Williams, D.E., Dashwood, R.D. Cruciferous vegetables and human cancer risk: epidemiologic evidence and mechanistic basis. *Pharmacol Res*. 2007;55:224–36.

Hill, E.E., Eisenmann, J.C., Gentile, D., Holmes, M.E., Walsh, D. The association between morning cortisol and adiposity in children varies by weight status. *J Pediatr Endocrinol Metab*. 2011;24(9–10):709–13.

Hillman, J.B., Dorn, L.D., Loucks, T.L., Berga, S.L. Obesity and the hypothalamic-pituitary-adrenal axis in adolescent girls. *Metabolism.* Mar 2012;61(3):341–48.

Himeno, A., Satoh-Asahara, N., Usui, T., et al. Salivary cortisol levels are associated with outcomes of weight reduction therapy in obese Japanese patients. *Metabolism.* Feb 2012;61(2):255–61.

Hjemdahl, P. Stress and the metabolic syndrome, an interesting but enigmatic association. *Circulation.* 2002;106:2634–36.

Ho, E., Clarke, J.D., Dashwood, R.D. Dietary sulforaphane, a histone deacetylase inhibitor for cancer prevention. *J Nutr.* 2009;139:2393–96.

Ho, S.M., Tang, W.Y., Belmonte de Frausto, J., Prins, G.S. Developmental exposure to estradiol and bisphenol A increases susceptibility to prostate carcinogenesis and epigenetically regulates phosphodiesterase type 4 variant 4. *Cancer Res.* 2006;66:5624–32.

Hoffman, P.R., Kench, J.A., Vondracek, A. Interaction between phosphatidylserine and the phosphatidylserine receptor inhibits immune responses in vivo. *J Immunol.* Feb 2005;174(3):1393–404.

Høj, L., Osterballe, O., Bundgaard, A., Weeke, B., Weiss, M. A double-blind controlled trial of elemental diet in severe perennial asthma. *Allergy.* 1981;36(4):257–62.

Holick, M.F. High prevalence of vitamin D inadequacy and implications for health. *Mayo Clin Proc.* 2006;81:363–73.

Holloszy, J.L. The biology of aging. *Mayo Clin Proc.* 2000;75(suppl):S3–8.

Horrobin, D.R. Fatty acid metabolism in health and disease: the role of delta-6-desaturase. *Am J Clin Nutr.* 1993;57(suppl):S732–37.

Hougee, S., Sanders, A., et al. Decreased pro-inflammatory cytokine production by LPS-stimulated PBMC upon in vitro incubation with the flavonoids apigenin, luteolin or chrysin, due to selective elimination of monocytes/macrophages. *Biochem Pharmacol.* Jan 15 2005;69(2):241–48.

Hsu, A., Wong, C., et al. Promoter de-methylation of cyclin D2 by sulforaphane in prostate cancer cells. *Clin Epigenetics.* 2011;3:3.

Hu, F.B., Stampfer, M.J., Manson, J.E. Dietary fat intake and the risk of coronary heart disease in women. *N Engl J Med.* 1997;337:1491–99.

Hu, Y., Ehli, E.A., et al. Lipid-lowering effect of berberine in human subjects and rats. *Phytomedicine*. Jul 15 2012;19(10):861–67.

Hypponen, E., Laara, E., Reunamen, A., Jarvelin, M.R., Virtanen, S.M. Intake of vitamin D and risk of type 1 diabetes: a birth cohort study. *Lancet*. 2001;358:1500–3.

IBD in EPIC Study Investigators, Tjonneland, A., Overvad, K., et al. Linoleic acid, a dietary n-6 polyunsaturated fatty acid, and the aetiology of ulcerative colitis: a nested case-control study within a European prospective cohort study. *Gut*. Dec 2009;58(12):1606–11.

Ika, T., Komori, N., Kuwahata, M., Hiroi, Y., Shimoda, T., Okada, M., et al. Pyridoxal 5'-phosphate modulates expression of cytosolic aspartate aminotransferase gene by inactivation of glucocorticoid receptor. *J Nutr Sci Vitaminol (Tokyo)*. 1995;41:363–75.

International Agency for Research on Cancer. Some drinking-water disinfectants and contaminants, including arsenic. In *IARC Monographs on the Evaluation of Carcinogenic Risks to Humans*. Lyon, France: IARC.

Ishigaki, T., Koyama, K. Plasma leptin levels of elite endurance runners after heavy endurance training. *J Physiol Anthropol Appl Human Sci*. Nov 2005;24(6):573–78.

Ishikawa, H., Saeki, T., Otani, T., et al. Aged garlic extract prevents a decline of NK cell number and activity in patients with advanced cancer. *J Nutr*. Mar 2006;136(suppl 3):816S–820S.

Issa, J.P. Cancer prevention: epigenetics steps up to the plate. *Cancer Prev Res (Phila)*. 2008;1:219–22.

Jäger, R., Purpura, M., Geiss, K.R., Weiss, M., Baumeister, J., Amatulli, F., et al. The effect of phosphatidylserine on golf performance. *J Int Soc Sports Nutr*. Dec 2007;4:23.

James, M.J., Gibson, R.A., Cleland, L.G. Dietary polyunsaturated fatty acids and inflammatory mediator production. *Am J Clin Nutr*. 2000;71(suppl):S343–48.

Janesick, A., Blumber, B. Obesogens, stem cells and the developmental programming of obesity. *Int J Androl*. Jun 2012;35(3):437–48.

Jang, H., Mason, J.B., Choi, S.W. Genetic and epigenetic interactions between folate and aging in carcinogenesis. *J Nutr*. 2005;135(suppl 12):2967S–2971S.

Janossky, E.D., Lester, G.E., Weinberg, C.R. Association between low levels of 1,25-dihydroxyvitamin D and breast cancer risk. *Public Health Nutr.* 1999;2:283–91.

Jayo, J.M., Shively, C.A., Kaplan, J.R., Manuck, S.B. Effects of exercise and stress on body fat distribution in male cynomolgus monkeys. *Int J Obes Relat Metab Disord.* 1993;17:597–604.

Jefferies, W.M. Cortisol and immunity. *Med Hypotheses.* 1991;34:198–208.

Jeong, D.H., Lee, G.P. Alterations of mast cells and TGF-beta1 on the silymarin treatment for CCl(4)-induced hepatic fibrosis. *World J Gastroenterol.* Feb 28 2005;11(8):1141–48.

Jezova, D., Duncko, R., Lassanova, M., Kriska, M., Moncek, F. Reduction of rise in blood pressure and cortisol release during stress by ginkgo biloba extract (EGB 761) in healthy volunteers. *J Physiol Pharmacol.* Sep 2002;53(3):337–48.

Jia-Shi, Z., Halpern, G.M., Jones, K. The scientific rediscovery of a precious ancient Chinese herbal regimen: Cordyceps sinensis—part I. *J Altern Complement Med.* 1998;4(3):289–303.

Jia-Shi, Z., Halpern, G.M., Jones, K. The scientific rediscovery of a precious ancient Chinese herbal regimen: Cordyceps sinensis—part II. *J Altern Complement Med.* 1998;4(4):429–57.

Jiang, X., Yan, J., West, A.A., et al. Maternal choline intake alters the epigenetic state of fetal cortisol-regulating genes in humans. *FASEB J.* Aug 2012;26(8):3563–74.

Jirtle, R.L., Skinner, M.K. Environmental epigenomics and disease susceptibility. *Nat Rev Genet.* 2007;8:253–62.

Johnson, T.E. Recent results: biomarkers of aging. *Exp Gerontol.* 2006;41:1243–46.

Jones, R.A., Baylin, S.B. The epigenomics of cancer. *Cell.* Feb 2007;128(4):683–92.

Julius, S. Effect of sympathetic overactivity on cardiovascular prognosis in hypertension. *Eur Heart J.* 1998;19(suppl F):F14–18.

Kaati, G., Bygren, L.O., Pembrey, M., Sjostrom, M. Transgenerational response to nutrition, early life circumstances and longevity. *Eur J Hum Genet.* 2007;15:784–90.

Kallio, P., Kolehmainen, M., et al. Dietary carbohydrate modification induces alterations in gene expression in abdominal subcutaneous adipose tissue in persons with the metabolic syndrome: the FUNGENUT Study. *Am J Clin Nutr.* May 2007;85(5):1417–27.

Kang, S.C., Lee, B.M. Methylation of estrogen receptor alpha gene by phthalates. *J Toxicol Environ Health.* 2005;68:1995–2003.

Karoutsou, E., Polymeris, A. Environmental endocrine disruptors and obesity. *Endocr Regul.* 2012;46:37–46.

Keller, U. From obesity to diabetes. *Int J Vitam Nutr Res.* Jul 2006;76(4):172–77.

Kelly, G. Clinical applications of N-acetylcysteine. *Alt Med Rev.* 1998;3(2):114–27.

Kelly, G.S. Nutritional and botanical interventions to assist with the adaptation to stress. *Altern Med Rev.* Aug 1999;4(4):249–65.

Kelly, G.S. Rhodiola rosea: a possible plant adaptogen. *Altern Med Rev.* 2001;6(3):293–302.

Kelly, J.J., Mangos, G., Williamson, P.M., Whitworth, J.A. Cortisol and hypertension. *Clin Exp Pharmacol Physiol.* 1998;25(suppl):S51–56.

Kelly, J.J., Tam, S.H., Williamson, P.M., Lawson, J., Whitworth, J.A. The nitric oxide system and cortisol-induced hypertension in humans. *Clin Exp Pharmacol Physiol.* 1998;25:945–46.

Kelly, T., Yang, W., Chen, C.S., Reynolds, K., He, J. Global burden of obesity in 2005 and projections to 2030. *Int J Obes (Lond).* Sep 2008;32(9):1431–37.

Keltikangas-Järvinen, L., Räikkönen, K., Hautanen, A. Type A behavior and vital exhaustion as related to the metabolic hormonal variables of the hypothalamic-pituitary-adrenal axis. *Behav Med.* Spring 1996;22:15–22.

Kemnitz, J.W., Roecker, E.B., Weindruch, R., Elson, D.F., Baum, S.T., Bergman, R.N. Dietary restriction increases insulin sensitivity and lowers blood glucose in rhesus monkeys. *Am J Physiol.* 1994;266:E540–E547.

Kempuraj, D., Madhappan, B. Flavonols inhibit proinflammatory mediator release, intracellular calcium ion levels and protein kinase C theta phosphorylation in human mast cells. *Br J Pharmacol.* Aug 2005;145(7):933–44.

Kendler, B.S. Taurine: an overview of its role in preventive medicine. *Prev Med.* 1989;18(1):79–100.

Khani, S., Tayek, J.A. Cortisol increases gluconeogenesis in humans: its role in the metabolic syndrome. *Clin Sci (Lond).* Dec 2001;101(6):739–47.

Kim, M.J., Aiken, J.M., Havighurst, T., Hollander, J., Ripple, M.O., Weindruch, R. Adult-onset energy restriction of rhesus monkeys attenuates oxidative stress-induced cytokine expression by peripheral blood mono-nuclear cells. *J Nutr.* 1997;127:2293–301.

Kleemann, R., Verschuren, L., et al. Anti-inflammatory, anti-proliferative and anti-atherosclerotic effects of quercetin in human in vitro and in vivo models. *Atherosclerosis.* Sep 2011;218(1):44–52.

Kloting, N., Bluher, M. Extended longevity and insulin signaling in adipose tissue. *Exp Gerontol.* 2005;40:878–83.

Knoops, K. Mediterranean diet, lifestyle factors, and 10-year mortality in elderly European men and women. *JAMA.* 2004;292:1433–39.

Kodama, M., Kodama, T. Vitamin C infusion treatment enhances cortisol production of the adrenal via the pituitary ACTH route. *In Vivo.* Nov–Dec 1994;8(6):1079–85.

Koo, S.I., Noh, S.K. Green tea as inhibitor of the intestinal absorption of lipids: potential mechanism for its lipid-lowering effect. *J Nutr Biochem.* Mar 2007;18(3):179–83.

Kraft, T.E., Parisotto, D., Schempp, C., Efferth, T. Fighting cancer with red wine? Molecular mechanisms of resveratrol. *Crit Rev Food Sci Nutr.* 2009;49:782–99.

Krähenbühl, S., Hasler, F., et al. Kinetics and dynamics of orally administered 18 beta-glycyrrhetinic acid in humans. *J Clin Endocrinol Metab.* Mar 1994;78(3):581–85.

Kremer, J.M. N-3 fatty acid supplements in rheumatoid arthritis. *Am J Clin Nutr.* 2000;71(suppl):S349–51.

Kuo, Y.C., Tsai, W.G. Cordyceps sinensis as an immunomodulatory agent. *Am J Chin Med.* 1996;24(2):111–25.

Laferrere, B., Abraham, C. Inhibiting endogenous cortisol blunts the meal-entrained rise in serum leptin. *J Clin Endocrinol Metab.* Jun 2006;91(6):2232–38.

Landis-Piwowar, K.R., Milacic, V., Dou, Q.P. Relationship between the methylation status of dietary flavonoids and their growth-inhibitory and apoptosis-inducing activities in human cancer cells. *J Cell Biochem.* 2008;105:514–23.

Lane, J.D., Pieper, C.F. Caffeine affects cardiovascular and neuroendocrine activation at work and home. *Psychosom Med.* Jul–Aug 2002;64(4):595–603.

Lanfranco, F., Giordana, R., Pellegrino, M., Gianotti, L., Ramunni, J., Picu, A., et al. Free fatty acids exert an inhibitory effect on adrenocorticotropin and cortisol secretion in humans. *J Clin Endocrinol Metab.* Mar 2004;89(3):1385–90.

Lang, I.A., Galloway, T.S., et al. Association of urinary bisphenol A concentration with medical disorders and laboratory abnormalities in adults. *JAMA.* Sep 2008;300(11):1303–10.

Larre, C., Rochat de la Vallee, E. *Rooted in Spirit: The Heart of Chinese Medicine.* Barrytown, NY: Station Hill Press; 1995.

Larson-Meyer, D.E., Heilbronn, L.K., Redman, L.M. Effect of calorie restriction with or without exercise on insulin sensitivity, beta-cell function, fat cell size, and ectopic lipid in overweight subjects. *Diabetes Care.* 2006;29:1337–44.

Larsson, B., Seidell, J., Svärdsudd, K., Welin, L., Tibblin, G., Wilhelmsen, L., Björntorp, P. Obesity, adipose tissue distribution and health in men—the study of men born in 1913. *Appetite.* 1989;13:37–44.

Lasikiewicz, N., Hendrickx, H., Talbot, D., Dye, L. Exploring stress-induced cognitive impairment in middle aged, centrally obese adults. *Stress.* Jun 2012.

Laughter: can it help keep you healthy? *Mayo Clinic Health Letter.* March 1993:6.

Law, C.M., Barker, D.J., Osmond, C., Fall, C.H., Simmonds, S.J. Early growth and abdominal fatness in adult life. *J Epidemiol Community Health.* 1992;46:184–86.

Le Gal, M., Cathebras, P., Strüby, K. Pharmeton capsules in the treatment of functional fatigue: a double blind study versus placebo evaluated by a new methodology. *Phytother Res.* 1996; 10:49–53.

Lee, J.H., O'Keefe, J.H., Bell, D., Hensrud, D.D., Holick, M.F. Vitamin D deficiency an important, common, and easily treatable cardiovascular risk factor? *J Am Coll Cardiol.* May 26 2009;53(21):2011–13.

Lee, K.M., Yeo, M. Protective mechanism of epigallocatechin-3-gallate against Helicobacter pylori-induced gastric epithelial cytotoxicity via the blockage of TLR-4 signaling. *Helicobacter.* Dec 2004;9(6):632–42.

Lee, S.J., Krauthauser, C., Maduskuie, V., et al. Curcumin-induced HDAC inhibition and attenuation of medulloblastoma growth in vitro and in vivo. *BMC Cancer.* 2011;11:144–57.

Leu, S.F., Chien, C.H., Tseng, C.Y., Kuo, Y.M., Huang, B.M. The in vivo effect of Cordyceps sinensis mycelium on plasma corticosterone level in male mouse. *Biol Pharm Bull.* Sep 2005;28(9):1722–25.

Lewis, J.G., Nakajin, S., et al. Circulating levels of isoflavones and markers of 5alpha-reductase activity are higher in Japanese compared with New Zealand males: what is the role of circulating steroids in prostate disease? *Steroids.* Dec 15 2005;70(14):974–79.

Li, Y., Zhang, T., Korkaya, H., et al. Sulforaphane, a dietary component of broccoli/broccoli sprouts, inhibits breast cancer stem cells. *Clin Cancer Res.* May 1 2010;16(9):2580–90.

Lillycrop, K.A., Burdge, G.C. Epigenetic changes in early life and future risk of obesity. *Int J Obes (Lond).* Jan 2011;35(1):72–83.

Liu, P.L., Tsai, J.R., Charles, A.L., et al. Resveratrol inhibits human lung adenocarcinoma cell metastasis by suppressing heme oxygenase 1-mediated nuclear factor-kappaB pathway and subsequently downregulating expression of matrix metalloproteinases. *Mol Nutr Food Res.* 2010;54:S196–204.

Loest, H.B., Noh, S.K., Koo, S.I. Green tea extract inhibits the lymphatic absorption of cholesterol and alpha-tocopherol in ovariectomized rats. *J Nutr.* Jun 2002;132(6):1282–88.

Lombard, C.B. What is the role of food in preventing depression and improving mood, performance and cognitive function? *Med J Aust.* 2000;173(suppl):S104–5.

Lovallo, W.R., al'Absi, M., Blick, K., Whitsett, T.L., Wilson, M.F. Stress-like adrenocorticotropin responses to caffeine in young healthy men. *Pharmacol Biochem Behav.* Nov 1996;55(3):365–69.

Lovallo, W.R., Whitsett, T.L. Caffeine stimulation of cortisol secretion across the waking hours in relation to caffeine intake levels. *Psychosom Med.* Sep–Oct 2005;67(5):734–39.

Lu, H.C., trans. *The Yellow Emperor's Classic of Internal Medicine and the Difficult Classic.* Vancouver, BC: Academy of Oriental Heritage; 1978.

Ludwig, D. The glycemic index. *JAMA.* May 3 2002;287(18):2414–23.

Ludwig, D.S., Majzoub, J.A., Al-Zahrani, A., Dallal, G.E., Blanco, I., Roberts, S.B. High glycemic index foods, overeating, and obesity. *Pediatrics.* 1999;103(3):E26.

Ludwig, H., Spiteller, M., Egger, H.J. Correlation of emotional stress and physical exertions with urinary metabolite profiles. *J Isr Chem.* 1997;16:7–11.

Ly, A., Lee, H., Chen, J., et al. Effect of maternal and postweaning folic acid supplementation on mammary tumor risk in the offspring. *Cancer Res.* 2011;71:988–97.

MacIntosh, A., Ball, K. The effects of a short program of detoxi-fication in disease-free individuals. *Altern Ther Health Med.* 2000;6(4):70–76.

Majid, S., Dar, A.A., Ahmad, A.E., et al. BTG3 tumor suppressor gene promoter demethylation, histone modification and cell cycle arrest by genistein in renal cancer. *Carcinogenesis.* 2009;30:662–70.

Maksymowych, A.B., Daniel, V., Litwack, G. Pyridoxal phosphate as a regulator of the glucocorticoid receptor. *Ann NY Acad Sci.* 1990;585:438–51.

Mali, P., Chou, B.K., Yen, J., Ye, Z., et al. Butyrate greatly enhances derivation of human induced pluripotent stem cells by promoting epigenetic remodeling and the expression of pluripotency-associated genes. *Stem Cells.* 2010;28:713–20.

Mandel, S.A., Avramovich-Tirosh, Y., Reznichenko, L., Zheng, H., Weinreb, O., Amit, T., et al. Multifunctional activities of green tea catechins in neuroprotection. Modulation of cell survival genes, iron-dependent oxidative stress and PKC signaling pathway. *Neurosignals.* 2005;14(1–2);46–60.

Manolagas, S.C., Provvedini, D.M., Tsoukas, C.D. Interactions of 1,25-dihydroxyvitamin D3 and the immune system. *Mol Cell Endocrinol.* 1985;43:113–22.

Mao, Q.Q., Bai, Y., Lin, Y.W., et al. Resveratrol confers resistance against taxol via induction of cell cycle arrest in human cancer cell lines. *Mol Nutr Food Res.* Nov 2010;54(11):1574–84.

Mao, T.K., van de Water, J., et al. Modulation of TNF-alpha secretion in peripheral blood mononuclear cells by cocoa flavanols and procyanidins. *Dev Immunol.* Sep 2002;9(3):135–41.

Marcu, M.G., Jung, Y.J., Lee, S., et al. Curcumin is an inhibitor of p300 histone acetylatransferase. *Med Chem.* 2006;2:169–74.

Markus, R., Panhuysen, G., Tuiten, A., Koppeschaar, H. Effects of food on cortisol and mood in vulnerable subjects under controllable and uncontrollable stress. *Physiol Behav.* Aug–Sep 2000;70(3–4):333–42.

Marsit, C.J., Karagas, M.R., Danaee, H., et al. Carcinogen exposure and gene promoter hypermethylation in bladder cancer. *Carcinogenesis.* 2006;27:112–16.

Martinez, J.A., Cordero, P., Campion, J., Milagro, F.I. Interplay of early-life nutritional programming on obesity, inflammation and epigenetic outcomes. *Proc Nutr Soc.* May 2012;71(2):276–83.

Mattsson, C., Reynolds, R.M., et al. Combined receptor antagonist stimulation of the hypothalamic-pituitary-adrenal axis test identifies impaired negative feedback sensitivity to cortisol in obese men. *J Clin Endocrinol Metab.* Apr 2009;94(4):1347–52.

Mayer, G., Kroger, M., Meier-Ewert, K. Effects of vitamin B12 on performance and circadian rhythm in normal subjects. *Neuropsychopharmacology.* Nov 1996;15(5):456–64.

McEwen, B.S. The neurobiology of stress: from serendipity to clinical relevance. *Brain Res.* Dec 15 2000;886(1–2):172–89.

McEwen, B.S. Protective and damaging effects of stress mediators. *N Engl J Med.* 1998;338:171–79.

McEwen, B.S. Stress, adaptation, and disease: allostasis and allostatic load. *Ann NY Acad Sci.* May 1998;840:33–44.

McEwen, B.S., Wingfield, J.C. The concept of allostasis in biology and biomedicine. *Horm Behav.* Jan 2003;43(1):2–15.

McGowan, P.O., Szyf, M. The epigenetics of social adversity in early life: implications for mental health outcomes. *Neurobiol Dis.* 2010;39:66–72.

McKay, J.A., Mathers, J.C. Diet induced epigenetic changes and their implications for health. *Acta Physiol (Oxf).* Jun 2011;202(2):103–18.

McNulty, H., Strain, J.J., Pentieva, K., Ward, M. C(1) metabolism and CVD outcomes in older adults. *Proc Nutr Soc.* May 2012;71(2):213–21.

Meeran, S., Katiyar, S. Cell cycle control as a basis for cancer chemoprevention through dietary agents. *Front Biosci.* 2008;13:2191–202.

Meeran, S.M., Ahmed, A., Tollefsbol, T.O. Epigenetic targets of bioactive dietary components for cancer prevention and therapy. *Clin Epigenetics.* Dec 2010;1(3–4):101–16.

Meja, K., Rajendrasozhan, S., Adenuga, D., et al. Curcumin restores corticosteroid function in monocytes exposed to oxidants by maintaining HDAC2. *Am J Respir Cell Mol Biol.* 2008;39:312–23.

Merton, T. *The Way of Chuang Tzu.* Boston: Shambala Press; 1992.

Michalsen, A., Schneider, S., Rodenbeck, A., Ludtke, R., Huether, G., Dobos, G.J. The short-term effects of fasting on the neuroendocrine system in patients with chronic pain syndromes. *Nutr Neurosci.* Feb 2003;6(1):11–18.

Milagro, F.I., Campion, J., Martinez, J.A. 11-Beta hydroxysteroid dehydrogenase type 2 expression in white adipose tissue is strongly correlated with adiposity. *J Steroid Biochem Mol Biol.* Apr 2007;104(1–2):81–84.

Millis, R.M. Epigenetics and hypertension. *Curr Hypertens Rep.* Feb 2011;13(1):21–28.

Milner, J.A., McDonald, S.S., Anderson, D.E., Greenwald, P. Molecular targets for nutrients involved with cancer prevention. *Nutr Cancer.* 2001;41(1–2):1–16.

Mischoulon, D., Fava, M. Docosahexanoic acid and omega-3 fatty acids in depression. *Psychiatr Clin North Am.* 2000;23(4):785–94.

Miyamoto, K., Kotake, M. Estimation of daily bisphenol A intake of Japanese individuals with emphasis on uncertainty and variability. *Environ Sci.* 2006;13:15–29.

Mochizuki, M., Hasegawa, N. Therapeutic efficacy of pycnogenol in experimental inflammatory bowel diseases. *Phytother Res.* Dec 2004;18(12):1027–28.

Monroe, J., Brostoff, J. Food allergy and migraine. *Lancet.* Jul 5 1980.

Monteleone, P., Maj, M., Beinat, L., Natale, M., Kemali, D. Blunting by chronic phosphatidylserine administration of the stress-induced activation of the hypothalamo-pituitary-adrenal axis in healthy men. *Eur J Clin Pharmacol.* 1992;42:385–88.

Monteleone, P., Beinat, L., Tanzillo, C., Maj, M., Kemali, D. Effects of phosphatidylserine on the neuroendocrine response to physical stress in humans. *Neuroendocrinology.* Sep 1990;52(3):243–48.

Morita, K., Matsueda, T., Iida, T. Effect of green tea (matcha) on gastro-intestinal tract absorption of polychlorinated biphenyls, polychlori-nated dibenzofurans and polychlorinated dibenzo-p-dioxins in rats. *Hukuoka acta medica.* 1997;88(5):162–68.

Moro, J.R., Iwata, M., Von Andriano, U.H. Vitamin effects on the immune system: vitamins A and D take center stage. *Nat Rev Immunol.* Sep 2008;8(9):685–98.

Muccioli, G.G., Naslain, D., Backhed, F., et al. The endocannabinoid system links gut microbiota to adipogenesis. *Mol Syst Biol.* Jul 2010;6:392.

Muhtz, C., Zyriax, B.C. Depressive symptoms and metabolic risk: effects of cortisol and gender. *Psychoneuroendocrinology.* Aug 2009;34(7):1004–11.

Muller, J.E., Tofler, G.H., Willich, S.N., Stone, P.H. Circadian varia-tion of cardiovascular disease and sympathetic activity. *J Cardiovasc Pharmacol.* 1987;10(suppl 2):S104–9.

Munger, K.L., Zhang, S.M., O'Reilly, E. Vitamin D intake and the inci-dence of multiple sclerosis. *Neurology.* 2004;62:60–65.

Murck, J., Song, C., Horrobin, D.F., Uhr, M. Ethyl-eicosapentaenoate and dexamethasone resistance in therapy-refractory depression. *Int J Neuropsychopharmacol.* Sep 2004;7(3):341–49.

Myzak, M.C., Dashwood, W.M., Orner, G.A., Ho, E., Dashwood, R.H. Sulforaphane inhibits histone deacetylase in vivo and suppresses tumorigenesis in Apc-minus mice. *FASEB J.* 2006;20:506–8.

Myzak, M.C., Tong, P., Dashwood, W.M., Dashwood, R.H., Ho, E. Sulforaphane retards the growth of human PC-3 xenografts and inhibits HDAC activity in human subjects. *Exp Biol Med (Maywood).* 2007;232:227–34.

Nanda, R. Food intolerance and the irritable bowel syndrome. *Gut.* 1989;30:1099–104.

Nandakumar, V., Vaid, M., Katiyar, S.K. (-)-Epigallocatechin-3-gallate reactivates silenced tumor suppressor genes, Cip1/p21 and p16INK4a, by reducing DNA methylation and increasing histones acetylation in human skin cancer cells. *Carcinogenesis.* 2011;32:527–44.

National Digestive Diseases Information Clearinghouse. Celiac disease. NIH Publication No. 08-4269, Sep 2008. http://digestive.niddk.nih .gov/ddiseases/pubs/celiac/.

National Institute of Mental Health. Anxiety disorders. www.nimh.nih .gov/ health/topics/anxiety-disorders/index.shtml.

Nestel, P.J. Fish oil and cardiovascular disease: lipids and arterial function. *Am J Clin Nutr.* 2000;71(suppl):S228–31.

Niculescu, M.D., Craciunescu, C.N, Zeisel, S.H. Dietary choline deficiency alters global and gene-specific DNA methylation in the developing hippocampus of mouse fetal brains. *FASEB J.* 2006;20:43–49.

Noreen, E.E., Sass, M.J., Crowe, M.L., et al. Effects of supplemental fish oil on resting metabolic rate, body composition, and salivary cortisol in healthy adults. *J Int Soc Sports Nutr.* Oct 2010;8(7):31.

Norris, P.C., Dennis, E.A. Omega-3 fatty acids cause dramatic changes in TLR4 and purinergic eicosanoid signaling. *Proc Natl Acad Sci USA.* May 29 2012;109(22):8517–22.

Nuttall, F.Q., Gannon, M.D. The metabolic response to a high-protein, low-carbohydrate diet in men with type 2 diabetes mellitus. *Metabolism.* Feb 2006;55(2):243–51.

O'Keefe, J.H., Gheewala, N.M., O'Keefe, J.O. Dietary strategies for improving post-prandial glucose, lipids, inflammation, and cardiovascular health. *J Am Coll Cardiol.* 2008;51:249–55.

Oberlander, T.F., Weinberg, J., Papsdorf, M., Grunau, R., Misri, S., Devlin, A.M. Prenatal exposure to maternal depression, neonatal methylation of human glucocorticoid receptor gene (NR3C1) and infant cortisol stress responses. *Epigenetics.* Mar–Apr 2008;3(2):97–106.

Ong, Z.Y., Muhlhausler, B.S. Maternal "junk-food" feeding of rat dams alters food choices and development of the mesolimbic reward pathway in the offspring. *FASEB J.* Jul 2011;25(7):2167–79.

Ornish, D. *Love and Survival.* New York: HarperCollins; 1997.

Ornish, D., et al. Changes in prostate gene expression in men undergoing an intensive nutrition and lifestyle intervention. *PNAS.* Jun 17 2008;105(24):8369–74.

Packer, L., Witt, E.H., Tritschler, H.J. Alpha-lipoic acid as a biological antioxidant. *Free Rad Biol Med.* 1995;19(2):227–50.

Palomer, X., Gonzalez-Clemente, J.M., Blanco-Vaca, F., Mauricio, D. Role of vitamin D in the pathogenesis of type 2 diabetes mellitus. *Diabetes Obes Metab.* Mar 2008;10(3):185–97.

Paluszczak, J., Krajka-Ku niak, V., Baer-Dubowska, W. The effect of dietary polyphenols on the epigenetic regulation of gene expression in MCF7 breast cancer cells. *Toxicol Lett.* 2010;192:119–25.

Pankevich, D.E., Teegarden, S.L., Hedin, A.D., Jensen, C.L., Bale, T.L. Caloric restriction experience reprograms stress and orexigenic pathways and promotes binge eating. *J Neurosci.* Dec 2010;30(48):16399–407.

Panossian, A., Wikman, G., Wagner, H. Plant adaptogens. III. Earlier and more recent aspects and concepts on their mode of action. *Phytomedicine.* Oct 1999;6(4):287–300.

Papandreou, M.A., Dimakopoulou, A., et al. Effect of a polyphenol-rich wild blueberry extract on cognitive performance of mice, brain antioxidant markers and acetylcholinesterase activity. *Behav Brain Res.* Mar 17 2009;198(2):352–58.

Papoutsis, A.J., Lamore, S.D., et al. Resveratrol prevents epigenetic silencing of BRCA-1 by the aromatic hydrocarbon receptor in human breast cancer cells. *J Nutr.* Sep 2010;140(9):1607–14.

Parillo, M., Rivellese, A.A., Ciardullo, A.V. A high monounsaturated-fat/low-carbohydrate diet improves peripheral insulin sensitivity in non-insulin-dependent diabetic patients. *Metabolism.* 1992;41:1373–78.

Park, L.K., Friso, S., Choi, S.W. Nutritional influences on epigenetics and age-related disease. *Proc Nutr Soc.* Feb 2012;71(1):75–83.

Patterson, D.G., Jr., Wong, L.Y., et al. Polychlorinated dioxins and furans, polychlorinated biphenyls (PCBs), and organochlorine pesticides. *Environ Sci Technol.* 2009;43(4):1211–18.

Pattison, D.J., Symmons, D.P. Dietary beta-cryptoxanthin and inflammatory polyarthritis: results from a population-based prospective study. *Am J Clin Nutr.* Aug 2005;82(2):451–55.

Paulose, C.S., Dakshinamurti, K., Packer, S., Stephens, N.L. Sympathetic stimulation and hypertension in the pyridoxine-deficient adult rat. *Hypertension.* 1998;11:387–91.

Pelsser, L.M., Frankena, K., Toorman, J., Savelkoul, H.F., Pereira, R.R., Buitelaar, J.K. A randomized controlled trial into the effects of food on ADHD. *Eur Child Adolesc Psychiatry.* Jan 2009;18(1):12–19.

Perera, F., and Herbstman, J. Prenatal environmental exposures, epigenetics and disease. *Reprod Toxicol.* Apr 2011;31(3):363–73.

Pledgie-Tracy, A., Sobolewski, M.D., Davidson, N.E. Sulforaphane induces cell type–specific apoptosis in human breast cancer cell lines. *Mol Cancer Ther.* 2007;6:1013–21.

Pogribny, I.P., Ross, S.A., Wise, C., et al. Irreversible global DNA hypomethylation as a key step in hepatocarcinogenesis induced by dietary methyl deficiency. *Mutat Res.* 2006;27:1180–86.

Pradhan, A.D., Manson, J.A.E., Rifai, N., Buring, J.E., Ridker, P.M. C-reactive protein, interleukin 6, and risk of developing type 2 diabetes mellitus. *JAMA.* 2001;286:327–34.

Prasad, K. Hypocholesterolemic and antiatherosclerotic effect of flax lignan complex isolated from flaxseed. *Atherosclerosis.* Apr 2005;179(2):269–75.

Prins, G.S., Tang, W.Y., Belmonte, J., Ho, S.M. Developmental exposure to bisphenol A increases prostate cancer susceptibility in adult rats: epigenetic mode of action is implicated. *Fertil Steril.* 2008;89:e41.

Ptak, C., Petronis, A. Epigenetic approaches to psychiatric disorders. *Dialogues Clin Neurosci.* Mar 2012;12(1):25–35.

Qin, W., Zhu, W., Shi, H., Hewett, J.E., et al. Soy isoflavones have an antiestroenic effect and alter mammary promoter hypermethylation in healthy premenopausal women. *Nutr Cancer.* 2009;61:238–44.

Radley, J.J., Kabbaj, M., Jacobson, L., et al. Stress risk factors and stress-related pathology: neuroplasticity, epigenetics and endophenotypes. *Stress.* Sep 2011;14(5):481–97.

Ravelli, A.C., van der Meulen, J.H., Michels, R.P., et al. Glucose tolerance in adults after prenatal exposure to famine. *Lancet.* 1998;351:173–77.

Ravindran, J., Prasad, S., Aggarwal, B.B. Curcumin and cancer cells: how many ways can curry kill tumor cells selectively? *AAPS J.* Sep 2009;11(3):495–510.

Reaven, G. Metabolic syndrome. *Circulation.* Jul 16 2002;106:286–88.

Resnick, L.M. Ionic basis of hypertension, insulin resistance, vascular disease, and related disorders: the mechanism of "syndrome X." *Am J Hypertens.* 1993;6:123S–134S.

Reynolds, R.M., Godfrey, K.M., et al. Stress responsiveness in adult life: influence of mother's diet in late pregnancy. *J Clin Endocrinol Metab.* Mar 6 2007;92(6):2208–10.

Rideout, C.A., Linden, W., Barr, S.I. High cognitive dietary restraint is associated with increased cortisol excretion in postmenopausal women. *J Gerontol A Biol Sci Med Sci.* Jun 2006;61(6):628–33.

Rigden, S., Barrager, E., Bland, J. Evaluation of the effect of a modified entero-hepatic resuscitation program in chronic fatigue syndrome patients. *J Adv Med.* 1998;11(4):247–62.

Rimm, E.B., Willett, W.C. Folate and vitamin B6 from diet and supplements in relation to risk of coronary heart disease among women. *JAMA.* 1998;279:359–64.

Riordan, A.M., Hunter, J.O., Crampton, J.R., et al. Treatment of active Crohn's disease by exclusion diet: East Anglian Multicentre Controlled Trial. *Lancet.* 1990;335:816–19.

Rivellese, A., Riccardi, G., Giacco, A. Effect of dietary fibre on glucose control and serum lipoproteins in diabetic patients. *Lancet.* 1980;2:447–50.

Rizvi, S.I., Zaid, M.A., Anis, R., et al. Protective role of tea catechins against oxidation-induced damage of type 2 diabetic erythrocytes. *Clin Exp Pharmacol Physiol.* Jan–Feb 2005;32(1–2):70–75.

Robinson, K., Arheart, K., Refsum, H. Low circulating folate and vitamin B6 concentrations: risk factors for stroke, peripheral vascular disease, and coronary artery disease. European COMAC Group. *Circulation.* 1998;97:437–43.

Roelfsema, F., Kok, P., Pereira, A.M., Pijl, H. Cortisol production rate is similarly elevated in obese women with or without the polycystic ovary syndrome. *J Clin Endocrinol Metab.* Jul 2010;95(7):3318–24.

Rosenman, R.H. Results of the multicenter antihypertensive treatment trials. Therapeutic implications and the role of the sympathetic nervous system. *Am J Hypertens.* 1989;2:313S–338S.

Rosmond, R., Björntorp, P. Alterations in the hypothalamic-pituitary-adrenal axis in metabolic syndrome. *Endocrinologist.* 2001;11:491–97.

Rosmond, R., Holm, G., Björntorp, P. Food-induced cortisol secretion in relation to anthropometric, metabolic and hemodynamic variables in men. *Int J Obes.* Apr 2000;24:416–22.

Ross, S.A., Dwyer, J., Umar, A., Kagan, J., Verma, M., Van Bemmel, D.M., Dunn, B.K. Introduction: diet, epigenetic events and cancer prevention. *Nutr Rev.* 2008;66(suppl 1):S1–6.

Roubenoff, R., Castaneda, C. Sarcopenia—understanding the dynamics of aging muscle. *JAMA.* 2001;286(10):230–31.

Rowland, I., Faughnam, M. Bioavailability of phyto-estrogens. *Br J Nutr.* Jun 2003;89(suppl 1):S45–58.

Rubin, B.S. Bisphenol A: an endocrine disruptor with widespread exposure and multiple effects. *J Steroid Biochem Mol Biol.* Oct 2011;127(1–2):27–34.

Rudel, R.A., Gray, J.M., Engel, C.L., et al. Food packaging and bisphenol A and bis(2-ethyhexyl) phthalate exposure: findings from a dietary intervention. *Environ Health Perspect.* Jul 2011;119(7):914–20.

Ruhe, R.C., McDonald, R.B. Use of antioxidant nutrients in the prevention and treatment of type 2 diabetes. *J Am Coll Nutr.* 2001;20:363S–369S.

Rushmore, T.H., Kong, A. Pharmacogenomics, regulation and signaling pathways of phase I and II drug metabolizing enzymes. *Curr Drug Metab.* Oct 2002;3(5):481–90.

Sabatino, R., Masoro, E.J., McMahan, C.A., Kuhn, R.W. Assessment of the role of the glucocorticoid system in aging processes and in the action of food restriction. *J Gerontol.* 1991;46:B171–B179.

Salmeron, J., Manson, J.E., Stampfer, M.J., Colditz, G.A., Wing, A.L., Willett, W.C. Dietary fiber, glycemic load and risk of non-insulin-dependent diabetes mellitus in men. *Diabetes Care.* 1997;20(4):545–50.

Salmeron, J., Manson, J.E., Stampfer, M.J., Colditz, G.A., Wing, A.L., Willett, W.C. Dietary fiber, glycemic load and risk of non-insulin-dependent diabetes mellitus in women. *JAMA.* 1997;277:472–77.

Sanchez-Fidalgo, S., Cardeno, A., et al. Dietary supplementation of resveratrol attenuates chronic colonic inflammation in mice. *Eur J Pharmacol.* 2010;633:78–84.

Sapolsky, R., Krey, L., McEwen, B. The neuroendocrinology of stress and aging: the glucocorticoid cascade hypothesis. *Endocrinol Rev.* 1986;7:284–301.

Schinner, S., Willenberg, H.S., Krause, D., et al. Adipocyte-derived products induce the transcription of the StAR promoter and stimulate aldosterone and cortisol secretion from adrenocortical cells through the Wnt-signaling pathway. *Int J Obes (Lond.).* Jan 9 2007;31:864–70.

Schwarz, N.A., Rigby, B.R., La Bounty, P., Shelmadine, B., Bowden, R.G. Review Article: A review of weight control strategies and their effects on the regulation of hormonal balance. *J Nutr Metab.* 2011, Article ID 237932, 15 pages. DOI:10.1155/201½37932.

Seeman, T.E., Singer, B.H., Rowe, J.W., Horwitz, R.I., McEwen, B.S. The price of adaptation—allostatic load and its health consequences: MacArthur studies of successful aging. *Arch Intern Med.* 1997;157:2259–68.

Shen, L., Kondo, Y., Rosner, G., et al. MGMT promoter methylation and field defect in sporadic colorectal cancer. *J Natl Cancer Inst.* 2005;97:1330–38.

Shi, J.H., Du, W.H., Liu, X.Y., Fan, Y.P., et al. Glucocorticoids decrease serum adiponectin level and WAT adiponectin MRNA expression in rats. Dec 2010;75(12):853–58.

Shibata, S. A drug over the millennia: pharmacognosy, chemistry, and pharmacology of licorice. *Yakugaku Zasshi* (journal of the Pharmaceutical Society of Japan). Oct 2000;120(10):849–62.

Shomori, K., Yamamoto, M., Arifuku, I., Teramachi, K., Ito, H. Antitumor effects of a water-soluble extract from Maitake (Grifola frondosa) on human gastric cancer cell lines. *Oncol Rep.* Sep 2009;22(3):615–20.

Sie, K.K., Medline, A., van Weel, J., et al. Effect of maternal and post-weaning folic acid supplementation on colorectal cancer risk in the offspring. *Gut.* Dec 2011;60(12):1687–94.

Siguel, E. Essential and trans fatty acid metabolism in health and disease. *Compr Ther.* 1994;20(9):500–10.

Siguel, E.N. Cancerostatic effect of vegetarian diets. *Nutr Cancer.* 1983;4:285–91.

Siguel, E.N., Lerman, R.H. Trans-fatty acid patterns in patients with angiographically documented coronary artery disease. *Am J Cardiol.* 1993;71(11):916–20.

Siguel, E.N., Schaefer, E.J. Aging and nutritional requirements of essential fatty acids. In: Beare-Rogers, J., ed. *Dietary Fat Requirements in Health and Disease.* Champaign, IL: American Oil Chemists Society, 1988;163–89.

Simopoulos, A.P., Salem, N., Jr. N-3 fatty acids in eggs from range-fed Greek chickens. *N Engl J Med.* 1989;32(20):1412.

Sinclair, H.M. Essential fatty acids—an historical perspective. *Biochem Soc Trans.* 1990;18:756–61.

Sinclair, K.D., Allegrucci, C., Singh, R., et al. DNA methylation insulin resistance, and blood pressure in offspring determined by maternal periconceptional B vitamin and methionine status. *Proc Natl Acad Sci USA.* 2007;104:19351–56.

Singh, R.B., Pella, D. Can brain dysfunction be a predisposing factor for metabolic syndrome? *Biomed Pharmacother.* Oct 2004;58(suppl 1):S56–68.

Siow, R.C., Mann, G.E. Dietary isoflavones and vascular protection: activation of cellular antioxidant defenses by SERMs or hormesis? *Mol Aspects Med.* Dec 2010;31(6):468–77.

Skantze, H.B., Kaplan, J., Pettersson, K., Manuck, S., Blomqvist, N., Kyes, R., et al. Psychosocial stress causes endothelial injury in cynomolgus monkeys via beta1-adrenoceptor activation. *Atherosclerosis.* 1998;136:153–61.

Smith, A. Stress, breakfast cereal consumption and cortisol. *Nutr Neurosci.* Apr 2002;5(2):141–44.

Sohal, R.S., Mockett, R.J., Orr, W.C. Mechanisms of aging: an appraisal of the oxidative stress hypothesis. *Free Radic Biol Med.* 2002;33:575–86.

Sohal, R.S., Weindruch, R. Oxidative stress, caloric restriction and aging. *Science.* 1996;273:59–63.

Sørensen, N., Murata, K., Budtz-Jørgensen, E., Weihe, P., Grandjean, P. Prenatal methylmercury exposure as a cardiovascular risk factor at seven years of age. *Epidemiology.* Jul 1999;10(4):370–75.

Spence, J.D., Thornton, T., Muir, A.D., Westcott, N.D. The effect of flax seed cultivars with differing content of alpha-linolenic acid and lignans on responses to mental stress. *J Am Coll Nutr.* Dec 2003;22(6):494–501.

Sreejayan, N., Rao, M.N.A. Nitric oxide scavenging by curcuminoids. *J Pharm Pharmocol.* 1997;49:105–7.

Stahlhut, R.W., van Wijngaarden, E., Dye, T.D., Cook, S., Swan, S.R. Concentrations of urinary phthalate metabolites are associated with increased waist circumference and insulin resistance in adult U.S. males. *Environ Health Perspect.* Jun 2007;115(6):876–82.

Starks, M.A., Starks, S.L., Kingsley, M., Purpura, M., Jäger, R. The effects of phosphatidylserine on endocrine response to moderate intensity exercise. *J Int Soc Sports Nutr.* Jul 2008;5:11.

Steptoe, A., Gibson, E.L., Vuononvirta, R., Williams, E.D., Hamer, M., Rycroft, J.A., et al. The effects of tea on psychophysiological stress responsivity and post-stress recovery: a randomized double-blind trial. *Psychopharmacology (Berl).* Jan 2007;190(1):81–89.

Steptoe, A., Kunz-Ebrecht, S.R., Brydon, L., Wardle, J. Central adiposity and cortisol responses to waking in middle-aged men and women. *Int J Obes Relat Metab Disord.* Sep 2004;28(9):1168–73.

Straus, D.S. Nutritional regulation of hormones and growth factors that control mammalian growth. *FASEB J.* 1994;8:6–12.

Su, L.J., Mahabir, S., Ellison, G.L., McGuinn, L.A., Reid, B.C. Epigenetic contributions to the relationship between cancer and dietary intake of nutrients, bioactive food components, and environmental toxicants. *Front Genet.* Jan 9, 2012;2(91):1–12.

Susiarjo, M., Hunt, P. Bisphenol A exposure disrupts egg development in the mouse. *Fertil Steril.* Feb 2008;89(suppl 1):e97.

Swaab, D.F., Bao, A.M. The stress system in the human brain in depression and neurodegeneration. *Ageing Res Rev.* May 2005;4(2):131–94.

Szyf, M. The early-life social environment and DNA methylation. *Clin Genet.* Apr 2012;81(4):341–49.

Szyf, M., Weaver, I.C.G., Cervoni, N., et al. Epigenetic programming by maternal behavior. *Nat Neurosci.* Jun 2004;7:847–54.

Tahiliani, A.G., Beinlich, C.J. Pantothenic acid in health and disease. *Vitam Horm.* 1991;46:165–228.

Takeda, E., Terao, J., Nakaya, Y., Miyamoto, K., Baba, Y., Chuman, H., et al. Stress control and human nutrition. *J of Med Investigation*. Aug 4 2004;51(3):139–45.

Tauchmanova, L., Rossi, R., Biondi, B., Pulcrano, M., Nuzzo, V. Palmieri, E.A. Patients with subclinical Cushing's syndrome due to adrenal adenoma have increased cardiovascular risk. *J Clin Endocrinol Metab*. Nov 2002;87(11):4869–71.

Tchantchou, F., Shea, T.B. Folate deprivation, the methionine cycle, and Alzheimer's disease. *Vitam Horm*. 2008;79:83–97.

Teitelbaum, J., Bird, B., Greenfield, R.M., Weiss, A., Muenz, L., Gould, L. Effective treatment of chronic fatigue syndrome and fibromyalgia: a randomized, double blind, placebo-controlled, intent-to-treat study. *J Chronic Fatigue Syndrome*. 2001;8:3–28.

Teperino, R., Schoonjans, K., Auwerx, J. Histone methyl transferases and demethylases; can they link metabolism and transcription? *Cell Metab*. 2010;12:321–27.

Thompson, C., Syddal, H., Rodin, I., Osmond, C., Barker, D.J. Birth weight and the risk of depressive disorder in late life. *Br J Psychiatry*. 2001;179:450–55.

Thompson, L.U., Chen, J.M., et al. Dietary flaxseed alters tumor biological markers in postmenopausal breast cancer. *Clin Cancer Res*. May 15 2005;11(10):3828–35.

Tomata, Y., Kakizaki, M., Nakaya, N., Tsuboya, T., Sone, T., Kuriyama, S., Hozawa, A., Tsuji, I. Green tea consumption and the risk of incident functional disability in elderly Japanese: the Ohsaki Cohort 2006 Study. *Am J Clin Nutr*. Mar 2012;95(3):732–39.

Torrecilla, E., Fernández-Vázquez, G., Vicent, D., et al. Liver upregulation of genes involved in cortisol production and action is associated with metabolic syndrome in morbidly obese patients. *Obes Surg*. Mar 2012;22(3):478–86.

Trichopoulou, A., Orfanos, P., Norat, T., et al. Modified Mediterranean diet and survival: EPIC-elderly prospective cohort study. *BMJ*. Apr 30 2005;330:799–805.

Tsao, A., Liu, D., Martin, J., Tang, X., Lee, J., et al. Phase II randomized, placebo-controlled trial of green tea extract in patients with high-risk oral premalignant lesions. *Cancer Prev Res (Phila)*. 2009;2:931–41.

Tuck, M., Corry, D. More on adrenal activity in the metabolic syndrome. *Curr Hypertens Rep.* Apr 2002;4(2):103–4.

Tully, D.B., Allgood, V.E., Cidlowski, J.A. Modulation of steroid receptor-mediated gene expression by vitamin B6. *FASEB J.* 1994;8:343–49.

Ursache, A., Wedin, W., Tirsi, A., Convit, A. Preliminary evidence for obesity and elevations in fasting insulin mediating associations between cortisol awakening response and hippocampal volumes and frontal atrophy. *Psychoneuroendocrinology.* Aug 2012;37(8):1270–76.

Uusitupa, M., Schwab, U., Makimattila, S. Effects of two high-fat diets with different fatty acid compositions on glucose and lipid metabolism in healthy young women. *Am J Clin Nutr.* 1994;59:1310–16.

Vaiserman, A.M. Hormesis and epigenetics: is there a link? *Ageing Res Rev.* Sep 2011;10(4):413–21.

Van Cauter, E., Spiegel, K. Metabolic consequences of sleep and sleep loss. *Sleep Med.* Sep 2008;9(suppl 1):S23–28.

Van Herpen-Broekmans, W.M., Klöpping-Ketelaars, I.A., Bots, M.L., et al. Serum carotenoids and vitamins in relation to markers of endothelial function and inflammation. *Eur J Epidemiol.* 2004;19(10):915–21.

Vanamala, J., Reddivari, L., Radhakrishnan, S., Tarver, C. Resveratrol suppresses IGF-1 induced human colon cancer cell proliferation and elevates apoptosis via suppression of IGF-1R/Wnt and activation of p53 signaling pathways. *BMC Cancer.* 2010;10:238.

van't Veer, P., Dekker, J.M., Lamers, J.W., et al. Consumption of fermented milk products and breast cancer: a case-control study in the Netherlands. *Cancer Res.* Jul 1989;49(14):4020–23.

Vardi, A., Bosviel, R., Rabiau, N., et al. Soy phytoestrogens modify DNA methylation of GSTP1, RASSF1A, EPH2 and BRCA1 promoter in prostate cancer cells. *In Vivo.* 2010;24:393–400.

Veith, I., trans. *Huang Ti Nei Ching Su Wen: The Yellow Emperor's Classic of Internal Medicine.* Berkeley, CA: University of California Press; 1949.

Verhulst, S.L., Nelen, V., Hond, E.D., Koppen, G., Beunckens, C., Vael, C., et al. Intrauterine exposure to environmental pollutants and body mass index during the first 3 years of life. *Environ Health Perspect.* 2009;117:122–26.

Verma, M., and Srivastava, S. Epigenetics in cancer: implications for early detection and prevention. *Lancet Oncol.* 2002;3:755–63.

Vessby, B., Uusitupa, M., Hermansen, K., et al. Substituting dietary saturated for monounsaturated fat impairs insulin sensitivity in healthy men and women: the KANWU Study. *Diabetologia.* 2001;44:312–19.

Vicennati,V. Response of the hypothalamic pituitary adrenocortical axis to high protein and high carbohydrate meals. *J Clin Endocrinol Metab.* 2002;87(8):3984–88.

Vicennati, V., Pasqui, F., Cavazza, C., et al. Cortisol, energy intake, and food frequency in overweight/obese women. *Nutrition.* Jun 2011;27(6):677–80.

Villardita, C. Multicentre clinical trial of brain phosphatidylserine in elderly patients with intellectual deterioration. *Clin Trials J.* 1987;(24):84–93.

Villareal, D.T., Apovian, C.M., Kushner, R.F., Klein, S; American Society for Nutrition; NAASO, The Obesity Society. Obesity in older adults: technical review and position statement of the American Society for Nutrition and NAASO, The Obesity Society. *Am J Clin Nutr.* 2005;82:923–34.

Villareal, D.T., Fontana, L., Weiss, E.P. Bone mineral density response to caloric restriction-induced weight loss or exercise-induced weight loss: a randomized controlled trial. *Arch Intern Med.* 2006;166:2502–10.

Viña, J., Perez, C., Furukawa, T., Palacin, M., Viña, J.R. Effect of oral glutathione on hepatic glutathione levels in rats and mice. *Br J Nutr.* 1989;62(3):683–91.

Vogelzangs, N., Beekman, A.T., Dik, M.G., Bremmer, M.A., Comijs, H.C., Hoogendijk, W.J., et al. Late-life depression, cortisol, and the metabolic syndrome. *Am J Geriatr Psychiatry.* Aug 2009;17(8):716–21.

Vogelzangs, N., Suthers, K. Hypercortisolemic depression is associated with the metabolic syndrome in late-life. *Psychoneuroendocrinology.* Feb 2007;32(2):151–59.

Volek, J., Sharman, M., Love, D., Avery, N., Gómez, A., Scheett, T., Kraemer, W. Body composition and hormonal responses to a carbohydrate-restricted diet. *Metabolism.* Jul 2002;51(7):864–70.

Vucetic, Z., Carlin, J.L., Totoki, K., Reyes, T.M. Epigenetic dysregulation of the dopamine system in diet-induced obesity. *J Neurochem.* Mar 2012;120(6):891–98. DOI: 10.1111/j.1471–4159.2012.07649.x.

Waalkes, M.P. Cadmium carcinogenesis. *Mutat Res.* Dec 2003;533(1–2):107–20.

Waldschläger, J., Bergemann, C., Ruth, W., et al. Flax-seed extracts with phytoestrogenic effects on a hormone receptor-positive tumour cell line. *Anticancer Res.* May–Jun 2005;25(3A):1817–22.

Walford, R.L., Mock, D., Verdery, R., MacCallum, T. Calorie restriction in Biosphere 2: alterations in physiologic, hematologic, hormonal, and biochemical parameters in humans restricted for a 2-year period. *J Gerontol A Biol Sci Med Sci.* 2002;57:B211–B224.

Walker, B.R. Cortisol—cause and cure for metabolic syndrome? *Diabet Med.* Dec 2006;23(12):1281–88.

Walker, B.R. Steroid metabolism in metabolic syndrome X. *Best Pract Res Clin Endocrinol Metab.* Mar 2001;15(1):111–22.

Walker, B.R., Andrew, R. Tissue production of cortisol by 11beta-hydroxysteroid dehydrogenase type 1 and metabolic disease. *Ann NY Acad Sci.* Nov 2006;1083:165–84.

Wallerius, S., Rosmond, R., Ljung, T., Holm, G., Björntorp, P. Rise in morning saliva cortisol is associated with abdominal obesity in men: a preliminary report. *J Endocrinol Invest.* Jul 2003;26(7):616–19.

Wang, J., Wu, Z., Li, D., et al. Nutrition, epigenetics, and metabolic syndrome. *Antioxid Redox Signal.* Jul 2012;17(2):282–301.

Wang, S., Chen, S. Genistein protects dopaminergic neurons by inhibiting microglial activation. *Neuroreport.* Feb 28 2005;16(3):267–70.

Warren, J.M., Henry, C.J., Simonite, V. Low glycemic index breakfasts and reduced food intake in preadolescent children. *Pediatrics.* Nov 2003;112(5):e414.

Waterland, R.A., Jirtle, R.L. Transpiosable elements: targets for early nutritional effects on epigenetic gene regulation. *Mol Cell Biol.* 2003;23:5293–300.

Watkins, B.A., Li, Y., Lippman, H.E. Omega-3 polyunsaturated fatty acids and skeletal health. *Exp Biol Med.* 2001;226(6):485–97.

Weber, M.A. Sympathetic nervous system and hypertension. Therapeutic perspectives. *Am J Hypertens.* 1989;2:147S–152S.

Weber-Hamann, B., Hentschel, F., Kniest, A., Deuschle, M., Colla, M., Lederbogen, F., Heuser, I. Hypercortisolemic depression is associated with increased intra-abdominal fat. *Psychosom Med.* Mar–Apr 2002;64(2):274–77.

Weindruch, R., Walford, R.L. *The Retardation of Aging and Disease by Dietary Restriction.* Springfield, IL: Charles C. Thomas Pub.; 1988.

Weinhold, B. Epigenetics: the science of change. *Environ Health Perspect.* 2006;114:A160–A167.

Weiss, E.P., Racette, S.B., Villareal, D.T. Improvements in glucose tolerance and insulin action induced by increasing energy expenditure or decreasing energy intake: a randomized controlled trial. *Am J Clin Nutr.* 2006;84:1033–42.

Widiker, S., Karst, S., Wagener, A., Brockmann, G.A. High-fat diet leads to a decreased methylation of the Mc4r gene in the obese BFMI and the lean B6 mouse lines. *J Appl Genet.* 2010;51(2):193–97.

Williams, J.K., Kaplan, J.R., Manuck, S.B. Effects of psychosocial stress on endothelium-mediated dilation of atherosclerotic arteries in cynomolgus monkeys. *J Clin Invest.* 1993;92:1819–23.

Williams, S.N., Shih, H., Guenette, D.K., et al. Comparative studies on the effects of green tea extracts and individual tea catechins on human CYP1A gene expression. *Chem Biol Interact.* 2000;128(3):211–29.

Wolstenholme, J.T., Edwards, M., Shetty, S.R.J., et al. BPA exposure in pregnancy linked to behavioral problems in offspring. *WorldHealth. net.* Jul 6 2012.

Wood, R., Kubena, K., O'Brien, B., Tseng, S., Martin, G. Effect of butter, mono- and poly-unsaturated fatty acid-enriched butter, trans fatty acid margarine, and zero trans fatty acid margarine on serum lipids and lipoproteins in healthy men. *J Lipid Res.* Jan 1993;34(1):1–11.

Worsley, J.R. *Classical Five-Element Acupuncture: The Five Elements and the Officials, Vol. III.* J.R. & J.B. Worsley, Pub.; 1998.

Xie, L., Li, X.K., Takahara, S. Curcumin has bright prospects for the treatment of multiple sclerosis. *Int Immunopharmacol.* Mar 2011;11(3):323–30.

Yan, M.S., Matouk, C.C., Marsden, P.A. Epigenetics of the vascular endothelium. *J Appl Physiol.* Sep 2010;109(3):916–26.

Yehuda, R., Seckl, J. Minireview: stress-related psychiatric disorders with low cortisol levels: a metabolic hypothesis. *Endocrinology.* Dec 2011;152(12):4496–503.

Yehuda, S., Rabinovitz, S., Carasso, R.L., Mostofsky, D.I. Fatty acid mixture counters stress changes in cortisol, cholesterol, and impair learning. *Int J Neurosci.* 2000;101(1–4):73–87.

Yehuda, S., Rabinovitz, S., Mostofsky, D.I. Mixture of essential fatty acids lowers test anxiety. *Nutr Neurosci.* Aug 2005;8(4):265–67.

Yuasa, Y., Nagasaki, H., Akiyama, Y., et al. DNA methylation status is inversely correlated with green tea intake and physical activity in gastric cancer patients. *Int J Cancer.* Jun 2009;124(11):2677–82.

Yun, J.M., Jialal, I., Devaraj, S. Effects of epigallocatechin gallate on regulatory T cell number and function in obese v. lean volunteers. *Br J Nutr.* 2010;103:1771–77.

Zadshir, A., Tareen, N., Pan, D., Norris, K., Martins, D. The prevalence of hypovitaminosis D among US adults: data from the NHANES III. *Ethn Dis.* 2005;15(4 suppl 5):S5-97–101.

Zaina, S., Lund, G. Epigenetics: a tool to understand diet-related cardiovascular risk? *J Nutrigenet Nutrigenomics.* 2011;4(5):261–74.

Zang, X., Ho, S.M. Epigenetics meets endocrinology. *J Mol Endocrinol.* Feb 2011;46(1):R11–32.

Zeisel, S.H. Epigenetic mechanisms for nutrition determinants of later health outcomes. *Am J Clin Nutr.* 2009;89:1488S–1493S.

Zhang, C., Browne, A., Child, D.F., Tanzi, R.E. Curcumin decreases amyloid-beta peptide levels by attenuating the maturation of amyloid-beta precursor protein. *J Biol Chem.* Sep 2010;285(37):28472–80.

Zhang, S., Rattanatray, L., McMillen, I.C., Suter, C.M., Morrison, J.L. Periconceptional nutrition and the early programming of a life of obesity or adversity. *Prog Biophys Mol Biol.* Jul 2011;106(1):307–14.

Zhang, X., Zhao, Y., Zhang, M., et al. Structural changes of gut microbiota during berberine-mediated prevention of obesity and insulin resistance in high-fat diet-fed rats. *PLoS One.* 2012;7(8):e42529.

Zhou, Y., Zhuan, W., Hu, W., Liu, G.J., Wu, T.S., Wu, X.T. Consumption of large amounts of allium vegetables reduces risk for gastric cancer in a meta-analysis. *Gastroenterology.* Jul 2011;141(1):80–89.

Zhu, J.S., Halpern, G.M., Jones, K. The scientific rediscovery of a precious ancient Chinese herbal medicine: Cordyceps sinensis: part I. *J Altern Complement Med.* 1998;4(3):289–303.

Zittermann, A. Vitamin D in preventive medicine: are we ignoring the evidence? *Br J Nutr.* 2003;89:552–72.

Zittermann, A., Frisch, S., Berthold, H.K., Götting, C., Kuhn, J., Kleesiek, K., et al. Vitamin D supplementation enhances the beneficial effects of weight loss on cardiovascular disease risk markers. *Am J Clin Nutr.* May 2009;89(5):1321–27.

INDEX

A

Acetyl-L-carnitine, 119, 123
Adaptation
  biochemistry of, 3–4
  capacity for, 3
  diet and, 22–31, 43, 173
  emotional states and, 6–7
  fats and, 74–76
  food allergies and, 57–58
  maintaining, 228
Adaptation Diet. *See also* Phase
  One; Phase Two; Phase Three
  components of, 24–25
  goal of, 24, 73
  health concerns and, 47–48
  phases of, 44
  stars of, 101–23
Adaptogens
  benefits of, 142–44
  botanical, 144–50
  definition of, 142
  nutrient, 150–52
ADHD (attention-deficit/
  hyperactivity disorder), 67,
  68, 139
Adiponectin, 13, 81
Adrenal glands, 5
Adrenaline. *See* Epinephrine
African Coconut Peanut Tofu,
  328–29
Aging
  of the brain, 116–19

  epigenetics and, 185
  premature, 10, 21, 97
Ahi, Sautéed, with Walnuts and
  Shiitake Mushrooms, 297
Alcohol, 47, 93
Aldosterone, 5
Allostasis, process of, 5
Allostatic load
  in children, 127
  definition of, 5
  markers of, 10
  reducing, 23–34, 47, 57–58, 69
Almond butter
  Celery Sticks with Almond
  Butter, 307
  Creamy Broccoli and Almond
  Butter Soup, 334–35
Almonds
  Coconut, Carrot, Squash Slaw, 306
  Nancy's Crunchy and Colorful
  Chinese Coleslaw, 335–36
  Oat Bran Muffins, 250
  Sweet and Sour Tempeh, 283–84
Alpha-carotene, 103
Alpha lipoic acid, 52, 118, 123
Alzheimer's disease, 10, 118, 120
American Academy of Anti-Aging
  Medicine, 349
American Academy of
  Environmental Medicine, 30,
  59, 63, 234, 349

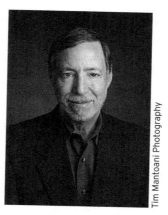

Tim Mantoani Photography

ABOUT THE AUTHOR

Charles A. Moss, MD, is a pioneer in the use of therapeutic nutrition in medicine. Since 1978 he has helped his patients regain health and manage their weight through dietary changes that reduce maladaptation (the long-term elevation of cortisol and other stress hormones that increases the risk for chronic disease). He has focused on nutritional therapy since his days in medical school in the late 1960s, when he embarked on a personal exploration of the effect of diet on health.

Over the past thirty-five years, through a combination of nutritional medical therapies, environmental medicine, and traditional acupuncture, he has successfully treated thousands of patients with the illnesses of maladaptation that include obesity, fatigue, chronic pain, headaches, allergies, digestive disorders, asthma, arthritis, anxiety, and depression.

Dr. Moss attended the State University of New York at Buffalo School of Medicine and completed a residency in preventive medicine and family practice at the University of Arizona College of Medicine in 1978. While in Tucson he developed the first holistic health course in the United States for medical students and residents.

In 1978 he established one of the first holistic health medical clinics in the United States. The Moss Center for Integrative Medicine is the oldest practice of its kind in San Diego. His unique approach to stress-induced and chronic medical problems has attracted patients from all over the United States, Mexico, and Europe. The clinic was the subject of the book *Caring and Responsibility* by June Lowenberg, PhD, published in 1989. She researched the groundbreaking methods that he employed as a model for holistic health practice. *Caring and Responsibility* is used as a textbook in several universities in departments of health policy studies.

Dr. Moss utilizes traditional Five Element acupuncture in his practice. He studied with J. R. Worsley in England in the 1970s and was the first American physician to combine the Five Element system with other areas of holistic health practices. He was an instructor at the UCLA School of Medicine Medical Acupuncture for Physicians postgraduate program, and in 1988 founded the Five Element Acupuncture Physician Training Program, which has trained physicians from throughout the United States and several other countries.

Dr. Moss is board certified in medical acupuncture, environmental medicine, and family practice, and is a fellow of both the American Academy of Environmental Medicine and the American Academy of Medical Acupuncture. He has served on the board of directors of the American Academy of Medical Acupuncture, the American Academy of Environmental Medicine, and the American Board of Medical Acupuncture. He is a member of the American Academy of Anti-Aging Medicine, the American Medical Association, the American College for Advancement in Medicine, and the Institute for Functional Medicine.

In addition to *The Adaptation Diet*, Dr. Moss is the author of *Power of the Five Elements: The Chinese Medicine Path to Healthy Aging and Stress Resistance,* which details how to improve adaptation and maintain health through knowledge of a person's unique Five Element adaptation type and mind/body medicine.

Dr. Moss resides in San Diego County with his wife. His two

sons live in Southern California. He continues to practice in La Jolla and teach physicians at medical conferences throughout the United States and abroad. For more information, visit:

www.MossCenterforIntegrativeMedicine.com
www.TheAdaptativeDiet.com